The Dieter's Dictionary
and Problem Solver

The Dieter's Dictionary and Problem Solver

An A to Z Guide
To Nutrition, Health, and Fitness

Victoria Zak and Peter Vash, M.D., M.P.H.

RUTLEDGE HILL PRESS
Nashville, Tennessee

To Deborah D. Reilly

With special thanks to

Patricia Downs
Joni Johnson
Theresa Bergen Carrigan
Neil Evans

Published in Nashville, Tennessee, by Rutledge Hill Press, Inc., 513 Third Avenue South, Nashville, Tennessee 37210. Distributed in Canada by H. B. Fenn & Company, Ltd., Mississauga, Ontario.

Typography by D&T/Bailey, Nashville, Tennessee

Library of Congress Cataloging-in-Publication Data

Zak, Victoria.
    The dieter's dictionary and problem solver : an A to Z guide to nutrition, health, and fitness / Victoria Zak and Peter Vash.
      p.   cm.
    Includes bibliographical references and index.
    ISBN 1-55853-172-6
    1. Reducing diets.   2. Reducing diets—Dictionaries.
3. Nutrition—Dictionaries.   4. Health—Dictionaries.   5. Physical fitness—Dictionaries.   I. Vash, Peter.   II. Title.
RM222.2.Z348   1992
613.2'5—dc20   92-11242
                                          CIP

Printed in the United States of America
1 2 3 4 5 6 7 8—97 96 95 94 93 92

Contents

Acknowledgments

I'd like to thank God, and others: Leona Zak, Judith Wagner, Kathy Zak, Katy Lembcke—my family; Sally McMillan—my special agent; all the people at Rutledge Hill Press, specifically Ron Pitkin and Larry Stone; Don Axinn for his remarkable heart; Stacey Chase and friends from Bread Loaf; Paul LaFramboise; and three people in weight management whom I'll never forget: George Blackburn, M.D., Mike Kenyon, and Cris Carlin.

—Victoria Zak

I'd like to thank George, Virginia, Barbara, and Stephen Vash.

—Peter Vash

Introduction

THE DIETER'S DICTIONARY AND PROBLEM SOLVER is the first resource of its kind for a new generation of dieters and fitness advocates. These are the people who want more from their diets than constant calorie counting and food deprivation and want better, healthier ways to slim down and shape up with the back-up that great bodies require—inner health and well-being that makes fitness worthwhile. It's for dieters who want to be good to themselves for a change.

This is the book for people who want it all, and something more. They want to be armed with facts so they can be smart eaters, smart exercisers, and wise consumers. They want to know what to look for and what to look out for. They don't want to be fooled about their health and weight anymore.

The Dieter's Dictionary and Problem Solver is also the bright promise of science, combining food and metabolism, exercise and behavior in a lifestyle program where the best success is achieved and endures. It's your personal resource, because you deserve the best. And your body will thank you for it.

PATTERNS, NOT POUNDS

The Problem Solver Motto is Today's Patterns Create Tomorrow's Health. This is an exhilarating, new approach to weight loss and total fitness based on *patterns*, not *pounds*.

People gain weight and develop weight-related problems through a series of behavior patterns that are learned and repeated day after day. A weight problem is a collection of small habits or patterns that add up to one big problem as it dominoes.

For instance, you may have a "sweet tooth" that attracts you to foods which are sugary. This problem can domino, because sugar

vii

and fat usually team up in foods so that when you eat sugary foods you also are eating more fat. The more sugar you eat, the less your natural palate can distinguish between higher fat mixes; therefore, the first problem—sugar—also becomes a fat problem. This dominoes again, since sweet/fat foods are also low fiber foods, and low fiber foods don't require much chewing. This speeds up your rate of eating and allows more calories to be absorbed and stored as fat. The first problem—sugar—has become a fat problem, a fiber problem, a rate-of-eating problem, an intestinal problem, and a fat storer problem. After that, it becomes an energy problem because high sugar foods don't give you the nutrition you need for daily work and activity. You might find that you tire more easily and often and that you're gaining body fat, which in turn slows you down and causes you to become less active. This reduces your metabolism, and you burn fewer calories; but you store more fat. The first problem—sugar—has escalated into a full-scale weight problem where larger issues now loom: body image problems, loss of mobility and range of motion, lack of self-esteem, and a new pattern of eating that is highly emotional and stressful.

The excess sugar you eat today will be the fat on your body tomorrow. It will affect your future health.

A similar result can occur with nonbreakfast eaters. You might skip breakfast as your first habit of the day. Then suddenly in midmorning, you start entering a pattern that is weight-gaining. Lacking nutrition for energy in midmorning, you reach for food, something easy to eat and acquire: a doughnut or a snack from a vending machine. Most of this energy comes from sugar, which provides a quick high, then a new low. By noon you're famished and eat a heavy lunch. By midafternoon you're sluggish (from your heavy lunch), and your energy needs another boost. You reach for candy or soda, lecturing yourself about control. Your moods can swing up and down with your energy because your brain needs nutrition too. You might cut back on dinner to try to make up for a bad day, and you're too tired to exercise, lacking balanced energy; so you promise yourself you'll exercise tomorrow. Suddenly—late at night—you eat the dinner you didn't have (or its equivalent in fat and calories), and you go to bed with a full stomach, when you metabolism is at its lowest ebb. During sleep, your body is in a "fasting state," meaning it will conserve its energy and store the late-night food you ate as fat. The next day you tell yourself, *Today I'll eat better*, and you start cutting calories and skipping breakfast. Snap, you're back in the same pattern again.

Patterns like these repeat, and, without being aware of it, *your future health is being written on automatic pilot.*

Excess weight is linked to more than fifty minor health problems and all of the major life-threatening diseases (*See* page 295–296: Risks in the dictionary for more details).

Excess weight is also a block to your enjoyment of life and to your natural potential. When you are too heavy, you change the clothes you wear, often disguising or hiding your weight. You find summer less fun, because of bathing suits and shorts; and always in the back of your mind your weight nags at you. Food is a constant preoccupation.

POUNDS vs. PATTERNS

When you go on a diet and are asked, "What have you got to lose?" you probably will answer in pounds. You go to the scale for the exact amount of pounds you want to lose, then decide to get them off by a certain day. This puts extra pressure on your mind, in addition to the feeling of weight you are carrying. Then you shake up your life to lose those pounds as fast as possible.

Most people try to eliminate their excess pounds by various eating patterns that are abnormal and unnatural. They try one or more of the following:

1. Stop eating for a few days or eat virtually nothing.
2. Rely on diet soda and melba toast to get through the day, then panic and eat late at night.
3. Cut out all sweets and desserts and long for them constantly, then have a sweet attack and binge, followed by starving to try to make up for it.
4. Cut down on everything for as long as they can handle it, then panic and switch back.
5. Try to cut out fat, and eat poorly as a result.
6. Join a get-the-weight-off-quick program, eating according to their plan, which usually provides less than 900 calories per day.
7. Take fiber pills, appetite suppressants, and formulas that are used in place of food.

None of these eating patterns work for successful weight loss. Why? They lead to muscle loss, not fat loss. If you never use one of these dieting patterns again, you will be leaner longer.

Diet patterns can reinforce your former unhealthy patterns. The

diet you choose in order to lose your pounds can affect your future
eating patterns and health.

Your foods/my foods. These diets divide the world into two kinds
of food: the foods you can eat for weight loss and the foods everyone else is eating (good food vs. bad food). You file *your* food in
Tupperware bowls in the fridge and strip your kitchen of all other
foods. You begin to fear going near places where everyday food
abounds—the kitchen, supermarkets, bakeries, delis, restaurants—and you begin to dread cooking for fear you'll eat. Out of
sight, out of mind becomes your pattern; and it's likely that you
will go out of your mind from food avoidance and break your diet.
These programs inadvertently teach you to fear food, using a good
food/bad food mindset that is not healthy thinking. It's ingrained
by repetition.

Chronic food restriction. These are very low calorie programs that
reduce food to the limit of safety and provide some form of substitute that you take like medicine. They've been shown to cause
rapid weight regain and greater hunger afterward, incidentally,
hunger that won't turn off. In addition, many test subjects developed eating problems they didn't have before the diet, such as
binge eating. These programs inadvertently treat food as your
enemy and you as a child who is unable to choose wisely and
therefore must be monitored. Weight loss becomes a form of
punishment that you somehow feel you deserve, just because you
gained excess fat. It's an extreme pattern that is unhealthy—mentally, emotionally, and physically—ingrained by repetitious denial.

No carbs, please. These are ketogenic diets where you measure
your fat loss with paper strips that turn different colors. It's like a
course in chemistry; but the formula is deficient, and it usually
means missing carbohydrates. These low-carbohydrate diets force
you to use anaerobic energy for exercise or activity, where you can
burn more muscle than fat. These programs inadvertently teach
you that there's a trick in science and some kind of magic in fat
burning that doesn't involve the food groups you learned about in
school. This teaches you to mistrust science and misuse food, until
you get to the point that you're not sure anymore what is or isn't
good for you. It's an unhealthy pattern that leads you to more
gimmicks for solutions, which only lead you further astray from
the real solutions.

If losing pounds were the solution to weight problems, everyone
in America would be slim by now. But weight problems are escalating. Diets alone have contributed a whole new population of mildly
obese people who got that way after dieting to lose pounds by a

certain date. Most repeat dieters will say, "I've lost and gained the same twenty to thirty pounds over and over for the last decade."

The fact is, repeat dieters are not losing the same pounds over and over. They're losing water and muscle and gaining back *fat*. Then on the second diet, they lose more muscle and water, and gain back more fat. It's a pattern of dieting that is too common to ignore; it ingrains failure—just like a habit—by repetition.

The pounds that are regained after a poor diet are fatter pounds than the pounds you had when you began it. Each time a diet fails, you get fatter internally, making the pounds harder to get off. Then you start to fear failure and blame it on yourself. It's a cycle of training for failure that we can't afford anymore.

HEALTHY PATTERNS CREATE HEALTHY LIVES

The next time someone asks you, "What have you got to lose?" think about your patterns and you will see that the solutions are within your reach. In the same way that small habits can trigger big problems with the domino effect, the situation can be reversed. Weight is a pattern that is learned and ingrained by repetition. Change your unhealthy pattern to a healthy one, and learn the healthy pattern by repetition. The result: weight gaining is *unlearned*, and health naturally follows, along with pound loss. You get the best of both worlds.

THE PROBLEM SOLVER DIET PROGRAM

The Problem Solver Diet program is a study of healthy patterns in *action*. You learn the program by doing it. You practice and repeat it, getting better with each repetition. Before you know it, the pattern is ingrained. This is behavior modification in action from the beginning.

The Problem Solver Diet was complicated to develop, but it's easy to use. You will notice that from the outset. It also begins to work from the first day you start because it's designed to enhance you on all fronts—body, mind, and food—for energy, health, and well-being.

The book is divided into three sections for your easy use:

Part One: The Top Twenty Problems and How to Solve Them
This gives you the most common weight problems and how to resolve them. You can check the list of problems and select your

most predominant one. The solutions are designed to help you break the patterns that are most common to the problem. These solutions are based on years of research and clinical trials in food science, physiology, and behavior. And they include something more—years of comments and complaints from dieters themselves, incorporated into the program as positive solutions.

Part Two: The Problem Solver Diet Program

This section gives you a complete pattern for total fitness, inside and out. It combines food, exercise, and behavior in a day-to-day plan to take you through a month of maximum results and performance.

It combines three ideal features:

The Problem Solver Calendar. This is your total fitness agenda for healthy weight loss, maintenance, food management, exercise, and behavior, all in one spot.

The Problem Solver Diet. This is your food pattern for ideal eating and ideal health while dieting. This is not an "eat this, don't eat that" food plan you find with most diets. It's a style of eating and dealing with food that is powerful and oriented toward pleasure. By practicing this eating style, you learn how to use food, instead of letting food use you. It treats you to a new relationship with food that is versatile and flexible, healthy and, yes, fun!

The diet accomplishes many things simultaneously:

1. It uses the strongest and healthiest fuel to burn fat. It's based on using foods that provide the best thermic energy (heat producing, therefore, calorie burning foods). They burn while you eat.

2. It's your best muscle insurance. It is based on the nutrient density of foods (the most nutrition in your calories).

3. It provides the best results. It's based on the full food groups, with optimum nutrition for overall health and disease prevention. It drives up your energy and stamina and meets all nutrient needs for body repair and maintenance. It builds up your health while it breaks down your fat.

4. It teaches the best pattern of eating. It's a pattern for eating that makes life pleasurable during and after your diet. When you eat right, you're satisfied. When you eat right, everything works better, including your metabolism, to burn fat. It's a lifestyle of eating that utilizes every positive principle of food including taste, texture, flavor, palatability, chewability, power, and total nutrition for energy. All you have to do is use it.

The Problem Solver Meals and Menus. This is your eating pattern in action, using common foods to show you how to balance your energy to create an ideal day. It keeps your energy stable and nutrients coming in at a steady rate. This balances your body and makes your food selections easy and practical, and it brings dieting back to the real world of food, with food choices that make fitness fun and easy for everyone.

You can follow this pattern exactly, or you can use the formula to experiment with your own recipes. As you practice the meals and menus, you'll find your old habits letting go and new, healthy ones emerging. It will give you a light feeling you can't get from any other style of eating, except healthy eating. You won't know how you lived without it.

Part Three: The Dieter's Dictionary

This is the backup for the plan that tells you everything you need to know about food, exercise, and fitness. It contains a wealth of "how-tos" to let you get on with the business of fitness on the spot.

For instance, when the Problem Solver Calendar recommends doing Relaxation exercises, you turn to the topic Relaxation to find out how to do state-of-the-art relaxation. You sit in a comfortable chair and practice. Each practice session improves your sense of well-being, and each practice becomes more perfect. Before you know it, you will have mastered the best behavior skills in the business.

In the same manner, you can find all of the skills you need to comply with the whole program. No other resources are needed. It's all between two covers.

To make your program easier, you might want to tab the book with Post-It notes to find your skills on the spot.

Today Is the Day to Start Creating Your Future Health

What have you got as a result of this combined-science approach? A top-drawer clinical program that you can do at home. The pattern for success that is the best in the field. Your ticket to future health and permanent weight control.

And you have even more. The dictionary section also includes many interesting facts about food, fitness, exercise, biochemistry, physiology, nutrition, and behavior.

It's *your* resource because you deserve the best.

Here's to your future health!

—The Authors

The Dieter's Dictionary
and Problem Solver

PART ONE

The Dieter's Problem Solver

The Top Twenty Diet Problems and How to Solve Them

Problem Number One

◆

TEN POUNDS THAT CLING

**You're not quite fit and not quite fat,
but always one step away from your ideal weight.**

TEN POUNDS OF EXTRA WEIGHT is generally regarded as a cosmetic weight problem, since your extra weight does not put you into a risk category for weight-related diseases. As a rule, you are healthy, and you may have learned to live with your extra fat, but you tend to face the same nagging problems every year in different variations:

- Every summer, you're uncomfortable wearing shorts or a bathing suit, trying to hide bumps and bulges.
- Before events like weddings, reunions, or your vacation, you're on a diet to fit into an outfit that seems to have shrunk.
- You don't regain weight immediately after you diet, but you slowly add pounds over six months to a year.
- Every January, you make a new resolution to lose those ten pounds, and you diet for a while, then slowly drift back to your old eating style.
- Your weight is constantly on your mind.

If you have ten pounds that won't let go, it means that your lean body weight (body muscle) is too *low*, and that thwarts your efforts to remove that extra fat. If you diet without addressing this specific problem, you can lose more muscle, increasing your problem, and adding more fat. Your original muscle losses may have occurred in the past on a poor diet or over a period of time when you didn't eat balanced nutrition and didn't stay active or exercise. If you eat well sometimes, and at other times slack off, undereating or skipping meals, over time this can cause muscle losses, which will in turn boost up your body fat. These factors combine to keep you at that weight just over your ideal, and it keeps those ten pounds clinging here and there in pockets of fat.

You may be able to hold down your weight to that extra ten pounds and never gain more, but the constant attention it requires and the nagging body dissatisfaction is a drain on your energy. It keeps you from being the best you can be, and it never lets you experience the total feeling of fitness that is just out of reach.

If you try to lose that last ten pounds by moderating your calories and becoming more active, your low muscle body will continue to thwart your results. Muscle is the most important factor for fat burn, and the less muscle you have, the slower you burn fat. In the case of ten pounds, a moderate approach isn't the best plan of action.

You need power on all fronts finally to renounce that fat.

Your last ten pounds is the crucial time to realign your body's fat and muscle content. Your goal at ideal should be high muscle, low fat. To accomplish that, your weight loss must be *only* fat (no muscle can be spared). That eliminates all rapid weight-loss diets and imbalanced food plans, since they will drain you of more muscle.

To get what you want, the last diet stage should be the one where you give it all you've got.

Do it once. Do it right. Do it all the way to ideal weight.

What kind of plan is right?

1. Maximum nutrition in your diet, to fuel your metabolism to burn fat better and to give you extra energy for exercise and the healthy glow that comes from total nutrition.

2. Maximum benefits from your exercise to build new muscle to replace what you've been missing, so you can have a fit, toned body inside and out.

3. An optimum behavior plan to defend you from stress, build your inner resources to achieve your desires and goals, and give you the skills you need to support your program and enhance the entire experience.

Where do you find that plan? Read pages 69–85: The Problem Solver Diet.

◆

OVERWEIGHT FOR A LONG TIME (OR OBESE)

You're a strong person because you have been carrying more weight on your body and mind than most people. You can use that strength differently.

IF YOU'VE BEEN OVERWEIGHT for a long time (or obese), you need a new outlook on dieting and health to spur you on to achieve your weight-loss goals.

To start, you might consider the value of step goals. This is a technique for setting closer goals and rewarding yourself when you achieve them.

How to Set Step Goals. Begin by weighing yourself and recording the total amount of weight you need to lose to be close to your ideal weight. Then take that total and divide it into five-pound increments, allowing yourself two weeks to lose each five pounds. Each time you reach a new five-pound goal, reward yourself with something positive and reinforcing which does not involve food. You might get tickets to a play you've wanted to see, learn a new art or craft, or spend a whole day pampering yourself.

By using step goals, you accomplish several important things simultaneously:

1. You don't become trapped by time or deadlines. Many overweight people make the mistake of jumping into a diet program with their final goal up-front: losing all of their weight in one swoop. When you have more weight to lose at the outset, this

4

means you are setting a goal that seems too far down the road. To combat the feeling of helplessness you get in the face of this long-distance dream, you set unrealistic time limits on yourself for the weight you have to lose, trying to squeeze as much visible success into the shortest time possible. This puts excessive pressure on you, and it makes your diet time obsessive, as you count every pound on the scale, agonize over every bite of food you put in your mouth, dread each new day, and live in fear of breaking your long-distance commitment. It ultimately leads to breaking your diet because of the stress and pressure to lose too much too fast.

It also makes you susceptible to trick diets that promise you can lose thirty pounds in a month. To do that you might accept a dreadfully restrictive program that separates you from the world of everyday eating, drinking formulas like a sick child, feeling you can't be trusted to deal with real food. This ultimately leads to breaking your diet, since that kind of regimen is based on punishment, and you don't need punishment to teach you what you need to know about food and fitness. Believe it or not, you can find pleasure and fun on a diet.

It's also vital to note that the rapid weight-loss diets and abnormal eating plans that remove you from food entirely or remove entire food groups like carbohydrates are also the plans that show the greatest weight regain and greater hunger afterward, hunger that can't be controlled. You don't need that kind of result from your diet.

2. You can stay in the real world for your diet with step-goal control. Many overweight people have been led to believe that they need diets that are different from real-world eating because their weight has been there since childhood, or because their weight issue is extreme. But this is not true, and is neither realistic nor healthy for you. The more overweight you are and the longer you've been that way, the better it is to learn how to eat healthfully *now*, since that will provide you with a new foundation for fitness that you can use for the rest of your life.

3. You don't chase the impossible dream. Five-pound step goals are really achievable, and right at the outset you know you can reach each step goal, whether you do it in two weeks, or need to take three weeks. Interestingly, this kind of planning is the pattern for achieving success in most endeavors in life, in any field.

4. You have much more health freedom. Five-pound step goals give you more freedom with the method you can use to reach your goal. Because you are not trying to take off all of your weight at once, you can breathe a sigh of relief and use the healthy method

for sure, steady weight loss. This gives you more food variety and pleasure every day, plus more energy and stamina as an immediate return. There is no weakness, starvation, or feeling cold all the time when you are dieting. You enjoy real food for real energy and balanced nutrition for your health foundation. You find energy you never knew you had, and it continues to increase as you reach each five-pound goal, because you are freeing yourself of your body fat, which slows you down and drags you out. It's a process that cycles upward to greater and greater health.

5. You see fitter results. The five-pound method also gives you something that will be thrilling in the short term and fulfilling in the long term: fitter, firmer weight loss and the ability to make it last.

Since you have the freedom to use the healthy method for your weight loss, you can trim down more firmly, burning fat and building your body muscle with each five-pound goal. You're going to be surprised at the difference in your appearance and health at each five-pound interval:

Five pounds of fat loss *looks like* ten pounds of weight loss.

Five pounds of fat loss *feels like* ten pounds of weight loss.

Overall weight loss can be water, muscle, or fat. But fat loss is only fat. It is a very definitive fitness builder, along with a body trimmer. It immediately shows in health, tone, and *inches*. Imagine five pounds of bacon fat in a bowl, and you'll see the benefits in your step goals. A five-pound loss is achievable, and it makes you feel terrific when you reach it, inside and out!

6. You get automatic behavior modification. Five-pound step goals provide a lifetime of benefits in behavior modification. Since you are using the healthy method for weight loss, you are utilizing your diet time to practice high-level eating and high-level activity, and as you practice, these eating habits and lifestyle habits begin to override your older, less healthy habits that led to weight gain. When you reach your last five-pound goal, not only will you be leaner and more toned, but you will have an automatic eating plan for weight maintenance for life. You will need no separate maintenance plan tacked on to the end of your diet, where you have to relearn how to eat and live healthfully. You learned it during your diet. You simply increase your food intake across the board and eat more food in the same style.

Believe it or not, healthy eating becomes addictive, just as fats and sweets were, and the key is simply to learn how to do it by repeating it over and over, until it becomes habitual. You'll find, over time, that your body won't feel as good if you shift back into your old eating habits, and that will be the incentive to forge ahead to success. The final benefit of learning how to eat healthfully, is that you get lean and feel good. You never have to return to your overweight state again.

How do you begin?

Step 1: Tap Your Inner Resources

You want to develop a fitness program that works forward from your strength. Your strength comes from within, so that's the place to begin.

Read page 304: Self-Esteem.

Read page 235: Inner Self.

Often, if you've been carrying weight for a long time, the burden of weight on your body drains your energy and makes you feel less strong, less sure inside. So your first goal is to take the weight off your mind to lighten up inside.

Read page 234: Imagery.

Practice the exercise for getting thin from within every day at the same time. Keep practicing, even if you don't think it is working. Suddenly, after the practice, one day you will experience the feeling of being light. Once you've got that feeling, you can call it up at any time to lift pounds of weight from your mind. The key here is *practice*.

Many overweight people come into a program with a negative body image, and it is vital for you to learn to like yourself as you are, before you start to change yourself. This has been clinically proven to lead to real success, since you first shed those deep-seated inner doubts and self-criticisms. Then they support your outside changes, and as you slim down, you accept yourself with more ease and comfort. The changes you make have a more lasting impact.

Read pages 264–267: Mirror Exercises.

Practice Creating a Positive Mirror Image until you start to feel the effect of being less critical of yourself. Continue to practice your imagery and mirror exercises daily, until you are comfortable with them and can do them as a regular routine.

Read page 214: Fear of Failure.

Do the notebook work for How to Combat Fear of Failure and use the information to identify areas that need more work. Move on to step two.

Step 2: Become a More Active Person

Continue to do your behavior exercises daily from step one, and combine that with a more active daily life. Move around more on a daily basis, walk more, stretch more, and try to gain more body flexibility.

Read pages 324–327: Stretching.

Practice a mild stretching routine every day. You can use our mild stretching routine, a video, or check your local library for reliable programs. The key to stretching is not to overstretch or stretch too far. You might begin by doing only the stretches you can do, relaxing through the others until you gain more flexibility and can do a more complete routine. Stretching elongates your muscles and increases the blood flow throughout your body.

Read pages 292–295: Relaxation.

Practice the Relaxation Initiator and the adjunct Full Body Release. Then try doing your imagery exercise *after* you do Full Body Release. The feeling of lightness will be greater and go deeper after you have learned the art of relaxation.

Your goal now is to add physical lightness to the inner lightness exercises you've been doing. Begin a regular walking program for one-half hour per day, three days each week.

Read page 348: Walking.

You want to begin your exercise routine with a low-impact one, such as walking. Low-impact exercises are ideal for beginners and people with more weight to lose. They don't cause strain or injury and they burn fat just as well as a more intensive routine. You need to exercise before you cut calories, since you need to build up body muscle on your diet, while you lose fat. The only way to insure that you will do that is to establish your exercise routine before you start to diet.

When you are comfortable with your exercise routine and walk on a regular basis, move on to step three.

Step 3: Eat for Leanness and Health

Read pages 69–85: The Problem Solver Diet.

Follow the food pyramid as your daily nutrition guide and design your own meals, or use the daily meals and menus we provide. Never eat less than the pyramid recommends on a daily basis, and always eat the full range of servings from the pyramid daily.

Practice this method of eating every day, until it becomes second nature. If you slip off the plan and make a mistake or two, don't let it deter you. Keep practicing the plan until it becomes a habit for healthy eating.

You can use the Problem Solver Calendar for a step-by-step plan for food, exercise, and behavior.

Follow the calendar to each five-pound step goal. Try to resist the temptation to stop doing a few of the exercises, since all of them in combination are giving you the inner support finally to achieve your goals.

Going the Distance!

When you lose five pounds of fat, reward yourself without food. Explore a new option for exercise. (Keep walking while you try it out.)

Keep these factors in mind while exercising:

- The more weight you have, the better it will be for you to exercise on a regular basis. *But stay within your capacity.* This means that you don't want to exceed your natural limits or try to do too much exercise at one time. For example, if you find that you can walk two miles with ease, walking two more miles will not be better for you. The first two miles is your capacity, and the second two miles would add too much stress on you. As you lose weight, you'll find that your capacity will increase. When more exercise becomes easy to do, that's the time to do a little more, but not before.
- If you find you have a hard time doing a full workout on an aerobic machine, don't push yourself to do it. Instead, use interval training.

Read pages 236–237: Interval Training.

This is the best method to use to adapt to more strenuous exercise, and it will give you the same benefits as a full workout.

We know you can do it!

Join the group of people who are success stories in spite of the amount of weight they had to lose. Do it slowly, surely, and use your inner resources to drive you forward, practicing your relaxation, imagery, and self-strengthing techniques all the way to ideal weight. When you've achieved it, don't let go of all the healthy habits you learned. Keep them on your side for a lean life!

◆

YO-YO SYNDROME

.

**Your weight goes up and down like a roller coaster.
After every diet, you regain weight rapidly,
often in excess of your original weight.**

THIS IS A VERY COMMON problem in weight control, especially for people who started out with more weight to lose and lost it too rapidly.

Many people, especially those who have been obese, believe that weight regain is inevitable in dieting and that somehow they were born to be fat, because their weight keeps coming back. But this simply isn't true. The biggest factor in weight regain is the diet you used to lose your weight in the first place.

The people who yo-yo the most are:

1. People who go on rapid weight-loss diets or imbalanced food plans.

2. People who don't exercise when they diet.

3. People who aren't given behavior modification skills that can be used to build a healthier permanent lifestyle. This doesn't mean behavior skills designed to get you to adhere to a very restrictive diet; rather it means behavior that will strengthen your inner resources to help you make healthy choices.

You can first start to yo-yo after a rapid weight-loss diet (less than 900 calories per day) or an imbalanced food plan that removes entire food groups for faster weight-loss results. These types of diets actually *cause* rapid weight regain because they let you lose too much body muscle and not enough fat. The programs hook you with slogans like "lose seven to ten pounds in one week," or "lose weight overnight." While that is possible, it's never desirable since your primary losses are body muscle and water.

Because your body muscle is vital for effective calorie burn, the less muscle you have, the fewer calories you will burn. If you go the distance on a rapid weight-loss plan from overweight to ideal weight, losing muscle all the way, you wind up with a body that is so low in muscle that it is preserving itself in a faminelike state and has been retrained to *exist on fewer calories*. Your body fat climbs higher when you introduce more calories after your diet phase because you have less muscle than before you started dieting.

If you've been thrust into the yo-yo syndrome by a rapid weight-loss diet, arm yourself with information before you proceed.

Read page 288: Rapid Weight Loss.

Read pages 355–357: Yo-Yo Syndrome.

Read pages 291–292: Relapse.

Read pages 191–193: Diets, Weight Loss.

The importance of a balanced diet cannot be overstated to a person who is locked in the yo-yo syndrome. It's better if you don't diet again than to take the risk of losing more body muscle with another poor diet. You deserve more for your future and your health.

Your new diet goal must be to eat *balanced* meals from the food groups and exercise to regain your lost muscle tissue. It's the only way you can repair the damage that was done.

When you exercise in conjunction with a balanced food plan, you build body muscle and force your metabolism out of its lethargic state. This sets you up with a higher body muscle content at ideal weight, in the right shape to maintain your new, lower weight. You'll be a better calorie burner because you dieted right.

Exercise is the only known way to build body muscle. That's why it's a must for anyone suffering from the yo-yo syndrome.

One more factor should be in place to ensure that your program for breaking the yo-yo syndrome succeeds on all fronts. You need to work on your inner self while you are dieting, to gain lasting skills for permanent lifestyle change. This is where behavior modification saves the day for yo-yo syndromers, especially those who have more weight to lose.

Contrary to popular belief, behavior skills aren't boring plans to make you stop eating and not want food anymore. The sophisticated skills give you techniques to enhance your own inner source of energy, a reserve you may not know you have. Before you proceed, tackle your fear of failure.

Read pages 214–215: Fear of Failure.

What kind of program combines all of these aspects to break the yo-yo syndrome once and for all? You need the best program you can get, in the right sequence to drive up your potential for success.

Here's how it works:

Step One: Break Your Old Habits and Ideas

If you're locked in the yo-yo syndrome, you have a number of leftover ideas and traps from very restrictive diets. Your first goal is to let go of these ideas, so you can open the door to real success. Spend the first few days reading and thinking about the information you read.

Read pages 329–330: Success.

Read page 280: Positive Thinking.

Read pages 301–303: Scale, Body Weight.

Read pages 242–243: Kitchen.

Read pages 175–176: Compliance.

Read page 174: Commitment.

Read pages 178–179: Control. This is important. Don't skip it!

On day three, begin to practice imagery to let go of your inner weight.

Read pages 234–235: Imagery.

Practice this skill until you actually feel the sense of lightness that it can create. When you are comfortable with this skill and can do it as a regular habit every morning, move on to step two.

Step Two: Begin to Exercise

If you're surprised that you aren't going to start dieting yet, don't be. Remember you have to *build* muscle as a main priority, so you don't want to start calorie reduction until you have developed an exercise routine and are comfortable with it. Take as much time as you need to develop a routine exercise program and avoid the diet plan until you are exercising on a regular basis.

Read pages 107–112: The Problem Solver Calendar. Follow the calendar with one exception: don't start dieting yet.

This is the most important aspect of your program to nail down before you start to strip out your body fat. When you are comfortable exercising as a routine and are still practicing your imagery every day, move on to step three.

Step Three: Begin the Problem Solver Diet

This is a totally balanced food plan that takes you to the maximum for fat burning. Never eat less than the minimum shown on the food pyramid. Eat from all of the food groups on a daily basis. Your goal is to practice this eating routine until it becomes a habit. If you want more food, feel free to eat more complex carbohydrates—grains, vegetables, and fruits. They will not add more fat, and they'll give you lots of needed energy for exercise.

Congratulations! If you've come this far, the rest will be a cinch. You have all the skills you need to rebuild your body and your inner resources for strength. If you break your program, see Break. When you are at ideal weight, see Maintenance. For further enhancement skills, you can practice the other relaxation adjuncts as well. We wish you a permanently lean life.

◆

GAINING WEIGHT
AS YOU AGE

**Every year you put on a pound or two
that you don't take off. Every decade it adds up
to ten pounds that you settle for as you age.**

THE TWO PRIMARY REASONS you gain weight as you age are: lack of regular exercise and lack of balanced nutrition on a regular basis.

Many of the so-called signs of aging may only be signs of low activity and low nutritional status. Consider these states of being, often attributed to age:

- Lack of energy and stamina
- Forgetfulness and lack of concentration
- Changes in sleeping habits
- Increased aches and pains in joints and bones
- More proneness to injuries and strain
- Back problems
- The blues or mild depression

All of these are signs of lack of exercise and all are reversed when you have a regular exercise routine.

Weight has also been attributed to aging. Averages show that women gain thirty pounds between the ages of twenty-five and fifty-five and men gain twenty-five pounds. But this is the case for people of all ages who don't exercise and eat too much fat. A teenager can gain thirty pounds in a year with the same two habits of no exercise and increased intake of fat.

You decide. Are you overweight because you are older, or have you settled for a fatter body as you've aged?

The old ideas of aging are passé. Every day new research shows that improving your exercise and diet will yield other health benefits as well, reversing the signs of aging:

- Arthritis symptoms are reduced with a regular exercise routine.
- Energy and stamina are increased with healthy nutrition and exercise.
- Digestive disorders and intestinal pressure are alleviated by routine exercise and increased fiber in your diet.
- The risks of all major lifestyle diseases, including hypertension, heart disease, diabetes, and cancer, are reduced with a combination of weight reduction and exercise.
- The risks of osteoporosis are decreased with regular exercise and improved calcium intake, particularly in women.

Your future health is being written now, in your lifestyle and habits. Now is the time to make those habits ones that will keep you young.

What do you need for a program?

- Weight reduction *by means of* balanced diet and exercise.
- Exercise for cardiovascular conditioning, calorie burn, and muscle building.
- Special exercises to prevent muscle shrinkage which can occur with aging, because of lack of activity.
- Special exercises for flexibility to prevent the loss of mobility that is associated with muscle losses and muscles not used.

New studies show that strength training is particularly important to prevent muscle shrinkage that comes with age because muscles have not been used. As you age, you lose a small amount of body muscle from hormonal changes, but most of your muscle losses come from lack of exercise.

People who use weights (resistance exercises) as part of their routine have been shown to be able to maintain their muscle mass, regardless of age. Studies comparing a thirty-five-year-old man and a sixty-five-year-old man doing resistance exercises found no major differences in their ability to perform equal tasks.

Muscle losses, particularly in your upper body and back, can affect your movement, flexibility, posture, and spinal strength. You can appear stooped or shorter, and you lose the ability to turn quickly in a crisis, leading to greater risk of strain or injury. You can appear older than you are.

Exercise changes the whole picture. Your muscle mass is increased with exercise. Your muscle strength is increased with resistance training (weights) and there's an antidote to loss of mobility with stretching routines that elongate your muscles and increase your range of movement. This protects your independence too, since loss of mobility in senior years leads to loss of independence—needing help from others to perform simple chores.

How do you start to reverse the direction of time?

Read pages 69–85: The Problem Solver Diet.

Follow the Problem Solver Calendar all the way to ideal weight, health, and muscle strength. Regain your youth while you lose your extra weight.

PROBLEM NUMBER FIVE

◆

ANOREXIA, BULIMIA

**You've experimented with extreme forms
of behavior for weight loss, such as self-induced
vomiting and use of laxatives. Now you're not sure
if you have an eating disorder.**

IT'S NOT UNUSUAL for a serious eating disorder to being with a bout of dieting. One-half of teenage girls are on diets by age thirteen, and at least 20 percent report that they've tried self-induced vomiting and laxatives for weight control. With the accent on thinness as the preferred image in our culture, eating disorders are escalating with every decade.

The main characteristics are:

Bulimia: Binge eating followed by self-induced vomiting, to the degree that the vomiting becomes an automatic reflex. The binge foods are usually sweets, starches, and fast foods that can be eaten in a hurry and in private, and the purging is kept private also.

Anorexia: Drastic reduction of body weight and food intake to the point of self-starvation.

The two disorders can overlap, with binging and purging, use of laxatives, and excessive exercise as weight-control measures. But the bulimic will usually stay within a normal weight range, while the anorectic will refuse to maintain normal weight, dropping to 25 percent below normal weight. These extreme muscle losses can be life-threatening.

If you think you might have one of these disorders in either the beginning stages or a later stage, please don't try to resolve the problem yourself. See your doctor, a registered dietitian, or a qualified psychologist for professional help.

Read page 127: Anorexia Nervosa.

Read pages 146–148: Bulimia.

◆

SLIM BUT NOT FIT

**You're at ideal weight, or very close to it.
But you wouldn't call yourself fit.**

SLIM PEOPLE HAVE fat problems too. See if you do:
- You look in the mirror and see pads of fat.
- You don't feel energized.
- Your body doesn't have the tone you desire.
- You haven't seen a muscle on your body since_____.
  (Fill in the date).

Recent Weight Loss

If you are slim but have lost weight recently and feel draggy and baggy, you need some body tuning. Your diet was not all you deserved for fitness. You need to add a little muscle (lean body weight), even if you don't have a lot of extra body fat. The muscle will keep you burning calories at a steady rate, and when you exercise, you'll strengthen your muscles and develop tone to give you a leaner, fitter appearance.

Read pages 107–112: The Problem Solver Calendar.

Follow the calendar for healthy eating, exercise, and behavior until you achieve the tone you desire.

Undereating for Slimness

If you are slim, are starving yourself to stay that way, or are using various gimmicks and pills for aid, you need to charge up your nutrition while learning the skills for healthy eating. If you are not exercising aerobically, you need to add that to your week, three times every other day, in conjunction with a healthy diet. If you are exercising regularly and undereating at the same time, stop exercising and start eating better before you begin exercising again. Exercising while undereating can lead to serious muscle losses or even an eating disorder.

Read page 315: Starvation.

Read pages 201–207: Exercise. Aerobic and Anaerobic.

Read pages 69–85: The Problem Solver Diet.

Use the Problem Solver Food Pyramid to create your new eating plan. Eat everything indicated on the pyramid, and *never less*. You can also use the Problem Solver Calendar for ideal exercise and relaxation. Your body muscle needs help, and strengthening will be beneficial. Don't skip the imagery exercises or mirror exercises. If you are starving to stay slim, that means you have a body image disturbance. The relaxation exercises and visualization will help you resolve your inner conflicts about your body. If it does not, it's worth a visit to a registered dietitian for help, or to a psychologist who deals with weight problems. It's important to understand that you're trying to be healthy, but undereating is the opposite, and you don't want to create greater problems. Give yourself the gift of nutrition. It will change everything!

Normal Weight

If you've never had a weight problem but need more energy and tone, you need to eat better and exercise more to bring that body into the modern age of fitness. The new method of cross-training is the problem solver you need.

You can be slim and exercising, but the results won't be what you desire if your exercise is only providing calorie burn and a half-body workout. For instance, if you are doing an aerobic routine such as calisthenics or Stairmaster at a club, running, or cycling, you aren't getting a full workout of all your muscle groups. You may be burning calories and staying slim, but you're missing upper-body strength and range of movement. In the case of running or calisthenics, your workout is putting a great impact on your lower body and if you are not stretching out your muscles as you should, you can have shorter, tighter muscles as a result. The addition of a full-body stretch will elongate those muscles and give your body more flexibility and grace.

Lower-body aerobics neglect the upper-body muscles, particularly the spinal muscles in the back. These can shrink if they are not exercised. Over time, you can lose the muscle tissue in this area, since muscles must be used to stay vital. You need a strength training routine to complete your workout.

When you add strength training (resistance exercises with weights) and stretching to your aerobic routine, you'll get a body that can't be beat. And you'll stay lean and younger looking as you age.

This kind of routine doesn't take much time. In only one-half hour each day, you can meet all of your muscle needs, while gaining the benefits of well-being, greater mobility, and grace.

Read pages 107–112: The Problem Solver Calendar.

Follow the calendar for two weeks in order to strengthen your exercise routine, eating habits, and behavior. When it has become a regular pattern, read page 252: Maintenance.

◆

CELLULITE

**You have lumps and bumps where you'd
rather have smooth planes, muscles, or curves.**

WITH APOLOGIES TO WILL ROGERS, we never met a
woman who didn't dread cellulite—those lumpy areas of fat that
seem to end up on derrières, hips, thighs, and knees. Dieters have
some of the best senses of humor and cellulite has been called
cottage cheese knees or spongecake thighs. Funny how most
things come back to food.

Men have cellulite too, centered around their stomachs and
spare tires. But somehow women are more forgiving when it
comes to cellulite on men. They call spare tires love handles. And
the most wished for man in the world for adults and children alike
is a man with a bellyful of cellulite—good old Santa Claus.

Product advertisements for cellulite removal may lead you to
believe that cellulite is a form of fat that is special and different
from ordinary fat. It's not. It's just plain fat. And there's only one
formula to get rid of fat, even the cellulite kind: healthy diet and
exercise.

If you are slim with cellulite, you should review your diet to see
if you are eating enough fiber to keep your system active and fat
resistant. Fiber flushes out wastes and increases the speed with
which food moves through your intestines, preventing food stagnation or excess fat storage.

Read pages 215–217: Fiber.

You also need eight glasses of water each day to keep toxins from
accumulating in your system. In addition, you may not be getting

enough oxygen pickup if you are not breathing properly from your diaphragm. Shallow breathing prevents the easy removal of toxins and byproducts of metabolism from your blood.

Read pages 142–145: Breathing.

Practice breathing from your diaphragm to increase the amount of oxygen picked up by your blood and the speed for it to reach your muscles and cells. This facilitates your natural body processes to remove that pocketed fat.

You need exercise to build muscle tissues to offset this last vestige of body fat. Even when you are slim, if you've lost too much muscle getting there or aren't staying active, you can still be too fat inside, and that will keep you fat in those bumpy areas that used to be larger fat cells, now reduced in size.

To do the job well and strip out that cellulite, you need three kinds of exercise: an aerobic exercise for cardiovascular conditioning, strength exercises to build muscle in weak areas of your body, and stretching for elongating your muscles and improving blood flow to these areas.

Choose an aerobic exercise that will work all muscle groups and be a full-body routine, such as rowing, Nordic track, or power walking with weights. Your strength training can be targeted to the areas with cellulite, such as leg exercises with weights for the lower body and arm exercises with weights for the upper body. Your stretching routine doesn't have to be extreme, just routine. It will lengthen your muscles, letting out lactic acid that can accumulate after exercise, causing muscle aches.

Your aerobic routine should be three times each week for one-half hour; strengthening, fifteen to twenty minutes two times each week; and stretching, two times each week. It's not really difficult to do this kind of cross training; it only takes a maximum of thirty minutes a day. And when you check the mirror and the cellulite has disappeared, you'll be glad you stuck to it.

If you have excess weight and cellulite on the side, take it off all at one time.

Read pages 69–85: The Problem Solver Diet.

Follow the Problem Solver Calendar to health and fat freedom, including the lumpy variety.

◆

COMPULSIVE EATING

Everything cues you to eat.

EATING HABITS PLAY AN IMPORTANT role in weight loss and weight gain. Many dieters have regained weight because old habits wouldn't let go.

Habits are behaviors that are learned and repeated until they become automatic responses.

Some of the most common compulsive eating habits are responses to thoughts and feelings.

- You're stressed by something. You eat.
- You're upset by someone. You eat.
- You think a negative thought about yourself. You eat.
- You feel you can't control your thoughts and feelings. You feel helpless. You eat.

There are as many cues for eating as there are thoughts, moods, and emotions. There are secondary cues as well: people who trigger bad moods in you; places that trigger fond memories of eating, like home for the holidays; situations that make you uncomfortable; celebrations where you let go. Even a diet can cue you to eat; because you think a diet means starvation, you eat to prepare for it.

If you tried to change all the moods, thoughts, emotions, people, places, and situations that cue you to eat, you'd need as many lives as Shirley MacLaine. So what can you do?

The key to changing an unhealthy habit into a healthy one isn't

24

to try to change the cause or apply your energy to everything. The trick is to change your response.

- You're stressed. You do relaxation exercises.
- You're upset. You take a walk.
- You think something negative. Change it to a positive.
- You're angry. You let it out on a rowing machine.
- You're tense. You do stretching exercises.

You can make your own list of positive responses, things that comfort and soothe you that don't involve eating fattening, sugary foods. Music to soothe you. Reading a great poem. Taking a ride on a merry-go-round. Be creative. However, the responses mentioned above have all been clinically proven to achieve the results you need: feeling a greater sense of well-being, reversing the stress symptoms, releasing anger and anxiety, easing depression, and calming a host of other emotions that cause you to eat. Relaxation exercises, aerobic exercise, stretching exercises, meditation, diaphragm breathing, positive thinking—all of these responses are substitution behaviors for negative health habits. Use them regularly and you've got compulsive eating beat.

Keeping a record of food and moods is also a marvelous way to unlock some of the thoughts, moods, and emotions that cause you to eat.

Read pages 187–189: Diary, Food.

Eat normally for a week and record your food and moods. Identify what caused you to eat, what you ate, how you felt eating it, how you felt afterwards.

Then, on the following week, practice changing your responses by using one of the substitution behaviors, and record how you felt. This will give you a wealth of information about yourself that you can use to improve your relationship with food.

Read pages 226–227: Habits.

Read pages 197–198: Eating Habits.

Read page 218: Food Cue.

Now that you've had a chance to review your eating habits, make the big change. Combine your new knowledge with a program to change your habit of holding on to your weight.

Read pages 69–85: The Problem Solver Diet.

Follow the Problem Solver Calendar to ideal weight.

Positive health responses are automatically built into the program. You emerge as a person who knows how to make your habits work for you, not against you. You emerge lean and know how to stay that way. You've made the crossover to a healthy lifestyle change. Go out and celebrate. Wait! Don't take that as a new cue to eat fattening foods. Do something active instead.

◆

YOU EAT TOO MANY SWEETS

You have a sweet tooth that you can't seem to control, and you may not realize how seriously that can affect your health, nutrition, and weight.

WE'VE ALL BEEN THERE, staring at the wrapper from some high-sugar snack we ate in a flash to satisfy hunger. And we've felt the outcome, a sudden rush of energy that makes us feel better, then boom, our energy level sinks and we feel suddenly tired, hungry again, and weak at the knees. If we do this repeatedly, we become the victim of energy swings, sugar urges and surges, and we have a compulsive eating habit that seems to drive us to sugary foods to ease an emotional need that we thought was hunger.

For you sugar lovers, this may come as no surprise, but sugar is the food most often associated with *emotional* hunger. You may be eating it for an emotional need that is not being satisfied. There is a difference between emotional hunger and real hunger, and sugar will never satisfy either hunger for long, not your psychological hunger (mind and emotions), nor your physiological hunger (body nutrient needs). Even real hunger is a signal for something you're not getting when you're eating sugary foods: solid nutrition. To make matters more interesting, did you know that your hunger signal will stay on until you get that solid nutrition you need? For this reason, even when you eat a lot of sugary foods, you can still feel hungry all day. Find out more information, before you proceed.

Read pages 128–129; 230: Appetite; Hunger, Psychological.

Read pages 132–133: Assertiveness. Take a little time to make a list of your wants and needs.

There are several reasons why that sweet tooth needs special attention if you want to feel better and lose weight too.

1. Sugars are empty calories. This means that they provide calories but no nutrition. If you're eating 300–400 calories a day as sugar, you're not gaining any nutrition or health benefits from those calories, and you can stay nutritionally needy.

2. Sugar minimizes your fat burn. You need maximum nutrition to burn fat effectively. If you're on a low-calorie plan for weight loss and are eating up your limited calories in sugar, you don't have enough calories left to eat as complex carbohydrates, the real fat-burning foods. Sugary foods tend to replace other, more valuable sources of energy in your diet.

3. You use sugar for quick energy. High-sugar foods give you a false sense of energy. Sugar is glucose, which causes your blood sugar level to rise quickly, then drop again quickly. These energy swings don't provide the stable nutrition you need on a daily basis to handle stress and meet your body's needs for repair and regeneration. Stress will deplete your nutrition faster, and your body will be left unarmed against disease and stress-induced illnesses. You'll tire easily, lack mental energy, and may experience mood swings. All of your systems will be operating at less than peak capacity.

4. There is a sugar/fat connection. Most high-sugar foods are fats in disguise. The combination of sugar and fat makes the food more palatable, especially processed foods that lack natural flavor and require longer shelf life. Because sugar and fat usually appear as a team in these foods, you are automatically eating more fat when you are eating high-sugar foods, and that leads to weight gain.

5. Sugary foods promote poor eating habits. The high-sugar foods are also the low-fiber foods. You don't have to chew them and can swallow them in a snap. They slide down easily, and you might not remember eating them. They promote the reverse of all the good habits of eating for weight loss, including chewing slowly in order to give your body time to turn off hunger (twenty minutes), and you are losing the natural appetite-suppressing mechanisms in digestion that keep you feeling full and satisfied all day. Instead, you're secretly hungry and you think you have to live that way to try to stay slim.

The good news is you'll feel immediate results by breaking your sugar habit. You'll have more true energy and more stable nutrition, and you'll find you have the stamina that always seemed to be lacking when it came to exercise. The results will also show in weight loss. Does this mean you have to give up all sugar and never touch the stuff again, feeling deprived and punished? Do yourself a favor and don't punish yourself for fitness because the results won't last. Start by cutting your sugar habit in half.

Here's how to do it:

Step One: Become a Sugar Sleuth

Using our sample form for making a food diary, record everything you eat for at least three weekdays and two weekend days. Specifically note your sugar habit by recording all sugar you add to coffee or tea, sodas you drink, cereals you choose, desserts, snacks, candy, cakes, artificial sweeteners in processed foods, and sugar added to recipes.

Please don't read anything about sugar before you make your diary, because that may change the way you eat and defeat your purpose. You want a real picture of your real sugar habit, so eat the way you usually eat, and eat what you want to eat.

Read pages 187–189: Diary, Food. This will explain how to keep your diary and give you the form to use. You might want to copy the form into a notebook to carry around with you, so you can record on the spot. This avoids the stress of having to remember what you ate and ensures that you record everything. Also make notes about your moods and emotions, because that will give you valuable information that you can work on later.

At the end of the week of recording, read the topic on Sugar, using the section "How Sweet It Is" to help you estimate the hidden sugars in your diet. One of the problems we face with sugar in our foods is that the amount of sugar isn't listed on each product. If you can't find the exact food you ate, use the average number of teaspoons of sugar in a similar item. For instance, you had a piece of chocolate cake, and cakes are listed as having five to ten teaspoons of sugar, so estimate that you ate ten teaspoons to allow for the chocolate. If you eat foods with artificial sweeteners, use our teaspoon measurement to judge their content of sugar, since artificial sweeteners are simply condensed sugars, meaning they are just as sweet as the real thing. Total up the number of teaspoons of sugar you ate.

Read pages 244–245: Label Reading.

Before you move on to step two, take one or two hours to have a supermarket adventure. You are going to the supermarket looking for sugar in foods. Don't combine this adventure with your grocery shopping. Go with your label clues and walk up and down the aisles, taking out the foods you most commonly buy to study the sugar content. If you get hungry, buy a fresh fruit and eat it while you study these products. It will be the best thing you ever did for your health.

After you complete your sugar adventure, stand in front of the vegetable and fruit section for a minute to remind yourself there are still foods you can eat. Don't be defeated by the amount of sugar you see. Your goal is to use this adventure to teach yourself how to choose the lower-sugar foods. When you choose the lower-sugar foods, you are making a big dent in your sugar habit.

Step Two: Halve Your Sugar Habit
Use the following guidelines to cut your sugar intake in half (or more if you feel committed).

1. Choose the foods that are lowest in sugar. If you find that you have a hard time adjusting to lower-sugar cereals, start by mixing your old high-sugar cereal with half of the lower-sugar cereal, and gradually ease out your old choice. Remember, a sugar habit is hard to break, so give yourself credit with every improvement you make.

2. If you drink sodas, switch to the other more natural drinks that are good for dieters.
Read page 85 for suggestions.

3. Take the number of teaspoons of sugar or packets that you use daily (from your diary) and divide the amount in half. Refill your sugar bowl and use that as your sugar maximum for the day. Think of the money you're saving, since you now have the same amount of sugar ready for tomorrow. If you have difficulty, eat a fresh fruit for natural sugar and wait a minute or two before adding more sugar to your food or drinks.

4. When you feel a sugar urge, eat a fresh fruit. It's natural sugar and filled with vitamins and fiber. A fabulous slimming food!

5. Experiment with spices to flavor your recipes instead of using sugar.

6. When it comes to desserts, don't eliminate, re-create them! For instance, if you love strawberry shortcake, have angel food cake with fresh strawberries and a dollop of vanilla frozen yogurt. It's delicious and nutritious, and it will make you lean.

7. Be creative with your food and meals, finding ways to cut sugar without sacrificing your pleasure.

Read pages 69–85: The Problem Solver Diet. You can use this program from the start to beat your sugar habit, since it is automatically a healthy low-sugar program. Use the food pyramid for your guide, but keep an eye on extra foods you might eat to be sure you're not letting your sugar habit creep back into your food plan.

Step Three: Step Up Your Activity

Now that you are eating a healthier diet, create a routine exercise program that you can combine with your new eating habits. Since you are not eating as much sugar, you will have more natural energy, and it will carry you through any exercise you want to do. Be creative with your program, including one machine (if you have access), one stretching routine to elongate and reshape that sugar-free body, and one weight-bearing exercise such as walking.

When in doubt, walk a half-hour every night. It will lighten your life.

Read pages 107–112: The Problem Solver Calendar. This will give you an automatic plan to follow for ideal exercise, eating, and behavior on the spot.

◆

YOU EAT TOO MUCH FAT

**The mere mention of the word *fat* can cause
a panic attack in people who eat too much fat.**

DO YOU KNOW THE FIRST thing people say when you ask
them, "Do you eat too much fat?"

No, but . . . I eat a lot of sweets. [Sweets are filled with fat.]

No, but . . . I eat a lot of ice cream. [Ice cream is rich with fat.]

No, but . . . I'm a pizza nut. [Cheese is chock full of fat.]

No, but . . . Don't ask me to give up butter.

For some reason, people have a hard time admitting that they
eat fat. Perhaps it's because admitting it will take off the blinders,
and when the blinders are gone, what has to follow? All those
desserts have to go out the window. All that cheese has to come off
the pizza. All that fat has to come out of your food. Because the fat
on your plate is your excess weight.

Butter lovers will say, "I'd rather die than use margarine."
Unfortunately, this is too close to the truth. Fat has been linked to
every major cause of death from heart disease and strokes to
diabetes and cancer.

On the opposite side of the fence are complex carbohydrates—
fresh fruits, vegetables, and grains—that make salads, pastas,
bread, cereals, desserts, sauces, and toppings that have almost no
fat; lean meats for stir-fry, beef kabobs, and entrées, or added to
pasta salads; and desserts that aren't dull, like raspberries with
vanilla frozen yogurt over angel food cake.

The list of fitness foods goes on and on, and the key to fat
freedom is finally to take the blinders off and see these foods as

pleasure-givers. Fat-filled foods aren't the only foods with taste. And the less fat you eat, the more taste you will gain for fresher, more nutritious foods.

Are you eating too much fat?

Here's the average to follow for fitness:

Women	*Men*
30–45 grams per day	45–60 grams per day

Take a look at butter: One pat of butter has 11 grams of fat. Eat four pats a day and you're right up there in fat maximum country at 44 grams for one food. And the rest of your food has fat too, especially the fatter meats.

Let's look at a cheeseburger: One cheeseburger has 37 grams of fat. That's an average cheeseburger. What about a quarter pounder? Or a double? Or a sub?

When you begin to look at fat grams in your favorite foods, it will be a rude awakening.

At first, you'll get depressed, because it won't look like there's anything left to eat, except vegetables.

That's a good start on a healthy diet. Vegetables have no fat. You can eat them without guilt.

And fruits. Fruits have almost no fat and a whole lot of fiber, which tends to remove fat from your body. So you can eat for sweetness.

And grains. You've got a lot of grains to choose, and they're very low in fat. You can eat pasta and bread. You can eat stuffed shells with cottage cheese and tomatoes, and you've got the same taste as you had in the past with fatter stuffed shells.

And dairy products. Don't forget them. A must for calcium. The low-fat varieties taste great and give you protein.

The lean meats are delicious, and there are hundreds of ways to make less go farther. This not only saves you fat, but money too. You can take a vacation on the savings in your meat budget alone.

When it comes to fat cutting, you can take the difficult road and try to count all the grams in everything you are eating. But who has time for that much fat?

You have better things to do with your life.

The easiest way to do it is to eat differently from the start. Eat a healthy diet first, meeting your nutritional needs for complex carbohydrates, protein, and dairy products in the leaner versions, then if you're still hungry and have to have fat, count that and tally the fat grams. Consider them the ones that are keeping you fat. Then gradually cut them back.

You can find out what you're eating in excess of daily fat by using the calorie counter at the end of this book to look up the fat grams in your daily food. Total it for the day.

Compare it to the fat gram averages we gave you to stay lean.

Take the extra grams off your day by cutting the one or two foods that give you the most fat. But don't cut nutrition in the name of fat. That could be a big mistake.

Eating less than you need for nutrition on a daily basis is one way of losing your body muscle. That will make you gain fat.

Take the fat out of your diet with foods that are *not* included on the Problem Solver Diet pyramid.

Do you need an easier way?

Read pages 69–85: The Problem Solver Diet.

Follow the food pyramid for your daily meal plans and don't eat extra fat. If you're hungry, eat fruit, vegetables, or grains as extras. Over time, you'll find that you have less desire for fat because you're eating nutritionally. Follow the Problem Solver Calendar to ideal weight. Not only will you shed your fat, but you will have learned how to eat low-fat for life.

PROBLEM NUMBER ELEVEN

◆

STRESS AND WEIGHT

You live a high-stress life and eat on automatic pilot.

STRESS PROBLEMS AND WEIGHT PROBLEMS go hand in hand to reinforce each other. When you have a high-stress life, with no outlets for your stress, you get caught in a stress/weight cycle that will make both problems escalate.

The following factors are common to the stress/weight cycle, and they show you how the cycle can escalate out of control.

One of the primary causes of overeating is *stress*. When you are tense, anxious, and experiencing stress symptoms, eating calms you down; your parasympathetic nervous system is activated during digestion, and this temporarily eases stress. But the problem is that you begin to use food as a coping response to stress. Food becomes a priority, and stress becomes your cue to eat, a habit on automatic pilot. When stressed, you reach for food, and this leads to weight gain.

The *style* of eating in response to stress also induces weight gain. To ease your stress, you eat fast, not taking time to chew; you may eat on the run, in your car—wherever you are—and take whatever is at hand for the quickest energy boost. Most often, these foods are high in sugar and fat: fast foods, prepackaged snacks, vending machine treats, processed foods. These foods are poor sources of nutrition and great fat storers, and they lead to weight gain.

As you gain weight, you begin to feel more stressed about your body and weight, and you start to feel guilty when you eat. All eating, even normal meals, becomes a source of concern, and

35

you're left without your former outlet of eating to ease stress. Eating now produces stress.

Excess weight is a stress on your body system, bearing down on your organs. Your clothes become tight and uncomfortable, and you seldom feel at ease. You may experience more digestive troubles and intestinal pressure, and your breathing becomes more shallow from tension in your midriff and diaphragm area. Shallow breathing is a stress symptom, and you will tend to breathe that way on a routine basis, because of your excess weight. This inhibits oxygen pickup in your lungs and limits blood flow to your body, resulting in a slower circulation and less comfort with activity.

Exercise and activity become more difficult because of excess weight, and you sit more and move less. The more you sit and the less you move, the more weight you gain, which causes more stress.

Family and friends may unwittingly add to your stress by pressing you to lose weight, and your interpersonal relationships become more strained. There is social pressure to be thin, and when you are not, you feel less at ease in social situations, especially when they center around food.

As you can see, this cycle continues to build, so that you are facing not only the everyday stresses common to everyone, but also the weight-related stresses that seem to meet you at every turn.

The good news is that you can take three steps to success for stress control and also have an automatic program for weight reduction. By dealing with your stress in the framework of a healthy diet, you will see dramatic benefits in your ability to handle stress, and you'll see your weight come down significantly.

Here's how to do it:

Step One: Build Your Inner Strength
Read pages 142–145: Breathing. Practice diaphragm breathing exercises for five minutes each morning when you wake. This breathing technique reverses the symptoms of stress caused by shallow breathing. It frees up trapped energy and gets your circulation moving again. It's unbeatable! Also, by learning this simple technique, you have an on-the-spot skill to use when stress besets you during the day.

Read pages 292–295: Relaxation. Practice the relaxation exercises for ten to fifteen minutes at the same time each night, until you master the skill. Start by learning the relaxation initiator, and when you've got it down, add on the adjuncts Finding Your Perfect Place, Stress, or Stressors. (Use only one adjunct at a time in each session.) Continue to practice these skills even if you aren't sure they are working. One day the effect will kick in, and you will be amazed how uplifted and stress-free you feel. The best times to do these exercises might be right after you come in from work or just before dinner. Your goal is to establish a routine, to make relaxation a habit. After you are comfortable with the relaxation skills, you can use them during the day when you are facing stressful situations. Often you won't have to use the initiator; you can simply step away from your desk or from the stress and picture your perfect place. It will immediately calm you and separate you from the stress.

For the first step, your only goal is to work on your inner self, trying to achieve a more relaxed state. Don't try to change your diet or routine at this point, since change is stress; and because of this, you should try to avoid too many changes until you have built up your inner reserves to handle stress better. When your breathing exercises and relaxation skills have become routine (a natural habit you do every day), move on to step two.

Step Two: Build Your Nutrient Defense

Read pages 320–324: Stress. Read about stress and see why you need a special kind of diet for your weight loss and stress defense.

Read pages 69–85: The Problem Solver Diet. Using our food pyramid as your daily nutrition slide rule, follow our eating program for superior fat burn and muscle protection. If you feel you want more food, eat all of your snacks in complex carbohydrates—vegetables, grains, and fruits. That way you will never feel you have to be hungry or deprived while burning fat, you will be getting the extra metabolic clout that complex carbohydrates give you, and you will receive a real energy booster and stress defense too.

Keep up your breathing exercises and relaxation skills every day, and you'll begin to feel the greater sense of inner strength and well-being that come from having better nutrition and better coping skills. Your goal in this step is to make balanced nutrition a routine that is comfortable and easy for you to do on a daily basis. When it becomes second nature and you're eating healthfully as a habit, move on to step three.

Step Three: Build Your Body Fitness

A regular exercise routine will not only give you new energy, strength, and tone, it will be a natural stress medication you can use for life. In regular doses, exercise will reduce your heart rate, reduce lactate production (associated with neurosis), reduce adrenalin circulation (associated with tension and anxiety), reduce your weight, and reduce your perception of effort (things that seemed difficult will seem easier to do).

There's a good reason why you saved your exercise routine for last, and it's this: High-stressed people tend to select high-stress exercise, and jump right in. This can cause strain and injury and defeat the purpose of your exercise, which was to reduce stress, not create more. The reason you learned your breathing and relaxation skills first was to give you a calmer outlook and quieter mind, and now that you have that on your side, you will have a clearer picture of the type of exercise that will best suit you.

Use your new inner strength to plan your exercise routine. At first, avoid high-stress programs like jogging or weight lifting and gradually advance your ability. You might choose a blend of stretching, walking, and strength training, repeating your activity three times each week. The stretching will elongate your muscles, continue to enhance your circulation, and give you more flexibility and mobility. The walking will burn off your fat, and the strength training will be the kick you need to work off that excess stress.

If you want a program that will put it all together for you, use the Problem Solver Calendar.

Read pages 107–112: The Problem Solver Calendar.

Congratulations! If you've come this far, you've now learned how to confront a challenge and overcome it. You're entitled to feel a new sense of well-being, self-esteem, and a great sense of accomplishment. You also have the skills you need for weight control and stress control for life. You can use this new energy to do something nice for yourself and move on to the other relaxation adjuncts or to meditation for greater self-enhancement.

◆

TOO MUCH SODIUM IN YOUR DIET

You need to break the salt habit for your heart's sake.

THE AVERAGE AMERICAN EATS three to six times the sodium he or she needs daily. This can cause high blood pressure, which leads to heart attacks and strokes.

Don't wait until you're told to cut back on sodium by your doctor, because by then you'll have reached a riskier state. Do it now and you will be protecting your future health.

Sodium that occurs naturally in food is not the source to cut back first. There are other more potent sources of sodium.

Most of your excess sodium comes from processed foods and salt added at the table or in cooking. Cut these sources and you've got your sodium under control.

Follow these sodium-smart guidelines:

- Diet with fresh foods, and use herbs and spices for flavor. That way, you can avoid the sodium in processed foods and gain other health benefits at the same time. Processed foods are low in fiber and high in fat and sugar. Fresh foods are everything you need for fitness and health.
- Cut salt in your recipes by one-half.
- Replace high-sodium condiments like steak sauce and soy sauce with low-salt varieties.
- Make an herbal shaker to use instead of salt in cooking and at the table.

- Make fresh soups and refrigerate them, instead of relying on canned soups with sodium.
- Spend an hour in the supermarket, identifying low-sodium varieties of your favorite foods, so you can shop with sodium-savvy in the future.

Read pages 308–312: Sodium.

This will give you a complete guide to sodium and the recipe for an herbal shaker. You can be salt-smart for life.

If you want to lose weight and cut sodium at the same time, use the Problem Solver Diet.

Read pages 69–85: The Problem Solver Diet.

Follow The Problem Solver Calendar to ideal weight and salt-sensible eating.

◆

CHOLESTEROL

**You've read countless articles on cholesterol,
but you still aren't sure you're taking the right road
to cholesterol control. You need an easier program.**

ONE OF THE MOST IMPORTANT studies to link coronary heart disease and strokes with cholesterol elevation in the blood was the Framingham Heart Study. Since that study, cholesterol has become the most talked about subject in health in the last few years, with special diets designed to lower it and a wide variety of programs designed to help you try to beat it. And yet, many people are still confused by the issue because it seems so complicated.

The three most important things you can do right away to keep cholesterol at bay are:

1. Decrease your total fat intake, specifically the high-cholesterol foods and cholesterol-raising fats (saturated fats). See our EZ Cholesterol Guide to find the high-cholesterol foods.

2. Increase your fiber intake, since this has been shown to have an even more dramatic impact on cholesterol control than cutting fat.

3. Increase your exercise, since this increases HDL (good cholesterol) and provides the cholesterol balance you need between HDL and LDL (bad cholesterol) in your body for a better cholesterol test.

Have your cholesterol checked regularly by your physician to find out your cholesterol range, since tests can change on different days. Don't rely on casual tests in malls or other nonmedical

41

settings, since the margin for error is greater with them. In addition, any heart-related issue such as cholesterol must be considered in the full context of your health and family history, and this is only known by your physician.

If you have a family history of heart disease and you eat a lot of high-fat desserts and use a lot of butter, have your cholesterol checked, since you are in a higher risk category.

To reduce your cholesterol, follow this three-step plan:

1. Make the necessary adjustments in your diet. Do as many as you can to reduce the cholesterol you eat:

- Switch from whole milk to low-fat milk or skim milk.
- Switch from butter to a low-cholesterol margarine.
  Tub margarines are the best choice, since they are not as hydrogenated (hard at room temperature). Land O Lakes Sweet Cream spread has the best taste.
- Limit egg yolks as much as possible. For every two eggs you cook, use one yolk, or use Egg Beaters.
- Avoid imitation creamers containing coconut oil and palm oil. Also check processed food labels for these oils.
- Choose lean meats and avoid the highest cholesterol meats: bacon, dark meat turkey, and all organ meats such as liver. Eat your poultry without skin.
- Limit high-cholesterol desserts, the ones with lots of butter, lard, cheese, cream, and more in the pie crust. The top seven are: custard pie, cheesecake, eclair, apple pie, lemon meringue pie, bread pudding, and sponge cake.
- Limit cheeses and cheese sauces.
- Switch from ice cream to low-fat frozen yogurt desserts. They taste just like ice cream and are very healthy for you.
- Switch from sour cream on your baked potatoes to whipped low-fat cottage cheese with lots of diced vegetables. This will remove a cholesterol offender while adding needed fiber to your diet.
- Increase your fiber intake. Eat plenty of fresh fruits, whole grains, and vegetables for complex carbohydrates.
- Substitute fresh foods for processed foods wherever possible.
- Use fresh fruits for quick snacks instead of candies, chips, and cheese snacks in bags.
- Cook with polyunsaturated oils instead of butter or margarine.
- In restaurants say, "Cook without butter. No cheese sauces, please!"

2. Exercise three times each week with an aerobic exercise of your choice. Regular aerobic exercise maintains your cardiovascular fitness and increases good cholesterol (HDL) to offset the bad cholesterol (LDL). The result is cholesterol balance.

3. Be sure your overall nutrition is balanced, to get the best total health benefits from your cholesterol control. Compare your daily diet against the food pyramid in The Problem Solver Diet.

Note: French studies show that a glass of red wine a day may keep arterial plaque away. Check this with your doctor.

Read pages 160–173: Cholesterol.

This will tell you everything you need to know about cholesterol. The EZ Cholesterol Guide will pinpoint how much cholesterol you're eating.

Read pages 215–217: Fiber.

This will show you an easy way to get the fiber you need daily.

If you want to lose weight while you cut cholesterol, follow the Problem Solver Diet and you'll do both simultaneously.

Read pages 107–112: The Problem Solver Calendar—A Month to Fat Freedom.

For total heart health, fix one other habit: if you smoke, stop.

◆

YOU DON'T EAT ENOUGH COMPLEX CARBOHYDRATES

**With all the confusion about carbohydrates
in the last decade, you're not sure if they're good or bad,
how to find them, which ones to eat.**

THERE ARE NUMEROUS BENEFITS from complex carbohydrates for dieting and health, but the three most important are:

The thermic effect of food
This is the heat your body produces as a result of eating. When you eat and digest complex carbohydrates, your body produces more heat (calorie burn) than it would if you were eating fat. Protein is also a heat-producing food, but the protein foods also come with hidden fats inside, so they aren't the leanest or easiest choice to drive up your heat by eating. Studies show, as we revealed in the *Fat-to-Muscle Diet*, that you can burn as much as 15 percent of your total daily calories simply by eating the "hotter" foods.

If you eat 1,500 calories per day on your diet, you can burn as many as 225 calories simply by eating thermically, which means eating more complex carbohydrates while you are eating less fat. If you look at it from the opposite point of view, it also means you can eat more calories with the confidence that they are burning off when you eat thermically. This is a very important eating lesson to learn when you are facing weight loss and the ideal weight maintenance for life; you want to be able to eat more calories without

44

gaining weight when you stop dieting. When you eat more complex carbohydrates while you are dieting, you are retraining your body to produce more heat and burn more calories, and you head into maintenance with the ability to increase your calories without regaining.

You can eat more complex carbohydrates without storing fat. This is the eating style to follow for dieting, since it drives up your calorie-burning power and allows you to eat more food during your diet. No starvation or deprivation and a better metabolism result. Since the complex carbohydrates—fresh fruits, vegetables, and whole grains—come stocked with vitamins and minerals, by eating more of these foods, you are also driving up your nutritional status and gaining better health. No nutritional deficiencies, no energy swings, great disease prevention status—all this while you are becoming a better fat burner.

The fantastic features of fiber

There are dozens of reasons you need more fiber in your diet for fat prevention and health status. Fiber is found in complex carbohydrates—fruits, vegetables, whole grains. Among the reasons you want more fiber are:

- It doesn't store as fat.
- It expands in your stomach to create fullness.
- It comes in all the low-calorie and low-fat foods, making it easy to choose extra foods for snacks.
- Fiber foods take longer to chew, which gives your hunger signal time to turn off.
- It is vital to your intestines to make them function properly. This keeps food moving through your system faster and better, meaning you store fewer calories overall.

Read pages 330–335: Sugar.

The section What Defines a Carbohydrate Food will show you the difference between a fresh complex carbohydrate and a processed one, which is actually a carbohydrate in a fat suit.

The energy you need

Complex carbohydrates break down during digestion to produce glucose, your body's preferred source of energy, the fuel for your muscles and brain. When you can give your body the best, why would you give it less?

Read pages 201–207: Exercise, aerobic vs. anaerobic.

This will explain the dangers of dieting and exercising when you don't eat enough complex carbohydrates.

How do you start to increase your complex carbohydrates?

If you have no weight to lose but you need to be sure you are eating enough complex carbohydrates, here's how to do it:

Read pages 215–217: Fiber.

- Meet your needs for the five best fibers on a daily basis, following the guide to determine where to find them and how to reintroduce them into your diet.
- Limit your use of processed foods.
- Eat *fresh* fruits, vegetables, and whole grains as much as possible.

If you have weight to lose, you cannot do it successfully without increasing your daily supply of complex carbohydrates. Here's how to do it the easy way, increasing your complex carbohydrates and losing weight simultaneously:

Read pages 69–85: The Problem Solver Diet.

Follow the Problem Solver Calendar all the way to ideal weight. By then, you will be eating balanced, healthy meals with all your fiber automatically worked in. It's a dream for total fitness.

◆

YOU HAVE A BLOCK AGAINST EXERCISE

**You have many reasons why exercise is a real problem
for you. As a result, you don't exercise regularly
and that keeps you out of shape and gaining weight.**

THERE ARE TWO PRIMARY REASONS why people gain weight: poor diet (high fat, low fiber, inadequate nutrition) and lack of activity.

You can lose weight by dieting alone, but the quality of weight loss will be inferior to the results that can be achieved by combining healthy dieting and exercising. In fact, when you are on a diet, if you don't exercise, the success of your program can be jeopardized for several important reasons.

Calorie burning power. One of the goals of dieting is to remove your fat from storage. To do this, you cut your intake of calories, forcing your body to take the fat from storage to burn for energy. But your body system is designed to protect itself and to perform its basic functions to build and repair tissues and cells. When you cut the calories you take in, your body reads this as a time for protection of its resources, and it in turn cuts down the amount of calories that are burned for energy. Your body preserves energy to be used in case of crises. The only way to force your system to burn more calories while you are cutting them is with exercise. If you diet without exercise, you don't burn calories as well and you lose weight slower.

Weight loss as fat. When you diet, you can lose body muscle along with fat, but your goal is to lose only fat. Exercise is the only way to ensure that your body muscle is protected so that you only lose fat.

Muscle for maintenance. Your goal should be a better body inside and out at the end of your diet. If you diet without exercise, you can't build more body muscle for maintenance, and you can reach ideal weight without sufficient muscle to keep your calories burning at a steady pace when you increase your food intake. Exercise gives you the muscle you need to eat more calories without gaining weight after you go off your diet. That means no yo-yoing and no regain.

Healthy intestinal tract. When you exercise, food moves through your system faster, and that means that fewer calories will be absorbed to store as fat. In addition, exercise helps to prevent digestive disorders that can be caused by intestinal blockage, including many diseases such as colon cancer.

Increased oxygen and circulation. Fat needs oxygen for an active burning process. Exercise not only increases the oxygen pickup by your blood, but it increases your circulation to deliver the oxygen faster. It makes every body process work better, including fat burn.

Appetite control. Studies show that a loss of appetite follows a good physical workout. If you don't exercise on a diet, you can be hungry longer, and your tendency to eat from boredom is increased.

Behavior modification. Exercise is the best substitute for eating and is a stress defense. It reverses the symptoms of stress, and that in turn prevents you from turning to food for calming or consolation in times of stress. It helps you take control over your emotional eating.

Euphoria and well-being. The modulators of pain and moods in your body are endorphins, and these are increased with exercise. This gives you a powerful, positive feeling that not only makes dieting easier and uplifting, but also eases anxiety and depression, major causes of overeating.

You reap many more benefits from exercise, including better muscle tone, agility, flexibility, and strength. Your weight loss looks better because of exercise. And yet, despite all this, you can't seem to get around to exercise.

What can you do?

Step One: Breaking the Block

Your mind plays a powerful role in the success or failure of your endeavors. But you have the ability to retrain your mind to ride right through obstacles caused by negative thinking and feelings that you *can't* or *won't* do something that's good for you.

Read pages 289–291: Rationalizations. This is an exercise in positive thinking, or how to turn your negative feedback into positive feedback to get you up and active. Read the list of typical "reasons" or excuses that people use for not doing something and the responses that show how to turn these excuses into positive feelings for action. Then make up your own list of reasons you don't exercise. Every time you find yourself expressing a negative reason, turn it around and express it as a positive thought. This will condition your mind to feel more positive about your fitness goals. You can use this technique on all negative feelings that come into your mind, in other areas than exercise. The more you erase your self-doubts and inner negative voice, the more energy you will free up to seek movement and exercise.

Read pages 292–295: Relaxation. A regular routine of relaxation gives you energy and stamina and frees your mind of clutter that can make your desires seem too complicated to pursue. Practice relaxation every morning for a week until it becomes comfortable and routine. First learn how to do the relaxation initiator, then use the adjuncts Exercise and Mental Rehearsal. Continue to use positive thinking and relaxation, until they become natural for you. When they become a habit, move on to step two.

Step Two: Walk While You Plan

Each night after work, take a one-half hour walk to clear your head and help you unwind from the day. As you are walking, think about the exercise program you will be developing for yourself, the choices of machines, sports, and activities that are available, and which possibilities are realistic for you.

Read page 248: Walking. If you prefer another time for walking, set that time and do it as a routine while you plan your future exercise workout. Set walking goals to keep you interested and to give your walks purpose, such as visiting a friend, dropping a letter at the post office, or walking to the store for a quart of low-fat milk. Find incentives that will keep you walking, such as tapes you can keep time with, walking a dog, or meeting a walking companion.

When you are comfortable with your walking routine and feel you are ready to create your exercise plan, make an exercise diary.

Read pages 185–187: Diary, Exercise. This will show you the form to use.

Read pages 201–207: Exercise. This will give you choices.

Select a few exercises that you think you'd like to try and list them on the column for type of exercise. Try out these exercises in the days ahead and write down how you felt about them, when you did them, why you stopped (if you did) in your exercise diary. Use your diary as a support system to keep you on track.

Continue to practice positive thinking and relaxation, combined with your walking, while you are trying out exercise machines and routines. Move on to step three.

Step Three: Team Up for Fitness

Start to eat according to the food pyramid for easy weight loss.

Read pages 69–85: The Problem Solver Diet.

Your goal is to create the most exciting exercise program you can think of to give you a total body workout. Since good nutrition is essential for creative thinking, it is vital to eat well as a routine. Continue walking while you make up your mind how you are going to set up this exercise program.

Consider cross training. This involves choosing one exercise for stretching, which will elongate your taut muscles and give your body new flexibility. Choose another exercise for strengthening, such as weight lifting, to build your upper body and skeletal muscles. Then choose a third exercise for cardiovascular conditioning, such as swimming, aerobic dance, or one of the aerobic machines.

And then there's walking. But you've already got that one beat, so just keep doing it.

Do you see how easy it is to overcome a block? All you have to do is walk it off.

Continue to practice your relaxation exercises and positive thinking while you are dieting with the pyramid, and before you know it, you will have mastered the art of staying lean for life.

When you get bored with one exercise, continue your walks while you plan which exercise to use for its replacement. Use your walks to do all of your creative thinking, such as planning your vacation this year. Instead of your old-style vacation, where you eat and drink and fall back into your sedentary style in two weeks, what about planning an active vacation, like a walking tour of the Swiss Alps?

◆

YOU EXERCISE BUT DON'T SEE RESULTS

**You know you're exercising, but your
mirror isn't getting the message.**

IF YOU ARE ALREADY EXERCISING but you find that you aren't losing weight or getting the tone you expected, you need to do a little backpedaling to find out what's going wrong with your diet and exercise program.

The most obvious place to turn for the answers would be your diet.

Ask yourself: Am I eating too much fat and not enough complex carbohydrates? How much fat am I eating? How many complex carbohydrates am I forgetting to eat each day?

Why are they important?

Fat will keep your body-fat content up, even when you exercise, if you are allowing too much fat to slip into your daily meals.

A common mistake exercisers make is to allow themselves more food because they are exercising. When that food contains too much dietary fat, you're thwarting your efforts to get lean and mean.

Fat is a common problem for weight lifters and body builders. They can work out every day, pumping up those muscles; but if they eat too much fat, their muscles are pumped up under a layer of fat, and it makes their bodies appear bulky and unflexible. To get the lean and muscular look, with well-defined outlines, you need to reduce your fat intake while you are lifting weights or

51

doing strenuous workouts, such as cycling, that accent certain muscle groups.

Women may find themselves getting that bulky look in their legs with machines or workouts that concentrate on lower-body muscle groups. To avoid this look, the fat content of your diet must be altered, and stretching exercises should be included to lengthen these muscles.

Women weight lifters will discover the same bulky look in their shoulders and backs, caused by pumping up muscles under a layer of fat. The solution is found in a lower fat diet and the addition of a stretching routine for the upper body.

But cutting fat isn't the entire answer for fitness. It's in the combination of fat and complex carbohydrates.

Complex carbohydrates provide your body with its preferred source of energy, glucose. This is the fuel for your muscles and brain and is the energy you use for sustained aerobic workouts. When you do not eat enough complex carbohydrates—whole grains, fresh vegetables, fruits—you are not providing your body with the energy it needs to get the best benefits from your workout. If you increase your complex carbohydrates while you cut fat, the results of your workout will begin to show *quickly.*

How do you do it without spending your life in nutrition and exercise books?

Step One: EZ Dietary Analysis

Take the time to find out what you're really eating and how that compares with what you should be eating to get the best effect from your workout.

Read pages 187–189: Diary, Food. This will give you the form to use.

Read pages 69–85: The Problem Solver Diet. This will give you the ideal nutrition pyramid. You can use this pyramid to compare what you are eating with what you should be eating.

Take five days to do this properly and record everything you eat on three weekdays and two weekend days. Don't forget that those weekend days can tally up a lot of dietary fat if you use them for a freewheeling time, eating and drinking and partying, even though you eat like a monk during the week.

Don't skip this step, thinking you can remember what you ate. Your food diary will give you important information about yourself, your tendency toward certain kinds of foods, what to watch for, and whether you are getting solid nutrition on a consistent basis.

Consistency is an important key in nutrition and fitness.

Step Two: EZ Diet for Best Effect

Start using the Problem Solver Diet to get your nutrition back in line the easy way. The food pyramid provides full nutrition in the form of the leanest fat, the strongest carbohydrate clout, and the leanest protein. If you need more food, increase your intake of complex carbohydrates. You won't be adding any extra fat, and you'll be getting an extra energy boost for working out. Continue to eat this way until it becomes a habit and use it as your bottom line for life. It will become so ingrained that when you start sliding off, you'll automatically know which groups you are overusing or underusing, and it will be easy to get back on track.

Weight lifters take note: Watch your protein intake, as excess protein can store as fat. While that can make you look bigger overall, it's not a wise course to be fatter inside in order to look bigger on the outside. In men, that can lead to early heart problems, primarly because men are upper-body fat distributors, and that's heart fat.

Read pages 283–285: Protein. Men who work out a great deal can eat from sixty to seventy grams of protein per day, but shouldn't exceed seventy grams to be on the safe side.

When you are comfortable with your new eating style and it has become a habit, move on to step three.

Step Three: EZ Exercise

Have you tried cross training to get the maximum body benefits and total fitness workout?

Use this easy formula:

Choose three exercise routines as the foundation of your cross training workout: one cardiovascular exercise, one stretching exercise, and one strengthening exercise.

The cardiovascular exercise is mandatory for heart health and overall body conditioning, but it often does not work all the muscle groups, specifically the skeletal muscles in the upper body. This can allow the upper body muscles to shrink or tighten over time.

The strengthening exercise (like weight lifting) is needed to pick up where the cardiovascular exercise left off. Strength training tends to use all the muscle groups that have been left out of the cardiovascular workout, especially the upper-back muscles and spinal muscles.

The stretching exercises are the most unappreciated exercises and the best for total effect. They elongate the spine and all muscle groups. They add grace and flexibility and give you the ability to turn fast or react easily in a crisis. They prevent injury, especially to the back and underworked muscle groups near the spine, and they give you more range of motion. People who tend to look bulky or hefty after exercise will see a real bonus of length and leanness when using stretches. Choose the best program you can get and introduce stretching into your regular routine. It also increases your circulation and acts as a form of simple meditation, which clears your mind and calms you. The best choice is callanetics, or you can begin with our at-home stretching routine.

To keep your workout interesting, keep up the variety of total body fitness that cross training can bring. See The Problem Solver Calendar for a complete follow-along cross-training workout.

Don't forget to work on your inner resources for strength, tone, and positive life goals. You can find many excellent techniques in the dictionary in articles that have the symbol ● in the left margin.

Here's to a total workout, for a new and vital you!

◆

PLATEAUS

Even when you diet, you reach a weight that you can't get below, and it's higher than your ideal.

WEIGHT PLATEAUS ARE A COMMON problem for certain dieters, and they can occur for the following reasons:

1. *Trying to lose weight too fast.* If you use a rapid weight-loss diet or starvation style of eating to try to lose weight fast, you lose too much muscle, which in turn causes your metabolic rate to drop drastically.

Normally on a diet, your metabolic rate will decrease by 15 percent, because you are decreasing your energy intake (calories). Your body responds to this calorie decrease by holding on to its energy (calories) to meet its need to keep all systems functioning. On a healthy diet, you can offset this metabolic decrease with exercise and thermic eating: eating to produce more heat (calorie burn). But on a rapid weight-loss diet, you are eating too little food and getting too little energy (calories), and often you don't have the energy or stamina to exercise, so you don't do it. In addition, when you do exercise, because the low-calorie diet might not be providing enough carbohydrates (and they usually don't), you aren't using the right energy for exercise. You're using ketone energy (anaerobic), and as a result you are more likely burning your muscle instead of fat. This form of exercise creates a drastic reduction in metabolism that does not occur on a healthy diet.

Rapid weight-loss diets can show more than 30 percent reduction in metabolism from loss of muscle and calorie reduction. This adds up to something you don't want: slower calorie burn and more retention of fat. As a result of dieting improperly, you can reach a point where you can't lose weight at all, even when you are cutting calories. Your body has retrained itself to exist on fewer calories.

A greater problem occurs when you stop eating at starvation calorie levels and try to go off your diet. You regain fat like a magnet is attracting it, and you don't regain your muscle. At the start, you were facing a weight plateau that you couldn't get below, but at the finish you're facing weight regain to a weight greater than your original weight.

This is the most dangerous reason for a plateau, the one to avoid at all costs. The others are less harmful.

2. *Too much fat is creeping into your diet.* If you are following a healthy diet and you reach a weight where you stop losing entirely, review your food intake to see if you are secretly eating too much fat. This increased fat intake will bring you out of calorie burn and begin to put fat back into storage.

3. *Too much fiber is falling out of your diet.* Check your fiber level to see if you are eating enough complex carbohydrates, since these are essential to removal of fat.

4. *You're not exercising regularly.* You may think you're exercising, but on review, you might find that you aren't doing it regularly three times each week or aren't doing it long enough (thirty minutes per session). If you're walking, are you meandering; if you're rowing, are you recovering more than rowing; if you're using Nordic track, are you simultaneously reading a book and forgetting to work hard? If you find that you are exercising diligently and it's still not working to take you off that plateau, you will have to change your exercise to a more intense workout, perhaps walking five nights a week instead of three. This will not exhaust you or harm you, since walking is low intensity. The slight boost in exercise provided by the two extra nights of walking will also boost your calorie burn, since you will be forcing your body to use more calories for the increased activity. You must do this in the context of a healthy, balanced diet such as the one shown in the food pyramid in the Problem Solver Diet.

You can also add an extra boost by becoming more active in your everyday life. Walk to the store instead of driving. Take more stairs instead of elevators. Try out a few sports activities that will be entertaining to do. The point is, don't accept the plateau as a block. Take it on as a challenge. The step afterward is worth it. It's ideal weight.

5. *You are accepting a higher weight.* This is not such an odd idea. It's a very real fact that many people are afraid to get below a certain weight for many personal reasons. Losing weight and being slim are not familiar states to many people who have been carrying weight for a long time. Slimness can be threatening, since it's unknown territory, something not experienced, therefore not safe.

Read pages 212–213: Fat Eyes.

Many people have spouses who also have weight problems, and they are afraid of the effect that slimness will have on the relationship. Many people have families who make comments like, "Don't get too thin, your cheeks will sink in." These comments can hold weight for a person who is trying to change a long-standing problem.

Whatever the reason might be for holding on to weight, it's something that must be changed from within, where it begins. To change your inner image of yourself, to support your goal as a slimmer person, take a little time to strengthen your inner resources. That way the changes you make will be real and more gratifying.

Read pages 234–235: Imagery.

Practice the exercise for Getting Thin from Within.

Read pages 264–267: Mirror Exercises.

Practice the exercises for body image approval. These will fill in the gap between your mental image and physical image, to help you let go of your weight.

If you need a diet that will accomplish all of the goals mentioned above in one combined program, use the Problem Solver Diet.

Read pages 107–112: The Problem Solver Calendar.

Follow the calendar to ideal weight. The combined method of healthy diet and exercise, supported by positive behaviors, will take you off the plateau and into the home stretch to fitness.

◆

SPECIAL EVENTS

**You want to diet, but you don't want
to feel ostracized from the rest of the world.**

SOMEHOW IT SEEMS THAT every time you make up your mind to lose weight, something comes up to spoil it. A party, a wedding, your vacation, business dinners all week, another graduation—these events are making you gain.

What can you do?

You have to expect that there will be special events in your life and plan your fitness goals in spite of them. In fact, if you eat healthfully and exercise, you can plan your fitness goals to include them.

If you see special events as threats, they will be, and the fat will keep coming in. If you see them as opportunities, they will be and you can get on with getting lean. If you try to avoid them, you'll feel stressed and disappointed. If you go with the fear of letting go, you'll be sorry when you get home.

Use the following guidelines to go with the flow of events without giving in to temptation:

1. *Identify your weaknesses in advance.* Make a list of the special events that occur regularly in your life: birthday parties, weddings, bar mitzvahs, vacations, graduations, dining out, and weekend getaways.

Using a looseleaf notebook, list these events, one to a page. Identify the foods you associate with these events, the ones you most commonly eat or look forward to as a reason to attend.

Using the calorie counter at the back of this book, record the fat content of the foods you listed next to each food. Be honest. If you tend to eat the largest slice of cake at a wedding, list it as two servings and double the fat content. Total the fat for the event. Compare your total to the average fat grams for a day's health:

Women	*Men*
30–45 grams per day	45–60 grams per day

If you usually eat twice your fat maximum at one event, you will have to cut your fat intake to at least one-half at the event.

You can do that by eating a hearty plate of fresh vegetables and fat-free dip before you leave the house. This will fill you with fiber and keep hunger at bay in the face of those fattening foods. At the event, choose the leanest meat selection and ask for sauces and salad dressings on the side to ration their use. Then add "tastes" of your old favorites—half- or quarter-sized portions. If you have a sweet dessert, cut it in quarters and leave three-fourths on the plate. With sweets, you can get the same emotional satisfaction from one-fourth of the sweet as you can from the whole portion. The rest of the sweet is just excess fat and sugar.

2. Focus on fun instead of food. Instead of sitting and eating, get on your feet when it's possible. At weddings and parties, dance. At barbecues, find sports to participate in. At graduations, walk around the campus. Before entering restaurants, take a walk around the block a few times and then go in and sit down.

Enjoy the company of people and watch them eat, instead of you. Drink water spritzers or nibble fresh vegetables to give the impression that you're one of the crowd. That way, you'll fit in and won't have to talk about dieting. And no one but you will know that you haven't been eating much fat.

3. Focus on fitness instead of feelings. If a panic attack for cheese fondue overcomes you, don't try to analyze it or talk yourself out of it. Take positive action. Do three minutes of diaphragm breathing to release the stress and move away from the food as you do it. Drink water or find a fresh fruit. In a pinch, a mint or a cough drop will do the trick. Congratulate yourself when the urge is gone and you've conquered it.

Read pages 142–145: Breathing.

This will show you how to breathe from your diaphragm to alleviate stress.

You can surmount any obstacle to fitness if you make up your mind that this time you'd rather feel healthy when you get home.

Plan active vacations to keep your level of fitness up to par all year. Do things out of the ordinary for a change of pace: learn a new sport or skill such as skin diving or hang gliding, go white-water rafting or hiking, or take a walking vacation in Saint Moritz where the slim and famous play. An active vacation will linger longer and happier in your mind than a list of restaurants and menus, or the image of a candy machine at midnight in the hotel.

If you're dieting diligently and an event comes up unexpectedly, use the maintenance pyramid as the guideline for a day's nutrition, since it will give you a few more options. Do the absolute best you can at the event without adding too much stress about food. Then return to your diet the next day and be sure you exercise to keep those calories burning. Remember that small lapses in food management will not stack on pounds of fat overnight. It's the big lapses which continue unabated that will add that extra weight. When you are eating healthily and exercising on your diet, you don't have to feel separated from the world of food and eating. You will have the skills you need to choose wisely and learn how to do an event without overdoing it.

Read pages 69–85: The Problem Solver Diet.

This will show you the healthy way to gain strength and self-sufficiency about food while you are losing your fat.

◆

HOLIDAY WEIGHT GAIN

Six short weeks can add six big pounds.

IF THOSE CURRIER AND IVES WINTER SCENES could come to life, think of what they'd say about the real story of the holidays.

It's a six-pound weight-gain season for the average American from Thanksgiving to New Year's Day.

Holidays are high-charged times where every threat to health is moving full speed ahead. Here are just a few of them:

- Emotions cue you to eat, and emotions run rampant over the holiday season.
- Eating patterns are learned in childhood, and holidays are times when the whole family gathers to eat again. All the old eating habits come right out of the closet with the holiday decorations.
- Food is abundant. The sight and smell of food are cues to eat.
- Parties and events are compacted into a short time frame. These are trouble times for dieters, even when they are spaced out over the year.
- The theme of the season is Eat, drink and be merry. The reality is that you eat, drink, and feel terrible—stuffed like the proverbial goose.
- Families are emotional triggers. They push panic buttons without meaning to. Tempers flare without warning; moods go up and down. These are cues to eat.

61

- Alcohol is flowing, as gifts and on buffets. It's socially expected that drinking is part of the holiday season. Alcohol increases your appetite and dulls your judgment. You eat without thinking. You eat to combat the effects of the alcohol.
- Stress is on every corner: shopping, overbuying, overtrying to please everyone with a present. You want everything to be perfect. It seldom is.
- Time is twice as precious. The days are shorter with less light.
- You never make time for yourself.

What can you do to defeat these holiday cues to eat and gain weight? Try these precautions:

1. Pay extra attention to nutrition during the high-stress holidays, since stress depletes your nutrients, making you more susceptible to flu and colds. Nutritional deficiency also can lead to mild depression and increased anxiety, doubling your stress.

Read pages 252–254: Maintenance, Ideal Weight.

Use the food pyramid for your daily food guide to defensive nutrition.

2. Use exercise for a tranquilizer. It's a natural antidote to stress, anxiety, and depression. A regular aerobic routine three times a week will help you burn calories, and it will increase the production of endorphins in your system to modulate your moods.

Read page 348: Walking.

It's the easiest to do.

3. Use relaxation exercises to keep you centered and in control. They remove you from chaos and give you a renewed sense of well-being and energy.

Read pages 292–295: Relaxation.

Use the adjuncts Full Body Release, and Finding Your Perfect Space.

4. Use stretching exercises to relax and relieve your muscles of stress and tension. This will make it easier to do all the carrying, decorating, and coping with additional body tension.

Read pages 324–327: Stretching.

5. Realize that you can't change the people or pressures that add cues to eat to your holidays, but you can change how you respond to them. With healthy nutrition, exercise, and relaxation on a regular basis, you can face the season with a new lease on life.

Read page 218: Food Cues.

6. Limit your use of alcohol by using wine and ginger ale, or bottled water and lime to expand your drinking time. You'll be glad you did when it's time to drive home.

Read page 125: Alcohol.

7. Change your focus from excess food to activities you can do that are enriching: attending concerts, taking walks to enjoy the decorations on homes in your neighborhood, or visiting public places to see the trees lit.

8. Limit the number of chores you take on by yourself. Trying to be perfect in everything you do will only add stress.

Read page 278: Perfectionist Thinking.

If you need a step-by-step guide to your nutrition, exercise, and self-enhancement for the holidays, use the Problem Solver Calendar as your fitness plan.

If you come out of the season without gaining weight, that's a holiday story you'll remember with joy. And just think, you won't have to make a New Year's resolution to lose your holiday weight.

◆

WEIGHT MAINTENANCE FOR LIFE

**You've lost weight, and now you
want to keep your old weight from returning.
You want to stay lean and feel light.**

MAINTENANCE IS A RE-ENTRY STATE. Just as the astronauts need an adjustment phase to go from weightlessness to a gravity plane, your body needs time to make the transition from a fatter state to a leaner one.

Give yourself time for the adaptation phase. If you skip it, thinking everything is now perfect in your life because you are lean, you are doing yourself a disservice. You put a lot of effort into dieting, and you don't need to repeat the effort again next year. You let go of your old weight, but you need time to let go of the old habits and beliefs that led to your overweight state.

You are now at ideal weight. Claim it as permanent.

How do you do it?

Maintenance after a poor diet

If you are coming off a diet where you lost weight fast and ate poorly to accomplish it, you will need more than a re-entry phase. You will need to learn how to eat healthfully and how to realign your body composition to avoid weight regain. Remember: The faster you lose weight, the faster you will regain it.

You will need to go on the Problem Solver Diet for at least two to three weeks before accepting that you are at maintenance, in order to adjust your body to a normal level of food after starvation calories. Be sure you're drinking eight glasses of water daily and are not oversalting your food.

The importance of regaining muscle in this fashion cannot be overstated. If you don't gain back some muscle, you will regain weight; and you may regain more than your original weight. You've come this far, give it another month if you must. Don't go back to being overweight because you chose a poor diet. It can be corrected. Your body is very forgiving. Read the facts.

Read pages 291–292: Relapse.

Read pages 10–13: Yo-Yo Syndrome.

Read pages 69–85: The Problem Solver Diet.

Follow the Problem Solver Calendar and do all the exercises. It's the only way to get your muscle back and into shape for real maintenance. Then use the regular maintenance plan to stay lean for life.

Maintenance after a healthy diet

If you are coming off the Problem Solver Diet or another plan where you ate balanced meals and exercised simultaneously, your goal is balance. You want to burn what you eat.

At the end of a diet, when you begin to introduce more calories into your body on a regular basis, you need to make sure that the new calories will burn off. In effect, you need to reset your metabolism to a higher flame.

You have several factors in place to achieve this goal:

- Because you used a healthy diet and exercise program, you now have more lean body mass and less fat. This is the internal body composition that keeps people lean. Studies show that dieters who ended their diets with more lean body mass were able to eat two times more calories than their fatter counterparts. But don't take this as permission to eat everything you see. You want to take the time to stabilize this new body composition.
- You have learned how to eat healthfully and you need no transitional skills to switch over to eating normally for a lean person. Lean people eat healthfully as a regular routine—low-fat, high complex carbohydrates, protein, and calcium maintenance for life.

Read pages 252–254: Maintenance.

Follow the food pyramid for healthy eating for maintenance. Use this as your guide to healthy eating for life.

- You learned how to exercise during your diet. You can't give it up now. You don't stop exercising because you stopped dieting. Keep up your aerobic program three times a week as the bottom line. However, now you might want to experiment with the wide variety of options that are available to you. You might want to work on a particular body area for supertoning. You can do circuit training with weights, take hiking trips, join cycling clubs, or a myriad of other activities that you resisted before. Now you can wear shorts without feeling uncomfortable.
- Water, water everywhere—why stop drinking it! Water balance is essential to your body. Keep enough water going in to equal half of your body weight in ounces. That's eight glasses a day. Don't stop drinking water because you stopped dieting.
- You have learned new behavior skills for self-enhancement. Keep these three skills for life:
  - relaxation exercises
  - breathing exercises
  - positive thinking

These are essential for routine stress control and self-appreciation from within, where it counts.

In the maintenance stage, you are stabilizing your new lifestyle. When you keep the skills you have learned on your diet—eating healthfully, exercising, and self-empowerment—you have an automatic plan for permanent weight control.

Then you can stop dieting for life.

Read page 177: Contingency Plan.
Read page 249: Lifestyle Change.

PART TWO

The Problem Solver
Diet Program

The Problem Solver Diet

A Month to Fat Freedom

IF YOU MAKE UP YOUR MIND that you're going to do it right this time, putting the energy where it counts, in food, exercise, and yourself, you're in for an exciting time.

This is no boring diet. It will be the healthiest time of your life. You'll feel more energy than you've had in years *while you're dieting,* more confidence in your abilities, and a whole new sense of purpose and direction that will open up new channels of energy for other achievements in your life. Isn't it time you did that for yourself?

How do you start?

Choose one month that you are going to dedicate to yourself.

Get excited about it. Focus your attention on it and give it all you've got.

You'll need three days before that month to set the stage for your program.

CHOOSING YOUR MONTH

The best decision is to start on the first day of a month and go to the end of the month without breaking your stride. If that is not possible for you, you can start midmonth and go to the next midmonth. But try to avoid starting in the middle of a week or on a weekend. Block it out as a visual month, to make it easier to stay dedicated.

Select a month that is as free as possible. Don't choose a month when company is coming for a two-week visit or one that includes weddings, graduations, and parties. This is a month in your life when you need to focus on yourself. Allow three days in the pre-

69

vious month or week to get yourself into the right state of mind to begin.

Once you choose your month, stick to it. Make up your mind that nothing will come between you and this decision. If a crisis occurs in your life that could set you off stroke, stay with the program. Say "Excuse me, but I have to exercise." This will give you the stress control you need and will help you manage the crisis more effectively, so your program will have double benefits. If a business trip occurs, remember there are supermarkets in every town, and that's where your food is. There are outdoor tracks at every high school in every town. There are workout rooms in most hotels. Travel doesn't have to break your stride or focus. You can do it: four weeks to a fitter, fat-free life!

THREE DAYS TO SET THE STAGE

Review the three areas you will be improving and the skills you will be using, so you will be familiar with the program before you start.

Diet

Prescreen the Problem Solver Diet and redesign your kitchen to be prepared for healthy eating. Stock your refrigerator and cabinets with healthy, low-fat foods. Select cereals with the least sugar and lowest fat, and choose crackers and grains that are low-salt and the least processed. One of your goals will be to eat food as fresh as possible, so keep fresh foods handy for cooking and eating. You don't want to be caught reaching for something to eat and having to go back to something sugary and fattening because you forgot to shop.

You never have to be hungry on this program, since you can eat more complex carbohydrates if you need extra food—fruits, whole grains, vegetables. Cut up fresh vegetables and store them in bowls with no-fat dips on the side, so you can have a veggie platter in a snap—and it adds no fat! You may want to make a pasta salad with vegetables the day before you start the program so you will have a low-fat side dish or entrée if you need one in a hurry. Make your refrigerator look inviting with colorful fruits and vegetables, water spritzers and seltzers, and low-sugar fruit juices. This will remove your old idea that dieting is a deprived experience.

Dress up your kitchen with jars of various pastas in all sizes, shapes, and colors. Make a colorful spice rack to have herbs and spices on hand for cooking. Put up pictures of fresh vegetables and fruits, and keep fresh fruits on hand in plain view. When you reach for something, reach for health. Use fresh fruits for snacks.

Familiarize yourself with the daily food requirements on the food pyramid and memorize or display it for daily use. You may want to write the requirements in a notebook to carry with you, in case you are away from home too long. Use the pyramid as your constant food guide. It is superhealthy, slimming food that will give you an energy boost.

Exercise

Preplan the exercise program that you will do for the month. The Problem Solver Program uses walking, but you may select another exercise as a substitute, as long as it is aerobic and, preferably, low intensity to begin. You may want to identify one other more intense, full-body exercise, such as one of the aerobic machines (rowing, Nordic track) to use along with walking as your selections for the month. Try not to use more than two different exercises, since too many options can lead to confusion, and you can wind up doing neither exercise. This is why we recommend that you start with walking and stay with it for the duration; it makes exercise simple.

You should buy a set of hand weights or strap-on weights for the strengthening part of your program. You can also use videos or audio tapes to support your program. However, if you use your own tapes or routine for your aerobic segment, be on guard. If your former routine had worked, you would still be doing it and losing your fat. You might want to *add* some of your former favorites to the existing program, rather than making substitues for walking.

We provide an at-home stretching and strength training program in the dictionary section of this book, including complete guidelines for walking, and how to do the behavior exercises you need for inner support. All you have to do is follow The Problem Solver Calendar for total success.

Get your gear ready. Put your sneakers and socks by the door, or keep them in plain sight in the same place every night. Get two workout suits ready, perhaps a set of sweats and one tighter suit with stretch pants so you're set like a pro. These will be your most important clothes for the month. You don't have to overdo your collection of workout suits. Often the simplest gear is the best, since it allows you to keep your focus on your goals.

Behavior

Prescreen the behavior skills recommended in the Problem Solver Calendar and consider putting tabs or Post-it notes in the book to make it easy to find these skills. Please don't skip this part of the program. These skills are vital. They take very little time, and they provide the foundation for all of the other work you will be doing. Later, you'll be amazed at the positive effect they have on your life. You can use them for many other problems besides weight.

Consider keeping a diary for every day of the month. Buy a small pocket notebook to carry with you. List your program days and requirements, then check them off each day as you complete them. Make any notes and comments in your notebook: how you feel, what you're learning, any blocks you may encounter, and how you overcame them. This is a time of great, positive change! Your diary will help you keep your focus, and it will be fun to look back on later. Each night for ten minutes, you might conclude your day with a few notes in your fitness diary.

Try to avoid making judgments as you glance over the program. If you have a block against exercise, see Block Against Exercise in Part One of this book. If you have doubts, see Rationalizations in the dictionary.

All of the exercises in The Problem Solver Calendar are described fully in the dictionary section, with guidelines for easy use. In addition, any special issue you may encounter can be found there. It is a complete system between two covers!

> *Go for it with everything you've got!*
> *You'll be glad you did.*

IS THERE MAGIC IN THIS PLAN?

Dieters love magic. It's part of their dreamers' streak. Rather than let it work against you, let it work for you.

Eating real, fresh food is the simplest, most powerful way you can get down to ideal body weight and stay there.

You might not realize that *what you don't eat* can be as fattening as what you do eat. When you don't get your daily nutrient needs met, nothing works right, least of all weight loss.

You can eat next to nothing and fail to lose weight because you don't have your daily nutrient needs in place. You can eat *more* calories and still lose weight when you have your daily nutrient needs in place.

It's the secret that lean people know and follow with pleasure. They like to eat for nutrition, because of the way it makes them feel, and it automatically keeps them lean.

The Risks: None. Anytime you use The Problem Solver Diet, you're doing yourself a favor.

The Extra Benefits: Name it, The Problem Solver Diet does it. Cholesterol is controlled. Sugar, fat, and sodium are regulated. It gives you the nutrient profile for disease prevention. It's the diet you need to handle stress. It is an automatic habit corrector—you don't have to wonder if you're getting enough behavior modification. The food groups are the pattern for automatic behavior adjustment. You're eating like a slim person. When you follow it regularly, it becomes a habit. And it doesn't do anything negative to you.

> The next time you see a field of grain,
> Think about the power of it.
> The next time you see fruit on the trees,
> Think about the power of it.
> Bring that power back into your life.
> You owe it to yourself to diet right!

HOW TO EAT SUCCESSFULLY
Fix Your Day with the Problem Solver Diet.

How do you start? Do you need special preparations, a food scale, kit of diet mixes, special formula foods?

No. Just start.

Do the best you can every day!

Then, when you get in the swing of eating healthy, do it straight out, take it to ideal body weight.

Any time you do, it's improving you.

Dieting doesn't have to be complicated. The Problem Solver pyramid is the key to fat-burning simplicity. All you have to do is follow the food pyramid daily, making sure you eat *everything* that's required, and you'll lose fat automatically.

You can use the food pyramid in two important ways:

1. If you want a day-by-day pattern to follow, use the Problem Solver Meals and Menus—it puts the pyramid into an eating plan that is easy and fun to do.

2. If you are away from home and are not sure what to eat, the food pyramid can act as your daily guide. Or, if you like to design your own meals for dieting, the food pyramid provides the healthy standard you need to select your own foods.

Strict: Follow the food pyramid daily and meet the requirements *no matter what.* Eat fresh food as much as possible. Avoid all extra fats. Cook with spray vegetable oil (unsaturated). Avoid processed foods and grains, except the whole grains that have at least the bran intact (and the germ where possible). Eat extra vegetables or fruits if you need more food, or if you are an active exerciser.

Moderate: Follow the food pyramid daily and meet the requirements *no matter what.* You can include extra fats, but keep an eye on them. More than two extra fats aren't recommended for superior fat burn. Moderate your use of processed foods, reading the labels for sugar, salt, and fat content. Realize that you aren't getting the fiber you need if you eat processed foods *instead of* more natural foods, so you might want to tack on an apple a day to be safe. Eat fresh food whenever possible. Eat all snacks in complex carbohydrates—fruits, whole grains, or vegetables. Your first job is to meet the minimum requirements on the food pyramid. Consider the rest extra.

Casual: Diet during the weekdays and take the weekends off. However, keep an eye on your food intake on the weekends, and try to moderate it. *Meet the requirements on the food pyramid on or off a diet.* Consider the rest of your food extra and use this as a guide to finding out about your food desires and habits. Read the sections on behavior and think about adding them to your life. Practice imagery and relaxation and use this as a foundation to give you the incentive to move to the stricter plan full-time for a boost in fat loss. Or you can continue with the more casual plan all the way to ideal weight.

Supercasual: Diet whenever you can, and don't feel guilty about it. The only requirement is to meet the food minimum on the daily pyramid, *no matter what.* The rest is your decision. The important point to remember about a real food diet is that it will always benefit you because you are getting your daily nutritional needs met. Even if you do it one week every month, over time you'll start to trim down, if you don't go overboard with food on a regular basis.

A NEW VIEW OF FOOD AND NUTRITION

Your Problem Solver Day

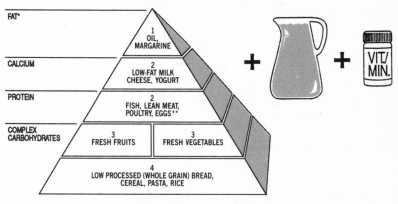

Nutrition at-a-Glance

The Food Pyramid

You need more than fifty nutrients, vitamins, and minerals daily in the presence of water for health and body balance. To make it easy for you to get them, ten leader nutrients were identified by science as the keys to the other nutrients. When you get these leader nutrients, you automatically get the rest of your vitamin, mineral, and nutrient needs met.

The Problem Solver food pyramid is based on the leader nutrient formula, targeting the foods that give you everything you need in nutrients, vitamins, and minerals daily.

The Problem Solver food pyramid provides the essential metabolic energy that everyone should eat daily. When you meet the requirements on a daily basis, something interesting happens that helps you lose weight. You're not as hungry for sweets. The water keeps your sodium in line. You feel more energy. The fiber keeps your fat mobilized and your cholesterol down. Everything feels better. Stress doesn't deplete you as it used to. By itself, the food pyramid trains you to eat correctly for life. Even when you eat more calories than you think are safe for dieting, you'll find that you burn your food better because your nutrients are balanced. That's the beauty of nature. Nothing can match it.

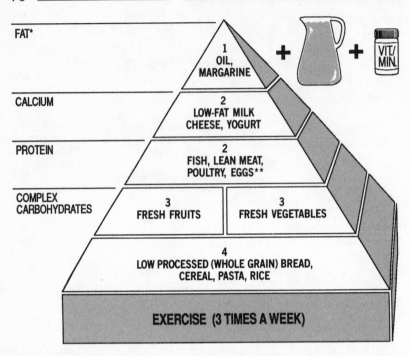

FAT*

CALCIUM

PROTEIN

COMPLEX
CARBOHYDRATES

1
OIL,
MARGARINE

2
LOW-FAT MILK
CHEESE, YOGURT

2
FISH, LEAN MEAT,
POULTRY, EGGS**

3
FRESH FRUITS

3
FRESH VEGETABLES

4
LOW PROCESSED (WHOLE GRAIN) BREAD,
CEREAL, PASTA, RICE

EXERCISE (3 TIMES A WEEK)

Water

A healthy, fit body and healthy fat-loss are not possible without water. It supplies oxygen to your muscles, which are the home of your fat burn. It removes wastes, which are increased during fat burn. None of your metabolic processes work as well without water balance. You naturally lose one-half gallon of water daily, and your goal for dieting and lifetime health is to replace the water you lose, to keep your body balanced for best effect.

Put two pitchers of water (two quarts) into the refrigerator daily, and make sure they're empty by the time you go to bed.

Vitamin/Mineral Supplement

A daily vitamin/mineral supplement is recommended during a diet, as a health booster, just in case you lose extra vitamins or minerals as you lose fat. It's that extra health protection you need.

Take one balanced vitamin/mineral supplement daily, preferably after you eat.

THE PROBLEM SOLVER SOLUTION

The easy way to deal with food is to start with the food indicated on the pyramid as *the bottom line* every day. Think about your food life this way:

> My first priority:
> Eat everything in the Problem Solver food pyramid daily.
> My second priority:
> Evaluate the foods I eat beyond that.

This makes your food life much simpler, especially on a diet.

When you are overweight and you begin eating everything in the food pyramid as the first priority, several benefits occur that begin to help you lose weight automatically. You are less hungry. You are getting fiber. You are more satisfied. You are getting all of your daily nutrients, vitamins, and minerals, and that makes everything work better, including your metabolism.

The Problem Solver Diet accomplishes many things simultaneously, and they are very important to a dieter.

- You get the protein you need for lean-muscle protection—that means *better fat burn.*
- You get the fiber you need for fullness and better intestinal transit time—that means *less calorie absorption.*
- You get the fifty essential nutrients automatically—that means *health and disease prevention.*
- You get the calcium you need to *prevent bone deterioration as you age.*
- You get the textures you need for chewing—that means *better appetite control.*
- You get pleasures from variety—*it's more palatable* and less likely to make you break your diet from boredom.
- You get an *automatic maintenance plan*—all you have to do is increase your calories across the board.
- You're set for *a healthy, slimmer life.*

When you choose all the lean varieties in food as shown in the food pyramid, you have the *most perfect* weight loss diet. Pure science.

But you also get a booster—*pleasure in eating* while you are dieting. To find out how to do it, see The Problem Solver Meals and Menus, a pattern for perfect eating.

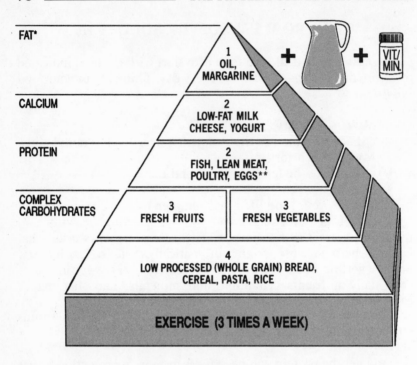

HOW MUCH TO EAT

Four grains a day (low-fat, low-sugar, low-processed)

1 serving grain	=	1 medium potato, waffle, pancake, roll, bagel, muffin
		1 cup cereal, pastas (cooked), rice (cooked)
		1 slice bread
		2 medium crackers, low-fat wheat or oat wafers

Three vegetables a day (fresh or frozen, eaten raw as much as possible)

1 serving vegetable	=	1 cup raw
		½ cup cooked

Three fruits a day (fresh, frozen, canned in light syrup)

1 serving fruit	=	1 medium fresh fruit
		½ cup canned fruits
		1 cup juice, fresh or frozen
		Try to eat one banana and one citrus each day.

Two dairies a day (low-fat or skim)

1 serving dairy	=	1 cup milk, yogurt, frozen yogurt
		1 slice cheese (low-fat)
		½ cup cottage cheese

Two lean meats a day (beef, poultry, fish)

1 serving meat	=	2 ounces

GRAINS ON THE PROBLEM SOLVER DIET

4 Servings Daily

This is the group that often tricks dieters because they mistake processed grains, cereals, breads, and pasta mixes for the real thing. They're not. Try to find as many whole-grain products as you can. Check cereals for excess sugar. Consider making your own muffins to freeze for superior whole-grain boosters. It will be worth the effort when you see the fat loss and health. Whole grains have trace fat, no cholesterol, and they're the complex carbohydrates you've been missing. Remember, the grains aren't fattening, it's what you put on them. Enjoy pasta salads, potato skins with vegetables, whole-wheat waffles with strawberries.

Eat any whole-grain or low-processed grain:

Barley
Bran
Bran flakes
Bread crumbs
Buckwheat
Bulgur
Breads, whole grain
Cornbread, muffins
Corn flakes
Cracked wheat
Crackers, whole grain
Cream of wheat (not instant)
English muffins
Farina
Flour, whole-wheat
Macaroni
Millet
Muffins, whole-grain
Oat flakes
Oatmeal

Pancakes (wheat or low-fat)
Pasta
Pita
Pizza, whole-wheat (sprinkle of
   low-fat cheese)
Pizza pitas (sprinkle of low-fat
   cheese)
Pumpernickel
Rice, wild, brown, converted,
   white, yellow
Rolls, whole-grain
Rye
Sesame
Shredded wheat
Spaghetti
Tortilla, yellow corn
Waffles (wheat or low-fat)
Wheat germ
Whole-wheat

VEGETABLES ON THE PROBLEM SOLVER DIET
3 Servings Daily

This is the best group for dieters. Versatile, pleasurable, power-ful, minimal fat, fabulous fiber. For salads, pasta salads, potato skin snacks, casseroles, soups, stews, entrées, sauces, snacks, and low-fat dips. Name it, vegetables can do it! Eat as many vegetables fresh as you can.

Avoid garbanzo beans (fat) and use soy beans as protein.

Eat any vegetable, legume, or drink fresh vegetable juice:

Alfalfa sprouts	Garlic	Shallots
Artichoke	Ginger root	Spinach
Asparagus	Kale	Squash
Bamboo shoots	Leeks	Sweet potato
Beans (any)	Lettuce (any)	Tomato
Beets	Mushrooms	Tomato juice
Broccoli	Mustard greens	(sugar-free)
Brussels sprouts	Okra	Turnips
Cabbage (any)	Onions	Turnip greens
Carrots	Parsley	Vegetable juice
Carrot juice	Parsnips	(not canned)
Cauliflower	Peas	Water chestnuts
Celery	Peppers (plain &	Watercress
Chard	hot)	Yams
Chives	Pickles (check	Yeast (bakers,
Collards	sodium)	brewers)
Corn	Pimientos	*Potatoes, baked or
Cress	Potato*	boiled. Avoid fried,
Cucumber	Pumpkin	dehydrated, hash
Dandelion	Radish	browns, or au gratin.
Dock	Rutabaga	Potato pancakes are
Eggplant	Sauerkraut	OK, with vegetable
Endive	Scallions	spray.

FRUITS ON THE PROBLEM SOLVER DIET

3 Servings Daily

FRESH FRUITS, FRESH FRUIT JUICES, FROZEN FRUIT, FROZEN JUICES (LOW-SUGAR), CANNED FRUIT IN LIGHT SYRUP

Fruits are low in fat, good fiber sources, high-vitamin foods. Use fruits in cereals, as a topping for a whole-grain waffle or pancake, and as desserts. In water, they make great diet spritzers. When you want something sweet, have a fruit instead of candy or cake. One apple a day makes good cholesterol sense, excellent for fat loss.

Omit these fruits: avocado (fat), dried fruits (sodium), fruits in heavy syrup (sugar), Greek olives (sodium), coconut (cholestrol, palm cholesterol).

Eat any fruit, fresh or frozen:

Acerola	Grapes	Prickly pear
Apple	Guava	Prunes
Apricot	Kumquat	Quince
Banana	Lemon	Raisins
Blackberries	Lime	Raspberries
Blueberries	Loganberries	Rhubarb
Boysenberries	Mango	Strawberries
Cantaloupe	Melon	Tangerine
Cherries	Nectarine	Watermelon
Crabapple	Olives	
Cranberry	Orange	Remember these fruit
Currant	Papaya	treats to spruce up
Dates	Peach	meals:
Elderberries	Pear	Applesauce
Figs	Persimmon	Cranberry sauce
Fruit cocktail	Pineapple	Apple butter
Gooseberries	Plums	
Grapefruit	Pomegranate	

Try making your own fresh fruit health booster with an extractor. Use the pulp for sauces.

DAIRY ON THE PROBLEM SOLVER DIET

2 Servings Daily, Adults

A MUST FOR CALCIUM AND PROTEIN

Fatter Dairy Products	Dieter's Choice Dairy
Whole Milk	2%, 1% or skim milk,
Creams	buttermilk, soy milk
Yogurt, whole	Low-fat yogurt, plain or fruit
Eggs	Egg whites or 1 yolk to two whites
Cheeses	Skim-milk or low-fat cheeses
Cottage cheese, whole	2 percent cottage cheese

Do not skip your dairy products.

Limit most cheeses except dieter's choice cheeses. Cheeses are the foods that can really add on fat. Two slices of an average cheese will give you 18 grams of fat, and 54 mg of cholesterol, plus a higher level of saturated fat than unsaturated. (You want to avoid that.)

If you drink coffee or tea with cream or an imitation creamer, train yourself to drink 2% milk in your coffee or tea. Use skim for cereals.

EXTRA FATS FOR A DIETER: Think about your fat cells before you add fats to your diet. Fats are already in your food. The rest is excess.

MEATS, POULTRY ON THE PROBLEM SOLVER DIET

Part of Protein Group
Total Protein—2 Servings Daily

Use meats in kabobs, as entrées, in stir-fry, on sandwiches. Use poultry in salads, casseroles, and soups. Avoid organ meats. They're superhigh cholesterol. Also high is turkey dark meat, cured ham, chicken (back), and frankfurters.

Poultry is lower in saturated fat than other meats. If you keep your red meat portions to 2 ounces, you can use the fatter proteins that are starred (★).

Fatter Proteins

Bacon
Braunschweiger
Bologna
Chicken (drum stick, thigh, wing)★
Corned beef
Duck
Goose
Ground beef, regular
Ham
Knockwurst
Lamb chop★
Pheasant
Porterhouse steak
Rib roast
Rump roast★
Sirloin steak
T-bone steak
Veal chuck

Leaner Proteins

Chicken white meat
Chuck roast
Flank steak
Ground beef, lean
Ground turkey, chicken, lean
Leg of lamb
Round steak
Turkey light meat
Veal cutlet
Veal rib roast
Venison

FISH ON THE PROBLEM SOLVER DIET
Part of Protein Group
Total Protein—2 Servings Daily

The standard serving size for the meat group is 2 ounces. But since fish is lighter and far less fattening than red meats, 3 ounces is acceptable for lean-muscle protection. Use fish as entrées, in fish kabobs, in stir-fry fares, in pita sandwiches, in fish salads. Broil or sauté with an unsaturated vegetable spray, with lemon and garlic, and your favorite spices.

Lower-Cholesterol Fish

Abalone
Anchovy
Bass
Bluefish
Carp
Catfish

Cod
Eel
Flounder
Frog legs
Haddock
Halibut

Perch, Ocean
Perch, Yellow
Pike
Pollock
Salmon
Sardines
Scallops

Shad
Smelt
Snails
Snapper
Trout
Wakame
Whitefish

Higher Cholesterol Fish
(Omega Oils)

Caviar
Clams
Crab
Herring
Lobster

Mackerel
Canned oysters
Shrimp
Tuna

Snacks

Snacks are energy boosters between meals. This can be a habit that adds a lot of sugar and fat if you choose low-nutrition snacks. But if you eat most of your snacks in complex carbohydrates—vegetables, fruits, whole grains—you'll have less hunger as a result. Complex carbohydrates are natural appetite suppressants.

The best snack: any fruit, vegetable, whole grain. You can find many snacks that give you pleasure and don't add fat. This is particularly important to a dieter, who tends to think of restricted calories as a dreadful situation. It doesn't have to be that way.

If you rate your snacks for their fat content, it will provide an easy method to keep your fat moderated. The average lean snack should be one to two grams of fat.

Safe Sweet Treats and Snacks

Toast with apple butter and cinnamon	1 gram fat
Frozen grapes	No fat
Jams, jellies	No fat
Popcorn, plain	No fat
Angel food cake	No fat
Sugar-free candies	No fat
Vanilla wafer	½ gram fat
Fig bar	½ gram fat
Ginger snap	½ gram fat
Mini chocolate mint patty	1 gram fat

Yogurt	Low fat
Popsicle	No fat
Bread sticks	No fat
Toast with jelly	1 gram fat
Any fruit (except avocado, coconut)	No fat
Any vegetable with no-fat dip	No fat
A cup of pasta salad with vegetables (No-fat dressing)	2 grams fat

There are numerous possibilities for nonfattening snacks that can make your dieting experience a pleasure. You do not have to starve yourself or deprive yourself of all pleasure to get slim. All you have to do is change habits like your high-fat snacking to lean-snacking techniques. You can be satisfied on a diet and still burn fat.

Beverages
The following beverages are listed in the order that provides the most value to a dieter.

1. Water. Necessary nutrient, no calories (includes water spritzers).
2. Low-fat milk drinks. Essential for calcium, excellent source of vitamins, minerals, low-calorie.
3. Fresh vegetable juices. (Canned have extra salt.) Excellent sources of vitamins, minerals, and essential nutrients, low calorie.
4. Fresh fruit juices. (Watch out for sugar in bottled and canned versions). Excellent sources of vitamins/minerals and essential nutrients, low-calorie.
5. Herbal teas. No nutrition, but positive therapeutic benefits.
6. Club soda. No nutrition, but low- or no-calories. (Includes club soda spritzers—lime, lemon, cranberry. The fruits add a bit of nutrition.)
7. Coffee. No nutrients, caffeine, water.
8. Tea. A tad of flouride, tannin, caffeine, water.
9. Fruit-flavored drinks. High-calorie, high sugar.
10. Carbonated soft drinks. High-sugar, contain acids to keep sugar in suspension.
11. Colas. 100 percent sugar, caffeine, additives.
12. Diet sodas. Artificial sugars, additives.
13. Alcohol. Calories, mood changers.

The Problem Solver Meals and Menus

A New Relationship with Food

THE PROBLEM SOLVER MEALS AND MENUS are designed to be easy and adaptable to any lifestyle or ethnic variety. They're based on real, fresh food, and tell how to prepare delicious lean meals in a snap.

The menus and meals also incorporate an eating style to show you how to develop a new relationship with food that's practical, versatile, and delicious. It's uncomplicated eating, and it will make you lean.

As you practice this style of eating, you will find that it makes you feel good about food and dieting. When you feel good, everything else seems brighter and newer. This positive view of dieting and eating can open up a whole new world of food pleasure and health for you. We know it will burn your fat, but wait until you see how satisfied you feel to eat this way. It's rejuvenating. It gives you energy you never knew you had.

What about extra food?

If you eat something extra, don't eliminate one of the foods on this plan to do it. Eat everything that's recommended as *the bottom line every day.* Practice bringing yourself back to that bottom line if you stray. Make this a habit, and you will be astounded at the change it makes. It takes away all the problems, questions, and doubts about food and frees you up to have fun with other things in your life. That's what eating healthy is all about.

THE PROBLEM SOLVER BREAKFASTS

Your problem: fat/lack of health and energy/low-level fitness.
Your breakfast solution:

1 grain = 1 cup cereal or
             1 slice bread
             1 muffin

1 fruit = 1 fresh or
             ½ cup canned or
             1 cup juice or nectar

1 dairy = 1 cup low-fat milk or
             1 cup yogurt

There are dozens of creative ways to start your day for fat loss and health. Choose any breakfast plan and use your own favorites in it. *Just eat it,* hungry or not, for the health of it. You burn fat better by eating this way. Include coffee or tea as desired (low-fat milk instead of creamers).

1	*2*
1 cup hot cereal 1 fruit or fruit juice 1 cup milk	1 muffin with any spread 1 fruit or fruit juice 1 cup milk or yogurt

IDEAS:
Hot oat cereal mixed with diced
  apples, raisins, cinnamon
Hot wheat cereal with diced peaches
Plain hot cereal with milk and fruit
  on the side
 	
Note: Add one-half teaspoon of fruit
juice to hot cereal for sweetener
instead of sugar.
	IDEAS:
	Bran muffin with raspberry spread
	Corn muffin with cranberry spread
	Raisin muffin with apple butter
	English muffin with jelly or
	  whipped cottage cheese spread
	Toasted muffin slices with fruit
	  spread medley
	
	Note: Spread isn't your one fruit.
	It's extra. Eat one fruit also.

3	*4*
1 slice toast with any spread 1 fruit or fruit nectar 1 cup yogurt or milk	1 cup dry cereal 1 fruit 1 cup milk
IDEAS:	*IDEAS:*
Super! Sliced bananas on toast. *Try it!* Toast with apple butter Toast with applesauce and cinnamon Toast with whipped cottage cheese sweetened with a teaspoon of favorite fruit juice	Wheat flakes with mixed fruits Oat or corn flakes with sliced bananas Puffed wheat with raisins, apples Cereal plain with milk, fruit on the side

5	*6*
1 slice French toast with lite syrup 1 fruit 1 cup milk Toast recipe: mix milk, cinnamon, egg white and a dash of margarine to cook *Note:* Oils are 14 grams fat per teaspoon. Many margarines are 5 to 7.	Fresh fruit shake 1 slice toast or 4 wheat crackers or muffin Mix your own fresh fruit shakes *Super fatless variety:* 　bananas, strawberries, milk, nutmeg 　raspberries, milk, banana, strawberries, milk, banana

Breakfast Spreads:

Any fruit spread
Any jam, jelly
Apple butter
Yogurt
Cottage cheese, whipped
Applesauce
Cranberry sauce as jelly
Any other no-fat spread

Your priority for breakfast is to learn to do without extra fats. The world of spreads is versatile, and it adds up to significant fat reduction.

It's so easy to spread a pat of butter or margarine on a muffin or toast, adding 10 grams of fat for butter and 7 to 10 for margarine each pat. Do it four times a day and you've topped your daily fat maximum, and you can't burn fat that way. Remove the problem, and you can strip out 10 to 20 grams of dietary fat *every morning!*

But this does not mean you should skip breakfast altogether. Eat breakfast, even if you don't want to. Eating this way will burn fat better, give you health, and start your day with a sense of real pleasure that only supernutrition can give you.

THE PROBLEM SOLVER LUNCHES

Problem: Energy slumps/fat habits/low-level nutrition
Your lunch solution:

2 grains	=	2 slices bread for sandwich or
		1 pita pouch (half of round) or
		1 cup any pasta or rice
		1 roll
		4 wheat crackers
1 vegetable	=	1 cup raw or 1 cup cooked
1 meat	=	2 ounces lean meat (or equivalent protein)
1 dairy	=	1 cup milk
		1 cup yogurt
		½ cup cottage cheese
★★★★ 1 fruit	=	(Save for afternoon snack or eat with lunch)

Your best strategy for lunch is to make a basic plan and stick to it. A lean eating style for lunch will be a tremendous boost for fat burning. Rely on standards to create a simple eating *pattern* that will minimize confusion.

Lunch Eating Pattern:
Lean meat sandwich with vegetable soup, fruit and dairy for dessert.
Pasta salad with lean meat and vegetables, fruit and dairy for dessert.
Hearty soup with everything inside, fruit and dairy for dessert.
Eat this kind of lunch *before* you think about anything else, and you'll find you don't want those chips, cheeses, fatter meats, and fattening snacks. *You really won't.* And you'll get lean automatically.

Special Lunch Strategy:
If you eat light at night, with a nonmeat dinner, you can have 4 ounces of lean meat at lunch. This is more similar to the portion sizes of average restaurant or deli sandwiches and burgers. *But don't have both!* Meat is a substantial source of fat, so keep your meat habit to 4 ounces per day.
Don't eat the same every day. Keep it varied.

Lunchtime/Work Strategy:
Salad Dressings: Keep a selection of no-fat dressings at work for salads, pasta salads, and sandwich spreads. You cannot rely on restaurant dressings, no matter how low calorie they say they are.
Snacks: Keep a supply of whole-wheat crackers or multigrain bread and a fruit spread or jelly. It will get you through any snack urge and give you a natural energy boost without extra fat.
Sugar: If you're craving sugar, instead of reaching for diet soda or candy, pick up a fresh fruit at the nearest store. It's natural sugar without the fat.

(1)
SANDWICH AND SOUP

2 oz./lean meat, fish, or poultry
2 slices bread
Any no-fat dressing
Any vegetable garnish
1 cup vegetable soup (*See* Soups)

DESSERT
1 fruit cup & cottage cheese

IDEAS:

• Chicken Breast Florentine Sandwich
2 oz. chicken breast topped with steamed spinach leaf, basted with any no-fat dressings (such as creamy garlic or Italian) between toast.

• Veal Florentine Sandwich use a V-8 baste, for variation.

• Burger (turkey or lean beef—lots of vegetable toppings and no cheese).

• Lean Roast Beef Sandwich (open face) with au jus gravy.

---

(2)
ALL-IN-ONE SOUP

Hearty soup with lean meat, poultry, or fish (2 oz.)
4 crackers or 1 slice bread to dunk into soup
See Soups

DESSERT
1 fruit

SNACK
1 cup milk or yogurt

(3)
SUPER SKINNY LUNCH

Sliced cucumbers and tomato on toast, any no-fat dressing (or plain)
Side of shrimp cocktail (4 shrimp)

DESSERT
½ cup cottage cheese and 1 fruit

(4)
ALL-IN-ONE PASTA SALAD

Super pasta salad with lean meat, poultry, or fish chunks
1 cup pasta
1 cup vegetables
2 oz. meat
No-fat dressing

DESSERT OR SNACK
1 frozen yogurt cone

(5)
SALAD SUPREME

1 cup vegetables (in addition to lettuce)
2 oz. lean meat, fish, or poultry
No-fat dressing
4 wheat crackers or croutons or 1 slice bread

DESSERT OR SNACK
½ cup cottage cheese and 1 fruit

(6)
VEGGIE LUNCH

Veggie pita sandwich or
Veggie pita pizzas (open face)
Stuff a pita pouch (½ round) with 1 cup mixed vegetables
(sautéed or stir fried) and ½ cup cottage cheese or
Spread vegetables on pita open-faced and bake, broil, or microwave
Baste with any no-fat dressing and ½ cup cottage cheese
(Skip the fatter cheeses on the pita to learn how to enjoy ultra-lean eating)
If you don't add the cottage cheese, don't forget your 1 dairy.
Save your meat, poultry, or fish (2 oz.) for dinner, and have 4 oz. of fish that
evening

DESSERT OR SNACK
1 fruit

THE PROBLEM SOLVER DINNERS

Problem: Late night eating/big dinners with heavy foods/often
the largest meal of the day.
Result: Fat stores easier when your metabolism is slower.
Solution: Eat *light* at night!

1 grain   = 1 cup pasta or rice or
               1 potato or
               1 slice bread or 1 roll

2 vegetables = 2 cups cooked or raw

1 meat   = 2 ounces lean meat, poultry, or fish
                 (or equivalent protein)

1 dairy   = 1 cup yogurt or milk
                 ½ cup cottage cheese

1 fruit   = 1 fresh or
                 1 cup juice or
                 ½ cup canned fruit (in light syrup)

Your difficulties with dinner will be over when you eat your breakfast and lunch the Problem Solver way. You won't be as hungry all day, and therefore you won't compensate by eating more, and eating higher fat foods at night, when your resistance is lower. Your lunch and dinner are approximately the same with an added cup of vegetables at night, which can give you a side salad or a vegetable sauce for entrées, side dishes, and casseroles. When you develop this lighter eating style as a nightly habit, you'll feel better, burn fat better, and sleep better too. You can always save your dairy for a glass of milk before bed, since studies have shown that calcium absorbs better when you are lying down. And remember, eating light doesn't mean eating less. It means eating better!

(1)
KABOBS & SALAD

> 2 oz. any lean meat, fish, or poultry
> 1 cup vegetables in chunks—zucchini, turnips, peppers, small whole
>   onions, cherry tomatoes, cauliflowerettes (even fruit chunks, such as
>   pineapple)
> 1 cup rice (white, converted, brown, wild, saffron)
> 1 side salad

DESSERT
Any fruit with dollop of frozen yogurt or no-fat topping

Kabobs: Make beef, fish, or poultry kabob sticks with vegetable variety. Baste with fruit nectar (apricot, peach, pear) or fruit juice for flavor. (Apricot nectar on lamb is terrific!) Bake in foil or microwave until meat is tender. Serve over rice. Consider adding small vegetables to rice, such as peas, corn, peppers, and making many rice varieties to keep kabobs constantly versatile and fun.

(2)
STIR-FRY

2 oz. any lean meat, fish, or poultry
2 cups mixed vegetables
(Use various combinations and spices for a wide variety of stir-fry
   options—Oriental, Mexicali, sweet and sour with fruits mixed in, hot
   and spicy, or use your chicken base for an all-American basic.)
Sauté or stir-fry with pear juice or any fruit. Serve with rice or pasta.
1 cup rice or pasta

DESSERT OR SNACK

Angel food cake with strawberries, a dollop of frozen yogurt or a dollop of
   Cool Whip Lite, or any frozen yogurt with fruit

IDEA

Island Chicken: Sauté chicken breast, onions, garlic, and basil. Make
sauce with one cup orange juice and 1 to 2 teaspoons whole wheat flour to
thicken. Pour sauce over chicken. Cook as is, or add raisins, pineapples,
and vegetable of choice. Simmer until chicken is tender, thinning sauce
with water as necessary. Serve with rice, potato, or pasta.

---

(3)
SPICY STEW OR CASSEROLE

2 oz. any lean meat, fish, or poultry—baste in V-8
1 cup vegetables—corn, red and green peppers, peppercorns, mushrooms,
   onion, garlic, chili powder, Tabasco sauce
Sauté meat and vegetables—add to one can whole tomatoes
Bake or microwave or simmer on stove top
1 cup rice, 1 baked potato, or 1 cup any pasta
Use stew sauce over rice, potato, or pasta (or leave out chili powder and
   Tabasco for a milder stew)
1 cup side salad or soup

DESSERT
Fruit Cup

SNACK

Root beer or cream soda float. 1 cup diet root beer or cream soda
with scoop of vanilla or chocolate frozen yogurt

(4)
ALL WORLD STANDARD
(Meat, Potatoes, Vegetables)

2 oz. any lean meat, fish, or poultry
1 potato baked or mashed (try mashed mix of turnips and potatoes)
1 side vegetable (any)
1 side salad or soup

DESSERT
Sliced peaches with peach frozen yogurt on top
(or any fruit and yogurt)

(5)
MEAT LOAF
(Eat one slice)

4–6 oz. lean ground beef
¼ cup V-8 or tomato juice
1 cup finely chopped celery, onion, pepper, garlic, and carrots
2 egg whites
Salt, pepper, and season to taste
Lightly sauté vegetables, add V-8, add to meat and eggs, and blend
(Thicken with bread crumbs if necessary)—bake or microwave
1 cup rice, pasta, or potato
1 side salad or soup

DESSERT
1 fruit

(6)
AD LIB

Use any lunch for dinner and add 1 cup of additional vegetables

---

IDEA

Chicken or Turkey Meat Loaf: Use bouillon base and above recipe. You might add diced mushrooms for an interesting variation.

Meatloaf Versatility: Use recipe for meatballs, stuffing for peppers, tacos, cabbage (with added rice)

PROBLEM SOLVER IN ACTION

The following recipe was originated by Marci Bruccoleri who typed part of the manuscript for *The Dieter's Dictionary and Problem Solver.* While reading and typing this book, Marci Bruccoleri came to realize that she was an oil addict and was using oil for pasta and garlic sauces. Soon she realized she was consuming three weeks' worth of fat in one dinner sitting.

From this realization came the beneficial changes to her favorite recipe, of course, substituting the fat and oil intake with one tasty ingredient—chicken broth.

Way to go, Marci!

(7)
PASTA BRUCCOLERI

2 cups broccoli, cauliflower, and carrots (steamed)
4 cloves of garlic
1 cup chicken broth
1 cup pasta
(Sauté garlic in ¼ cup of chicken broth—add steamed vegetables, pasta, and
    remainder of chicken broth to garlic)
Sprinkle grated parmesan over pasta to serve

DESSERT
1 fruit and gelatin with dollop Cool Whip Lite

THE PROBLEM SOLVER SOUPS

Problem: No time to cook/fast lane life/need easy, healthy meals/need to lose fat

Solution: Hearty, fresh soups that you can eat for appetizers, snacks, or main courses. *But wait!* That's not all. You can convert these soups to sauces for side dishes, quick meat or veggie casseroles that can be baked or microwaved.

Soups are a marvelous way to get everything you need in one meal for health, nutrition, and super fat burn. Your soup strategy is to make your own—as lean as can be—stocked with fresh vegetables, super low-fat, and none of the excess sodium found in the canned or pouch versions of soup.

Make a soup base each week to take you through the program. Refrigerate in glass containers to keep the ingredients fresher. You can turn our two Problem Solver soup bases—chicken base and tomato base—into dozens of easy meals to make food management easy on your diet. Here's how it works:

Problem Solver Tomato Base
    1 can whole tomatoes in juice
    1 cup vegetables (different medleys for each soup)

Add any pasta or rice, and you've got a super soup.

Add any meat or fish, and you've got a main course that can't be beat for leanness.

Spice your soups to taste the way you like them, using different herbs and spices for variety.

How to turn this simple tomato base into a bonanza of soups and sauces:

(1)
Minestrone Like Magic

1 can whole tomatoes
1 cup vegetables—diced celery,
    carrots, peas
1 cup pasta twirls
Spice to taste

• Add chunky chicken or lean beef and you've got an entrée

(2)
Creamy Tomato Soup

1 can whole tomatoes
½ cup finely diced celery, parsley,
    carrots, peas
½ cup low-fat milk

• Add rice for old-fashioned tomato rice
• Use green fettuccine and shrimp for a soup entrée

(3)
Tomato and Elbows Soup

1 can whole tomatoes
1 cup vegetables—diced celery,
   pepper, onion, mushrooms
1 cup elbow macaroni
Spice to taste

- Add lean ground beef sautéed in its own juice and you've got macaroni and beef

- Use pasta shells instead of elbows and a topping of bread crumbs, and presto! A casserole!

- Layer on lasagna pasta for vegetable or meat lasagna

(4)
Cheese and Tomato Soup

1 can whole tomatoes
½ cup low-fat cottage cheese

- Cook over low heat—cottage cheese will blend in

- Spice with Italian seasoning or oregano, parsley, or basil

- Add diced vegetables—onions, mushrooms, celery, garlic—and you've got another soup

- Add vegetables with extra mushrooms for a very lean pasta sauce with the cheese taste you long for

- Add any pasta and you've got a casserole (vegetable)

- Add any meat, and you've got a casserole entrée complete

(5)
Ratatouille Soup

1 can whole tomatoes
1–2 cups chunky vegetables—
   onions, celery, zucchini,
   cauliflower, broccoli, etc.
Season to taste, mild or hot

- Make this thicker with more vegetables and use it as a sauce over rice, pasta, or meat, fish, and poultry

(6)
Soup to Sauces and Casseroles in Seconds

- Spaghetti sauce—Use the cheese and tomato soup recipe. Sauté vegetables in their own juice, add to soup. Make it thick, spice to taste.
(Skip the Parmesan on top)

- Thicken any of the soups with extra mushrooms, wheat flour, or bread crumbs to use for casserole with meat, fish, or poultry

- Thicken any soup and use as a topping for rice, pasta, baked potatoes, tacos, meat loaf, and stuffed peppers

- Make a Mexican variety with peppers, corn, peppercorns, rice, and lean ground beef or chicken to stuff tomatoes and peppers

- Make a bean or lentil version with chili powder and Tabasco, chili, or bean stuffing for tacos

- Experiment with possibilities. They're unlimited!

THE PROBLEM SOLVER CHICKEN BASE

This takes a bit longer, but it's worth it. Once a week, bake a chicken or turkey to use for sandwiches and entrées *and to get your low-fat soup base.*

Soup base: Break up the carcass of poultry and cover with cold water in a big pot. Add diced celery, carrots, parsley, ½ lemon, peppercorns, and 1 to 2 bay leaves (don't forget to remove the bay leaves later). Cook over medium heat until the mixture boils. Just before boiling, skim off top residue, then bring to boil. Cover and simmer for two to three hours to a gel. Strain off any extra fat. Refrigerate in glass jars or freeze in single soup pouches to be ready in a minute. Skim off extra fat from cold version, and you've got a chicken soup base that can be used for many soups, as a sauté base, or as a gravy base.

(1)
Lemon Chicken Soup

2 cups base—thin with water
½ cup rice
2 egg whites
3 tablespoons lemon juice
2 oz. chunky chicken
Spice to taste (if preferred)

(2)
Chicken Vegetable

2 cups base
1 cup vegetables—chunky, fresh medley, mushrooms, celery, carrots, water chestnuts, etc.
2 oz. chunky chicken
Spice to taste

- Make thick for chow mein sauce

(3)
Chicken Noodle Soup

2 cups base
1 cup noodles
1 cup vegetables—celery, carrots, onions
2 oz. chunky chicken

(4)
Barley or Lentil Soup

2 cups base
1 cup vegetables (any)
1 cup barley or lentils
Spice to taste

• Use rice instead for chicken rice soup
• Use turkey instead for turkey noodle.
Add extra vegetables if you like.

• Add 2 oz. lean beef for beef barley or lentil

(5)
Ad Lib

2 cups base
1 cup any leftover vegetables
(Shred leafy vegetables)
1 cup rice or pasta
Spice to taste

(6)
Sauce, Gravy and Soup to Stew in Seconds

• Thicken with whole wheat flour for gravies or sauces
• Use mushrooms and onions for mushroom gravy with base
• Pot roast or stews. Use base, add extra vegetables
• Use as bouillon for any recipe, or as sauté
• Creamy mushroom or celery—use base, vegetables, and low-fat milk; make it thick

PROBLEM SOLVER BROCCOLI SOUP
with Unbelievable Ease

Steam 1 full bunch of broccoli with stems, cutting off only the rougher bottom of stalks. When tender, put broccoli chunks in blender (half full). Add water and blend to purée. As blend thickens, take top off to let air into purée. Add a dash of low-fat milk for creamy broccoli or a teaspoon of wheat flour for extra thick soup. Season with oregano or basil (or your favorite spices).

Make the whole bunch into soup this way. Refrigerate and heat as needed. _A no-fat dream soup!_ Superthinning and the extra disease prevention assets of broccoli. Try it with celery, carrots, cucumbers—a whole range of soups.

Special Occasions: Sprinkle grated Parmesan cheese over broccoli soup to serve.

With these fabulous soups as your problem solver base, you never have to go hungry or lack nutrition. Have a bowl of soup for a daily boost.

THE PROBLEM SOLVER DESSERT SOLUTION

Problem: Too. many options cause confusion/need something sweet

Solution: Fruit and dairy/natural sweetness and super low-fat

Think of your desserts as your fruit and dairy servings and create tasty variations. This one change in your habits will sub-tract a *lot* of fat.

Examples (These are sweet and delicious):

Any Fruit with Fruit Nectar and Cool Whip Lite Blend or
Fruit Nectar and Frozen Yogurt Blend

- Mandarin oranges and pineapples topped with apricot nectar blended with Cool Whip Lite
- Peaches and pears topped with peach nectar blended with Cool Whip Lite
- Melon balls topped with pear nectar and vanilla yogurt blend

Any Fruit Topped with Frozen Yogurt

- Peaches with peach frozen yogurt topping (or vanilla)
- Blueberries and blackberries with raspberry frozen yogurt topping
- Strawberries with vanilla frozen yogurt topping (serve over angel food cake for strawberry shortcake that's lean)
- Bananas with chocolate, vanilla, and strawberry frozen yogurt (a split!)

Any Fruit with Sherbet
(less frequently—more sugar than the other toppings)

- Oranges and bananas topped with orange sherbet
- Any fruit topped with dollop of sherbet

Any Low or No-Fat Cream Pop

Can be whipped in your blender with water or skim milk for a mousse or parfait! The chocolate cream pop (no fat) is like mousse when whipped. How about the strawberry cream pop whipped with raspberries and strawberries mixed in!

Special problem solver note: Please be sure that you get your two servings of dairy daily. If you forget, drink milk alone, as you might take a vitamin. It's so essential for healthy bones and teeth. Don't even consider skipping it. It will maximize your health!

SUCCESSFUL DIETING STYLE

If the rigid rules and standards of most American diets were successful, everyone would be thin by now. Every twenty minutes, someone is going on a diet. Often one dieter will go on and off a diet in twenty minutes. Punishment, self-denial, deprivation, and restriction are adding up to weight regain. When you aren't comfortable with what you're doing, you won't keep doing it for long, and most diets are based on deprivation. That makes them something to be dreaded.

If you are a former dieter, you have to shake some old diet ghosts out of your closet. Good foods and bad foods. Guilt, blame, and self-recrimination. A head war with food on a daily basis. Starving to get thin. Feeling like you're being punished because you are dieting. The list goes on and on. You know what the problems are.

Just because you are dieting, you don't have to treat yourself as though you're not worth a normal life. You don't have to adopt abnormal eating patterns, eating foods you don't like and wouldn't eat unless you thought you had to.

Isn't it possible to create a world of food for yourself that will be thrilling and still be fat-free? There are hundreds of foods to choose from to fashion a new world of food.

Here are some hints that might help you get started on the right track.

Eat for Pleasure
There are dozens of ways to get gourmet pleasure without cooking with fat.

- Tomato juice with lemon and herbs makes an excellent cooking sauce that tastes salty, but isn't.
- Garlic, lemon, and basil make an excellent base for sauté.
- Whole-grain flours with herbs and spices make healthy gravies, with the fat skimmed off.
- You can stir-fry with pear juice or other fruit juices. Fruit nectars make excellent basting sauces for meats.
- You can top a waffle with fresh strawberries and juice.

- Mushrooms make a marvelous meaty gravy that is fat-free.
- Wine vinegar and herbs add juice and flavor to meats.
- Ratatouille vegetables with spices make a fabulous sauce.
- Soups can be fabulous fitness boosters, and they can become cooking sauces in a snap. See The Problem Solver Meals and Menus for great soup recipes.

Use your imagination. You don't have to cook with butter or margarine to eat fabulously.

Chocolate Urges

What about a panic attack for something chocolate? If you've been dieting for a few weeks, or even on the first week, is something chocolate going to throw your whole system out of balance? No. Is it going to make you lose weight slower? No, not if you don't eat the whole cake. And your odds of eating a whole cake are greater if you try to deny yourself constantly and lust after it in every window. Dieting is an art of moderation. Have a small mint patty to satisfy your chocolate urge, or take a vanilla wafer and dot it with chocolate syrup. If you're going to hit the ceiling if you don't have a piece of chocolate cake, have a small piece, then continue with your diet the next day. Exercise regularly and you'll still be in good shape.

Dining Out

What about eating out? Should you carry a bag of *your* food and refuse to look at the menu? Should you sit there and not eat, and talk about not eating throughout the entire meal? What happens then? You go home and eat to compensate. You can eat successfully in a restaurant without feeling like an ostracized child. Choose from the leaner offerings, and add side dishes of vegetables. Ask for your sauces on the side, and moderate their use. Ask the waitress to have your meal cooked without butter. Drink plenty of water and eat slowly. Don't tell yourself you'll never be able to enjoy eating in a restaurant again, because you'll believe it. If you choose poorly this time and eat a basket of onion rings, try again the next time to eat more nutritiously. Keep up your regular eating with the food wheel as a guide and keep up your exercise. You'll make it. Believe it and you will.

Lean Atmosphere

Learn to enjoy dieting. When you eat real food and learn to have fun in the kitchen experimenting with recipes, you get a renewed sense of food pleasure. Food pleasure is a vital part of life. A microwave diet dinner deprives you of more than fiber. It takes away the smell of food cooking and the sensory pleasure of food. You don't have to cook with fat for that pleasure, and you don't have to dread going into the kitchen because you have excess fat. Adapt your kitchen to a leaner, healthy fare, and fill your refrigerator with healthy foods instead of stripping it down to metal shelves with celery and cottage cheese looking lonely in there.

Fast Food Health

TV and microdinners. Make your own variety of quick-cook dinners that you can heat up in a snap. Cook batches of soup, pasta salads, low-fat casseroles and stews, and freeze them in one-meal packs. That way, you won't be caught without a healthy choice some night when you're extra hungry.

The Super Snack Habit

Learn to eat your snacks in carbohydrates instead of sweets. Before you reach for the chocolate cream pie, eat an apple or a bowl of strawberries. Before you take the cheesecake, eat a bagel with jelly. Not only will this save you a lot of excess fat, but it will provide nutrition and satisfaction. And it is the best lean habit you can learn. Extra carbohydrates aren't going to layer on fat. They're long chain molecules, and they take a long time to digest. Many studies indicate that they never get to fat. You'd have to eat a lot of them to equal the calories and fat in one piece of cheesecake, and halfway through, you'd be full.

Enhance Yourself

Use your dieting time to learn relaxation exercises, practice meditation, and read self-supportive materials that help you create a new view of life. Use positive self-talk as a booster every night and morning. Learn to look at the good things that happen to you every day instead of focusing on the bad ones. Dieting can be a resource for self-renewal that is far greater than the one-note goal of weight loss. You can lose the weight you've been carrying in your mind. That makes you lighter inside, where it really counts.

FOOD SHOPPING

Each diet has its own shopping list for foods, and many are not foods you can find easily in your supermarket; or you have to shop in the diet sections. However, when you choose a natural food diet that uses the food groups, more options are available to you, but that also means making careful choices. It can be educational and fun, and it makes you a wise consumer.

1. Give yourself a little more time for shopping when you use the food pyramid system for dieting. Let yourself enjoy the process, and explore the food varieties, especially in the vegetable and fruit sections.

2. Read labels on processed foods to determine which ones have the least fat, sugar, sodium, and additives. Select the best possible versions of these foods (or limit them as much as possible).

3. If you shop when you're hungry, it makes sweets and bakery goods irresistible. If you find yourself getting hungry while you shop, buy an apple and eat it while you select foods. It will give you sweetness and fiber, and those urges will be dramatically decreased.

4. Make your shopping list an educational system for foods by drawing it in five columns, headed by the food group divisions shown on the food pyramid. Each time you list a food you need during the week, list it under the food group heading. You'll automatically see the group or groups you neglect. Fill in the missing groups with healthy selections, and you'll be rounding out your diet regularly.

5. Buy fresh food whenever possible and as many whole grains as you can find.

6. Don't neglect your desserts (on the light side). When you plan these into your daily diet, you do not feel deprived or dissatisfied. Fruit pops, frozen grapes, a mini mint patty, angel food cake—you can allow yourself to have a dessert each day and still burn fat. That way, you won't be fooled by the candy rack that's always next to the checkout counter—it's there to grab you at the last minute. You'll be fortified with food pleasures that won't make you fat.

The Problem Solver Calendar

A Month to Fat Freedom

BELOW IS YOUR STEP-BY-STEP CALENDAR for fat freedom and fitness. It includes the Problem Solver Diet for healthy eating; an exercise routine for muscle building, cardiovascular conditioning, and better calorie burn; and behavior exercises for program support and personal well-being. It's everything you need on a daily basis to gain fitness while you lose your fat.

All you have to do is follow the program, making sure you complete each requirement by the end of the day, and you have an automatic plan to achieve your weight-loss goals, tone your body and mind, and combat all of the eating problems that keep you out of shape and overweight. It's low-sugar, low-sodium, low-cholesterol and nutrition-packed for disease prevention. It's an energy builder and a no-hunger program for superior results in all areas of health. As you practice it and learn to use it as a habit, it will show you that everything works right when you do it.

You will find that it is easy to use and is teaching you all of the lifestyle habits you need for stress prevention and weight maintenance for life.

The Problem Solver Exercises: The exercise program is designed to limber you up and increase your capacity, endurance, and strength gradually. The exercise we've chosen as the mainstay of your program is walking. We show you how to take one exercise and develop it into a stronger and more intense workout as you adapt. It's a skill you can carry over to other forms of exercise.

You can use another aerobic exercise for your routine instead of walking, such as swimming, cycling, trampoline, or any aerobic machine. You might want to choose an alternative to take you through the month (so that you have two options). But try to avoid

107

switching exercises midstream, since this could lead to confusion and will break your stride.

The best course is to use walking as your foundation and to use your other exercise as an alternative for variety.

Enjoy your program! It will be the healthiest time of your life!

THE IDEAL DIET WEEK

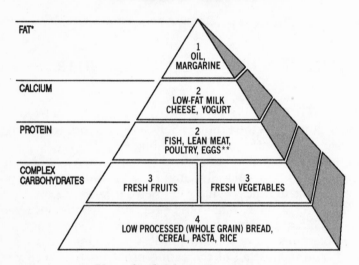

Your *food* drives up your *energy*
Your *activity* drives up your *calorie burn*
Result: Your *output* exceeds your *input*
You burn more than you eat

Your food burns calories too from thermogenesis—the heat of eating. The pyramid provides the fifty essential nutrients you need to feed your metabolism, to activate its chemical action to repair, rebuild, and maintain all your body processes, from the largest organ to the smallest cell. When you take the pyramid to its low-fat format, the result is fat burns and burns.

Your thirty-minute aerobic routine, three times per week, drives up your metabolism to burn more calories (15 percent plus). It also builds muscle, the vital body protein you lose from poor dieting but need to rebuild, in order to be a better fat burner for life. These factors combine to revive your sluggish metabolism, align your body composition, and set you up with the status you need to stay lean after your diet.

Overall result: While fat is burning, muscle is restored. You get superior weight loss and a body composition to match. In maintenance, you will be able to raise your calorie level without regaining weight.

Your goal: To get back in balance

THE PROBLEM SOLVER CALENDAR

A Month to Fat Freedom

THIS IS YOUR MONTHLY fat-burning calendar, with everything you need for nutrition, muscle building, and self-enhancement. You will find how-to-do keys to the recommended exercises in the dictionary section.

WEEK ONE

Day 1:   Eat the Problem Solver Diet.
Do one cardiovascular exercise for one-half hour: Walking.

Day 2:   Eat the Problem Solver Diet.
Do one behavior exercise for ten to fifteen minutes: Imagery.

Day 3:   Eat the Problem Solver Diet.
Do one cardiovascular exercise for one-half hour: Walking.

Day 4:   Eat the Problem Solver Diet.
Do one behavior exercise for ten to fifteen minutes: Relaxation and the adjunct Full Body Release.
Do one stretching routine for fifteen to twenty minutes: Stretching.

Day 5:   Eat the Problem Solver Diet.
Do one cardiovascular exercise for one-half hour: Walking.

Day 6:   Eat the Problem Solver Diet.
Do one behavior exercise for ten to fifteen minutes: Relaxation and the adjunct Finding Your Perfect Space.
Do one stretching routine for fifteen to twenty minutes: Stretching.

Day 7:   Eat the Problem Solver Diet.
Do one behavior exercise for ten to fifteen minutes: Mirror Exercise—Creating a Positive Mirror Image.

WEEK TWO

Day 1:   Eat the Problem Solver Diet.
Do one cardiovascular exercise for one-half hour: Walking (intensified by extending your distance and increasing your speed).

Day 2:   Eat the Problem Solver Diet.
Do one behavior exercise for ten to fifteen minutes: Breathing (practice breathing from your diaphragm).

Day 3:   Eat the Problem Solver Diet.
Do one cardiovascular exercise for one-half hour: Walking (intensified).

Day 4:   Eat the Problem Solver Diet.
Do one behavior exercise for ten to fifteen minutes: Relaxation and the adjunct Exercise.
Do one stretching routine for fifteen to twenty minutes: Stretching.

Day 5:   Eat the Problem Solver Diet.
Do one cardiovascular exercise for one-half hour: Walking (intensified).

Day 6:   Eat the Problem Solver Diet.
Do one behavior exercise for ten to fifteen minutes: repeat Breathing.
Do one stretching routine for fifteen to twenty minutes: Stretching

Day 7:   Eat the Problem Solver Diet.
Do one behavior exercise for ten to fifteen minutes: Fear of Failure.

WEEK THREE

Day 1: Eat the Problem Solver Diet.
Do one cardiovascular exercise for one-half hour: Walking, briskly (keeping a stronger pace throughout, using your breathing technique).*

Day 2: Eat the Problem Solver Diet.
Do one strength routine for fifteen to twenty minutes: Strength Training.

Day 3: Eat the Problem Solver Diet.
Do one cardiovascular exercise for one-half hour: Walking briskly.

Day 4: Eat the Problem Solver Diet.
Do one behavior exercise for ten to fifteen minutes: (repeat Relaxation and the adjunct Full Body Release).
Do one stretching routine for fifteen to twenty minutes: Stretching.

Day 5: Eat the Problem Solver Diet.
Do one cardiovascular exercise for one-half hour: Walking, briskly.

Day 6: Eat the Problem Solver Diet.
Do one behavior exercise for ten to fifteen minutes: Mirror Exercise—Whole Self Appreciation.
Do one strength routine for fifteen to twenty minutes: Strength Training.

Day 7: Eat the Problem Solver Diet.
Do one stretching routine for ten to fifteen minutes: Stretching.

*Here you can switch to any other aerobic workout, such as rowing, Nordic track, or swimming. Use Interval Training to adapt. Avoid joining a club at this point if you didn't start with that program for exercise. The dramatic shift in focus could break your stride. Your goal is to be independent and able to do everything you need at home or on your own. That way, if a sudden business trip comes up, your workout can go with you. If it's stressful to think about changing your routine at this time, just keep walking.

WEEK FOUR

Day 1:   Eat the Problem Solver Diet.
Do one cardiovascular exercise for one-half hour: Power Walking (add hand weights to your walk or use varied terrain by climbing hills, walking on gravel, grass, or sand without slowing down).

Day 2:   Eat the Problem Solver Diet.
Do one behavior exercise for fifteen to twenty minutes: Imagery (thin-within).
Do one strength routine for fifteen to twenty minutes: Strength Training.

Day 3:   Eat the Problem Solver Diet.
Do one cardiovascular exercise for one-half hour: Power Walking (or varied terrain walking).

Day 4:   Eat the Problem Solver Diet.
Do one behavior exercise for ten to fifteen minutes: Relaxation and the adjunct Mental Rehearsal.
Do one stretching routine for fifteen to twenty minutes: Stretching.

Day 5:   Eat the Problem Solver Diet.
Do one cardiovascular exercise for one-half hour: Power Walking (or varied terrain walking).

Day 6:   Eat the Problem Solver Diet.
Do one behavior exercise for ten to fifteen minutes: your choice. Don't skip this step. When in doubt, use Finding Your Perfect Place.
Do one stretching routine for fifteen to twenty minutes: Stretching.

Day 7:   Eat the Problem Solver Diet.
Do one behavior exercise for ten to fifteen minutes: Mirror Exercises—Creating a Positive Mirror Image. Note the changes!

That's the end of your perfect month. If you have more weight to lose, repeat. If you're at ideal, see Maintenance in The Top Twenty Problems and How to Solve Them.

PART THREE

The Dieter's Dictionary

Introduction to the Dictionary

THIS DICTIONARY IS THE FIRST resource that gives you everything you need to know about weight loss, maintenance, food management, and fitness in one easy reference. It includes diets, exercise, behavior modification, nutrition education, food cue control, lifestyle training, physiology, biochemistry, and psychology.

With more than 400 diet books giving you conflicting information, more than 500 exercise books featuring their own programs, and more than 500 nutrition books focusing on different foods, as a health-conscious consumer, you face difficult decisions when you are trying to sort out facts from fads. Here you can find the basic science that is the foundation of diet, exercise, health, nutrition, and fitness. It's the resource you can trust.

As an education aid, the dictionary is both a guide to good health and a self-empowering resource. It gives you the information you need to make healthy, effective choices.

With knowledge comes power. When you have science on your side, you have the knowledge you need to make sound choices and take an active role in your own program for health and well-being. When you are armed with information, it makes you less susceptible to faddish programs and imbalanced food plans that can undermine your fitness goals.

The Dieter's Dictionary is keyed for your easy use:

Food Questions	See Food Keys ▲
Behavior Questions	See Behavior Keys ●
Exercise Questions	See Exercise Keys ◆

You can find easy ways to take charge of your own program with many behavior modification and food management skills. These are indicated by arrows.

How To's	See ⇒

115

We also included a key to topics that are particularly vital for heart health. These are keyed with a heart.

Heart Health   See ❤

Today is the day to start creating your future health.

A

ABSORPTION, CALORIE

The process between digestion and metabolism where nutrients are absorbed by your blood. During digestion, your food nutrients are broken down into smaller and smaller molecules to convert them into the form that your blood can absorb. Carbohydrates are broken down into glucose, fat into fatty acids and glycerol, protein into amino acids. This process starts in your mouth and ends in your small intestines where absorption takes place. When the nutrients are in the form that your blood can pick up, they pass into the cells of your intestinal lining. From there, they are absorbed into your bloodstream and lymphatic system. Some nutrients go to your liver for storage, to be meted out when you need them. Other nutrients go to your adipose tissue to be stored and metered out when you need them. The rest go to all the cells of your body for the process of metabolism. *See* Digestion; Metabolism.

ACIDITY

An acidic system. This is often the result of gastric juices that are not neutralized after digestion. It can be prevented by eating a more fibrous diet, rather than by taking a medication. Fiber binds with bile acids and excess bile is excreted. The double benefit for a dieter is better weight loss, since high-fiber diets lead to less fat storage. *See* Fiber.

ADDITIVES

Chemical, synthetic, or natural ingredients added to foods for a variety of purposes, such as coloring, flavoring, sweetening, preserving, emulsifying, thickening, and chelating.

Excess additives aren't good for anyone, but particularly not for dieters. When you are on a calorie-limited plan, your system is more susceptible to foreign substances, and you can experience symptoms you might not have otherwise. Real, fresh food is the best way to burn fat, protect your body muscle, and revitalize your

---

▲ Food Skills   ● Behavior Skills   ♦ Exercise Skills

health. Foods with additives are typically low-nutrition food with added fats, sugars, salt, and little or no fiber. That's the combination that leads to weight gain. So you'll find that a nonadditive diet is also a fat-prevention technique that's automatic.

To choose the best foods, look for products with natural additives that are safe or even beneficial. For instance, beta carotene, used as a coloring agent, is a valuable source of vitamin A, and lecithin, used as an emulsifier, is a good source of choline.

Overprocessed foods need additives to try to fix the problems created by processing: loss of color and texture, lack of stabilization, loss of appeal. Often they need additional additives to counterbalance harmful effects inherent in one of the additives used. For instance, sodium nitrate and nitrite in bacon, ham, and cured meats are known to form potent carcinogens called nitrosamines. To prevent nitrosamines from forming, ascorbic acid is needed as an additive. It makes sense chemically, but you don't need to take the risk with your body.

When you start tracking additives on your supermarket shelves and see the overwhelming number of foods that use long lists of additives, it will give you a new respect for the companies that had your welfare in mind when they opted for natural or safe additives.

ADDITIVES: WHAT TO LOOK FOR ON FOOD LABELS

ANTIOXIDANTS: Prevent rancidity, loss of color, and flavor.

_____ CHEMICAL _____

Butylated Hydroxytoluene (BHT)	Cereals Gums Chips	Avoid May promote cancer, allergies
Butylated Hydroxyanisole (BHA)	Cereals Gums Chips Oils	Avoid Not enough tests
Propyl gallate	Soup bases Meat products Oils	Avoid Not enough tests

⟶ How-to Skills   ♥ Good for Heart

_____ NATURAL _____		
Alpha Tocopherol (Vitamin E)	Wheats Rices Oils	Beneficial
Ascorbic Acid (Vitamin C)	Cereals Meats Sodas Oily foods	Beneficial
Lecithin	Baked goods Margarine Chocolate Ice cream	Beneficial

CHELATORS: Trap metal atoms that cause food to spoil.

_____ NATURAL _____		
Citric acid	Ice cream Sherbet Fruit drinks Candy Instant Potatoes	Safe
EDTA	Salad dressings Margarines Mayonnaise Processed fruit Processed vegs Soft drinks Canned shellfish	Safe

_____ NATURAL _____		
Phosphoric acid Phosphates	Baked goods Cured meats Sodas Cereals Cheese	Avoid Excess can lead to osteoporosis

COLORINGS: To make food look palatable.

_____ CHEMICAL _____		
Blue #1	Sodas Candy Baked goods	Not safe Poorly tested

▲ Food Skills   ● Behavior Skills   ◆ Exercise Skills

Blue #2	Sodas Candy	Not safe Tumors in rats
Red #2	Some Florida orange skins	Not safe Cancerous
Red #3	Cherries Candy Baked goods	Not safe Cancer
Red #40	Sodas Candy Baked goods Sausage	Questionable
Green #3	Sodas Candy	Not safe Tumors in rats
Yellow #5	Candy Baked goods Gelatins	Not safe Poorly tested May promote cancer, allergies
Yellow #6	Sodas Candy Baked goods Sausage	Appears safe, but watch allergies

———————————————— NATURAL ————————————————

Beta carotene	Margarine Shortening Creamers Butter	Beneficial
Ferrous Glutonate	Black olives Pills	Beneficial
Dextrose Glucose	Breads Baked goods	Safe Empty calories

EMULSIFIERS: Keep oils and water from separating.

———————————————— CHEMICAL ————————————————

Polysorbate 60	Baked goods Imitation dairy Frozen desserts Pickles	Not pure Can contain carcinogenic compounds

| Sorbitan | Desserts
Candy
Icings | Safe |

_____ NATURAL _____

Bromated vegetable Oil (BVO)	Soft drinks	Avoid Not tested enough
Lecithin	Margarine Baked goods Ice cream Chocolate	Beneficial
Monoglycerides Diglycerides	Baked goods Peanut butter Candy Margarine	Safe
Phosphoric acid Phosphates	Cereals Sodas Baked goods Cheese Processed foods	Excess can lead to osteoporosis

FLAVORINGS: Chemicals that imitate natural flavors. Often many chemicals are needed to make one flavor.

_____ CHEMICAL _____

More than 100	Sodas Candy Cereals Gelatins	Can cause hyperactivity in children
Ethyl Vanillin	Ice cream Baked goods Chocolate Candy Gelatins	Needs testing
Quinine	Tonic waters Bitters	Can cure malaria: not for pregnant women; poorly tested
Sodium Nitrate Sodium Nitrite	Cured meats Lunch meats Bacon Ham Hot dogs	Promotes cancer-causing nitrosamines

_____

▲ Food Skills   ● Behavior Skills   ◆ Exercise Skills

——————————————— NATURAL ———————————————

Citric Acid	Ice cream Sherbet Fruit drinks Candy Carbonated drinks Instant potatoes	Safe
Sodium Citrate	Ice cream Candy Jams	Safe
Fumaric Acid	Powdered drinks Puddings Pie fillings Gelatins	Safe Not great Needs detergent-like additive to dissolve in cold water
Ethyl Vanillin	Ice cream Baked goods Sodas Chocolate Candy	Safe
Hydrolyzed Vegetable Protein (HVP)	Instant soups Hot Dogs Sauces Stews	Beneficial
MSG Monosodium Glutomate	Processed foods Soups Stews Poultry Seafood	Avoid Affects nerve cells in brain MSG syndrome
Sodium Chloride	Most processed foods	Excess can cause high blood pressure

PRESERVATIVES: Prevent mold and bacteria.

——————————————— CHEMICAL ———————————————

Sulfur Dioxide	Processed fruits Instant potatoes Wine	Safe but destroys vitamin B-1

──────────────── NATURAL ────────────────

Calcium Propionate Sodium Propionate	Baked goods	Safe
Heptyl Paraben	Beer	Safe but poorly tested
Sodium Benzoate	Fruit juices Pickles Preserves	Safe but excess causes high blood pressure
Sodium Nitrate Sodium Nitrite	Bacon Lunch meats Cured meats	Not safe Carcinogenic Nitrosamines Created
Sorbic Acid	Cheese Baked goods Syrups Dried fruits Wines	Safe

SWEETENERS: Add sweet taste.

Brown sugar, Caramel, Corn syrup, Corn syrup solids, Dextrose, Fructose, Glucose, Honey, Lactate, Maltose, Malitol, Mannitol, Raw sugar, Sorbitol, Sucrose, Turbinado, Xylitol. *See* Sugar.

THICKENERS: Absorb water in foods, keep compounds mixed.

──────────────── NATURAL ────────────────

Alginate Propylene glycol Alginate	Dairy products Frostings Candy Beer Sodas	Safe
Carrageenan	Ice cream Chocolate milk Jelly	Small amounts safe Large amounts can harm colon
Casein Sodium Caseinate	Ice cream Sherbet Creamers	Beneficial

──

▲ Food Skills   ● Behavior Skills   ◆ Exercise Skills

Corn syrup	Candies	Empty calories
	Syrups	Tooth decay
	Snack foods	
	Imitation dairy	
Gelatin	Dessert mixes	Safe
	Dairy products	
	Beverages	
Gums:		
Arabic	Ice cream	Poorly tested
Funcelleran	Puddings	
Ghatti	Salad dressings	
Guar	Dough	
Locust bean	Cottage cheese	
Tragacanth	Candy	
	Drink mixes	
	Fast-food burgers	
Sodium	Ice cream	Safe
Carboxmethyl-	Pie fillings	
cellulose	Icings	
	Diet foods	
	Candy	
	Beer	
Sorbitol	Diet drinks	Safe
	Diet foods	Doesn't raise
	Coconut	blood sugar
	Candy	as fast as
	Gum	other sugars
Starch	Soups	Safe
Modified starch	Gravies	

ADRENALINE

The stress hormone. Increased adrenaline causes your system to speed up, and that includes your metabolism. While this may seem like a good thing to a dieter who wants a faster metabolism, the after-effects are not. Stress causes nutrient depletion and anxiety that leads to eating. One of the major causes of overeating is stress. *See* Stress.

● AFFIRMATIONS

Positive self-statements. This is a behavior technique to change the way you view yourself and the world. Essentially it means rethinking and rephrasing the negative statements you make to yourself in order to gain a more positive framework for succeeding with weight loss and lifestyle change. For instance, you might say, "I never do anything right." While you might mean this in good humor, or you might think you don't seriously believe this, by saying it, you are making a judgment about yourself. To be self-affirmative, you don't have to go to the opposite extreme and say, "I do everything right." You want to think of the things you did right and succeeded with in the past and call them to mind when you doubt your own abilities or put yourself down verbally. If you only see the mistakes in your efforts, you need to shift your point of view to find the value in your efforts. It's there. You just have to look. When you're dealing with food and eating, rather than look at what you can't do, the self-affirming position would be to look at what you can do. *See* Mirror Exercises and Rationalizations for examples.

▲ ALCOHOL

A depressant with calories. Alcohol is a double-edged sword. The first drink acts as a stimulant, making you feel relaxed and more outgoing. The second drink acts as a depressant, slowing your system down, dulling your reaction time. Alcohol withdraws water from your tissues and cells. In excess, this destroys brain cells. A low amount of alcohol can be neutralized by your liver, but when you have food in your stomach, your liver can only neutralize one drink per hour. If you drink too much alcohol, your liver adapts by increasing its tolerance, but it becomes fatty and in severe cases, scarred. Two drinks per week are considered safe for a dieter, but not the sweet ones. A glass of wine every other day will not create problems. But you have to watch out! Alcohol dulls your senses and you forget that you're dieting. The foods you reach for when you're drinking alcohol are usually sugars, fats, and salts.

● ALL-OR-NOTHING THINKING

A behavior term for thinking in extremes. Also called black and white thinking. Either/or thinking; to a dieter, this means either you are on a diet feeling deprived of all pleasure, or you are off a diet giving in to food whims, telling yourself you'll start another diet next month. This pattern of thinking is failure-bound. It's based on negative input for both extremes—a lose/lose situation

---

▲ Food Skills   ● Behavior Skills   ♦ Exercise Skills

(everything but fat). When you're not on a diet, you feel guilty and critical of yourself. When you're on a diet, you want fast results to make up for lost time. You get disappointed easily if a client doesn't provide major weight loss right away. This is a difficult mindset to maintain, because it provides you little personal pleasure and keeps your head-war going about weight.

To change this pattern, you must first change the way you perceive a diet. A diet isn't a short-term affair where you can starve yourself to ideal body weight, then somehow magically maintain it. Successful dieting is a gradual *process* where you earn leanness through sound nutrition, using behavior skills to change weight-gaining habits into supportive lean ones. You can change an all-or-nothing approach to food by learning moderation—eating smaller portions of a wide variety of foods and substituting low-fat foods for their high-fat equivalents. In this way you avoid the good food/bad food extremes regarding your body's fuel. One dish of ice cream won't add pounds of fat, but a dish every night will add weight over time. When you deal with your food and eating attitudes from a more moderate perspective, you steadily ingrain less extreme patterns you need to get lean and stay lean. The positive effect flows over into other decision-making areas of your life.

▲ AMINO ACIDS

Nutrient components of protein. Approximately twenty-two amino acids occur in protein foods, in different combinations. They are broken down in your body to make other combinations. Your body can manufacture some of its own amino acids, but it cannot make eight of the amino acids. These are called essential, since you must get them from your food. The eight essential amino acids are: isoleucine, leucine, lysine, methionine, phenylalanine, threonine, tryptophan, and valine. You wouldn't need this list of essential amino acids if it were not for tryptophan and phenylalanine, the more commonly known amino acids. Phenylalanine is often used as an ingredient in diet aids or so-called "magic pill" formulas sold as a cure for weight. Tryptophan was used as a sleeping aid until it was linked to a rare blood disease. It's important to realize that your amino acids must be provided in the right proportions for your body to use them. If they are not, it can throw off your metabolism of protein. Taking any amino acid in isolation is not a healthy idea and one of which you should beware. *See* Protein; Tryptophan.

ANOREXIA NERVOSA

An eating disorder characterized by reduction of food intake to the point of self-starvation.

Anorexia is a chronic condition that requires medical intervention and often hospitalization. It is easily recognizable as excessive thinness to an emaciated state, or loss of at least one-fourth of normal weight. The individual is malnourished and usually refuses to maintain normal weight. Severe losses of muscle mass become life threatening. Other complications include: breast atrophy, thin hair, dry skin, edema of legs, a layer of fine hair over the body, intolerance to cold, slow heart rate, low blood pressure to the degree of dizziness, menstrual disturbances, abdominal pain, and bloating.

Anorexia is particularly difficult to treat because the individual usually resists treatment and is reluctant to enter therapy. The disorder involves unresolved family conflicts making the person feel powerless in his or her own life. Control is exercised over food and the body as a way to feel power.

Treatment is long term and includes dealing with nutritional deficiencies, medical conditions, body image distortions, assertiveness behavior, and exercise patterns.

If you or anyone you know suffers from this disease, don't feel that it can be resolved with an at-home plan or a change in diet. Find medical help without delay, for life's sake.

ANTHROPOMETRIC MEASUREMENTS

Traditional tests to determine body fat and muscle composition; clinical pinch-an-inch. Anthropometrics takes into account weight, height, mid-upper arm circumference, skin-fold thickness in the triceps, and mid-upper arm muscle circumference. The measuring device for skinfold thickness is the caliper, which resembles a large metal pincher or tweezers. The mid-upper arm muscle circumference is an indirect result of the other tests and is based on hundreds of clinical averages, using a formula to arrive at this number. The tests measure subcutaneous fat tissue. *See* Scale, for the recommended levels of healthy body fat content.

● **ANXIETY**

Fear or uncertainty about the future. *See* Relaxation, to let it go.

▲ Food Skills   ● Behavior Skills   ◆ Exercise Skills

APPETITE

Your body's internal nutrient regulator, with cues for hunger and satiety. Your appetite originates in your brain, in the hypothalamus. Both aspects of eating are controlled there, hunger and satiety. Various chemicals stimulate this area, creating hunger pangs or the urge to eat, and ending hunger with fullness or a chemical cue for nutrient satisfaction. Scientists are not sure of the exact causes for hunger and satiety, or exactly what triggers the process. However, they have identified some of the key chemicals that are involved.

Glucose is an important factor in hunger. When blood glucose is low, the cue to eat is signaled. Glucose is the nutrient from carbohydrates, derived in the digestive process. It's the primary source of energy for your muscles and brain. Scientists believe that the brain contains a glucose receptor, a gauge for blood levels. When glucose levels rise from eating carbohydrates, the cue to stop eating is given. An easy way to stop hunger would be to eat complex carbohydrates. They're low-fat, satisfying, and fibrous. Carbohydrate snacks during the day would keep glucose levels stable.

Insulin is another important factor in hunger and satiety, and it's also related to glucose. When glucose levels are high in your blood, insulin is released. According to researcher Judith Wurtman, the insulin increases the amount of tryptophan that goes to your brain. Tryptophan stimulates the production of serotonin, a neurotransmitter in your brain. Serotonin turns off hunger.

Neurotransmitters are brain chemicals that transmit messages through your nerves to your muscles. When your brain has high levels of the neurotransmitters serotonin, norepinephrine, epinephrine, and dopamine, appetite is reduced. Exercise increases the production of epinephrine and norepinephrine. Stress on your body, such as exercise, leads to an increase in the neurotransmitters. This is one of the reasons why exercise is an excellent substitute for eating.

Cholecystokinin is a hormone in your small intestines, produced after eating. Researchers believe that it can act on the hypothalamus to produce satiety.

Fiber has been credited with a decrease in hunger by creating fullness in the stomach. But many researchers feel that the stomach has no direct effect on hunger or satiety. Rather, the stomach fullness creates a sense of satisfaction, or a feeling of fullness, which causes the individual to stop eating. Fiber is also a component of carbohydrates.

⮕ How-to Skills   ❤ Good for Heart

The biochemical factors in hunger are only part of the picture. People eat for many reasons, even when they don't feel hungry. Regulating these hungers falls into the domain of habit control, and taking charge of the emotional appetite. *See* Habits; Hunger, Psychological.

APPETITE SUPPRESSANT DRUGS

Anorectic agents that chemically reduce hunger. Many experts say that amphetamine-type agents (but not amphetamines) can be helpful in the early stages of a diet, particularly for people who have severe hunger problems and a history of diet failure. But they recommend that these agents only be used for the first two to three months in conjunction with a sound diet and exercise program, and only in the care of your doctor.

The downside of appetite suppressants involves more than the stated risks or side effects. While these chemicals do not *directly* cause nutritional imbalance, they can lead to it, because of what they do: suppress your natural appetite. Your appetite is the regulator of your nutrient needs. Without it, you won't get a reading on nutritional depletion. When your appetite is suppressed, you may not eat balanced meals, you may eat very little or nothing at all, thinking less food is better, that less food will let you lose weight faster. This can result in the opposite effects you were striving for: inferior weight loss caused by muscle wasting and inferior health brought on by nutrient deficiency. This will cause weight regain.

While a chemical may be judged safe, this safety exists in isolation, not in the user's framework. The users of appetite suppressants are people with weight problems—and that means habit problems—often addictive food habits. These are the most likely people to become emotionally dependent on the pills or overuse them. Many dieters misuse the pills, thinking more is better, regardless of the recommended dose. It's like getting a free credit card in the mail when you have a habit of overextending.

The best course is to forget the pills and use a sound diet and exercise program alone. That way, you get the results without risks. The list below shows you some of the most common chemical agents used to curb appetites. Many of them are the main ingredients in over-the-counter aids you can get without a prescription. Always check with your doctor before using any chemical aid or adjunct to your diet to be on the safe side. After the list of chemical suppressors, we've developed a list of *natural* appetite suppressors that are your body's best defense against weight problems. You can weigh the difference.

APPETITE-SUPPRESSING CHEMICALS

Amphetamines. They're prescription anorectic agents which stimulate your nervous system. They were widely used for weight loss years ago, until the side effects were catalogued. These include nervousness, irritability, insomnia, blurred vision, dizziness, palpitations, sweating, nausea, vomiting, and sometimes hypertension. They also lead to dependency. They stimulate your hypothalamus (brain center for appetite), which decreases your appetite. They are now prohibited in many states for use in weight control.

Phenylpropanolamine (PPA). This is the ingredient in most over-the-counter appetite suppressants. It's chemically related to amphetamine and stimulates your central nervous system, but in a lower degree. The side effects include nervousness, insomnia, headaches, nausea, and tinnitus (ringing in your ears). They stimulate your hypothalamus, which decreases your appetite. You should check with your doctor before using PPA. *Not for use by people with high blood pressure, thyroid, kidney, or heart disease.* You don't need to risk side effects like these for weight loss.

Benzocaine. This is the ingredient in most over-the-counter candies, lozenges, and gums for weight control. It's a topical anesthetic that numbs your tongue, reducing your ability to taste food. It's presumed that if you can't taste food, you won't desire it as much, or eat as much. This could mean that you become nutrient deficient, because you're not eating. Or it can have the opposite effect than intended. You eat more high-sweet foods, without realizing how sweet and fattening they are.

Methylcellulose. This is the ingredient in bulkers, such as fiber tablets, laxatives, and fiber cookies. It absorbs liquid in your stomach, creating a feeling of fullness. It can absorb up to fifty times its weight. There's no harm in these adjuncts, providing that you eat a balanced diet simultaneously and take a vitamin/mineral supplement, since you can suffer loss of minerals. But be sure to check for sodium content. Don't see these as a cure for weight gain or rely on them for a major part of your day, since they are only aids. *Never use them instead of food, since that will lead to muscle losses, which causes fat gain.*

⟾ How-to Skills   ❤ Good for Heart

NATURAL APPETITE SUPPRESSANTS

Cholecystokinin. This is a hormone that is produced in your intestines after you eat. It stimulates your hypothalamus, which suppresses hunger. If you eat lean, you get your hunger suppressed and excellent fat burn, with *no risks*.

Glucose. This is the nutrient created from digestion of carbohydrates. When it reaches your brain, hunger is terminated. When your daily diet is high in complex carbohydrates, your hunger is naturally abated all day. And you get the double benefits of better fat burn, with *no risks*. If you eat your snacks as carbohydrates, you can have your hunger terminated, along with a boost of natural energy.

Insulin. This is the hormone produced by your pancreas to regulate your glucose metabolism. It increases the amount of tryptophan that gets to your brain, which in turn produces a neurotransmitter called serotonin, which turns off your hunger. This is a natural part of digestion of carbohydrates.

Exercise. Sustained aerobic activity produces endorphines, which are neurotransmitters in your brain that stimulate your hypothalamus to turn off hunger. One aerobic workout also depletes your body's carbohydrate stores, so you're ready for another carbohydrate boost, which will turn off hunger again.

The cycle of healthy eating and regular exercise is the best appetite suppressant you can find. *See* Appetite.

ARTERIOSCLEROSIS

Cholesterol buildup in artery walls. Also called hardening of the arteries, because the arteries harden with the plaque deposits. *See* Cholesterol.

ARTIFICIAL SWEETENERS

Imitation sugar: aspartame, saccharin, cyclamates. Of the three synthetic sweeteners, only aspartame is considered safe so far and is still being tested. The others have been linked to cancer, although recent studies of saccharin refutes that. There is an issue you should consider regarding aspartame. Since it contains a synthetic version of one of the essential amino acids, phenylalanine, and since the amino acids must be balanced to work properly, excessive use of one amino acid, without the presence of the others, doesn't suggest safety. Studies indicate that imbalanced amino

---

▲ Food Skills ● Behavior Skills ◆ Exercise Skills

acids can inhibit protein synthesis by your body. Until more is
known about the intricate workings of the amino acids in tandem
and in isolation, it's best to play it safe. When in doubt, do without. The calories you save by using artificial sweeteners can be
saved a better way, by cutting fats. *See* Sugar.

● ASSERTIVENESS

The ability to act definitively in your own behalf. Many diets talk
about assertiveness as the ability to say no—to food that makes
you fat, to habits that promote fat, and often they mean saying no
to foods and habits that aren't on the *particular* diet plan. You've
got to be very careful about the choice you make for weight loss,
because assertiveness is really about *choosing for yourself.* Lack of
assertiveness is generally associated with overweight and obesity. A
combination of improper eating and lack of exercise, along with a
number of environmental and emotional factors, causes weight
gain. And once weight is gained, you become less assertive.

What does that actually mean? Does that mean you can't be
trusted with food? Does it mean you can't be trusted to stand up
for yourself in situations where food is involved? If you choose a
diet that makes those choices for you, giving you lists and rules
and only certain foods you can eat, are you learning to be assertive?

One of the primary keys to being assertive is to *know* what you
want and need. That's not as easy as it sounds. Many people don't
take enough time to explore their *real* needs and feelings, let alone
express them. Nonassertive people tend to let everyone else express their needs, and they also try to help everyone else with their
problems, leaving little time for themselves.

If that sounds like you, you might buy a small pocket notebook
and begin to jot down feelings you have about yourself and needs
you have that don't seem to be met. Your diary can start with cues
like:

"I like_____" Make a list of the things you like and give
yourself more of them.

"I need_____." Make a list of the things you need and
think about how to meet those needs.

"I was confused by_____." If a situation makes you feel
put down or ineffective, describe what it was and what came about
to make you feel that way. Then do a few mental rehearsals to set
that situation up again in your mind, and resolve it in a way that

---

would make you feel good. You'll find examples of mental rehearsals in the topic Relaxation.

Assertiveness is acting definitively for you. That also means acting positively for you. Wanting to lose weight is a decision. Wanting to lose weight *effectively* is an assertive decision.

EFFECTIVE WEIGHT LOSS AND MAINTENANCE

How do you make a self-supportive diet and health decision? Choose safe weight loss, because that's the kind that's effective for both weight loss and maintenance.

1. Your weight loss should be slow and steady.
2. The best choice is real food.
3. The program should fit into your lifestyle, so you'll keep doing it. That means you have to ask yourself who you are, how you live, and what you can live with. (And you should expect to live better because of a diet, not worse, after it.)
4. Go for the maximum, not the minimum.
   The *minimum* is weight loss at any price.
   The *maximum* is a healthy, balanced diet, plus exercise, plus self-enrichment.

Lack of assertiveness is choosing *not to choose*, letting choices be made for you, doing what other people think is best for you. This year, choose yourself. Choose to concentrate on what you *can* do, not what you *can't* do. Say yes to yourself. You have far more power over everything when you take it.

B

● BEHAVIOR MODIFICATION

The science of self-enhancement. Behavior modification is a branch of psychology, but it differs from clinical psychology in its approach to problem solving. While psychology goes after deep-seated causes for problems in childhood and past experiences, behavior modification tackles problems in the present, as they express themselves in your attitudes and responses to situations. It is based on changing the things you *can* change, instead of dwelling on things you can't change, such as the past. For instance, if your response to a family crisis is to eat and feel guilty, you may not be able to change your family or the cause of the crisis, but you can change how you react to it. You can do relaxation exercises or go for a walk instead of eating. Both of these skills help you handle stress better and help you stay more centered in crisis.

More than one hundred clinical tests have demonstrated the effectiveness of behavior modification for weight control and maintenance. *See* all Behavior topics ●.

▲ BEVERAGES

Thirst quenchers. *See* Beverages in The Problem Solver Diet section.

◆ BICYCLING (STATIONARY)

An aerobic exercise.
Benefits:
- Great cardiovascular training.
- Excellent calorie-burning exercise, if you pedal at sufficient speed and tension.
- Easy to use with minimal instruction.
- Easily exchanged with outdoor bicycle fun.
- Strengthens leg and back muscles.
- Readily available at most health spas.
- Very appropriate exercise for advanced pregnancy since the extra "baby weight" is not a prohibiting factor when sitting on a bike.

- Advanced technology, with computerized Lifecycles and fan bicycles (Airdyne), adds another dimension of challenge. (*Lifecycles* are computerized cycles, incorporating an interval-training workout, that enable you to individually program pace, duration, and degree of difficulty along any desired incline. *Fan cycles*, which are relatively uncommon on the heath spa scene, have long arm bars that move up and back as you pedal, giving you an upper-body workout as well. In addition, the front wheel of the bicycle has a fan generated by pedaling, to keep you cooled off as you work out.)

Guidelines:
To adjust your seat height properly to avoid leg cramps, knee strain, and leg fatigue:
- Sit on the seat and rotate the right pedal to the down position.
- Place the ball of your foot on the pedal. Your leg should be fully extended. Test for a slight knee bend rather than a knee lock and adjust the height of the seat.
If you cycle outdoors with a conventional bicycle:
- Use a standard bicycle or adjust the gears on your ten-speed to pedal with some tension.
- Keep your speed comfortable and steady. Avoid too much gliding when the bike is working without you.
- Invest in safety gear such as a helmet, reflectors, rear view mirror, lights, and reflective clothing for night riding.

BILE

An enzyme produced by your liver, used in digestion to break up fats. *See* Digestion.

● BINGE

A bout of excessive eating. To dieters, this usually means breaking a diet by eating foods not listed on the plan—cheating eating. Or eating anything you want for a period of time away from your diet, especially sweets and fats. In some cases, such as during starvation diets, binges occur because your body cannot sustain itself on low nutrition, and the binge provides needed energy. Many very low-calorie diets have been known to provoke cycles of binging, because of lack of adequate nutrition.

In nonstarvation situations, binges occur because you *want*

▲ Food Skills   ● Behavior Skills   ◆ Exercise Skills

something you feel you can't have, such as chocolate cake. This is common to dieters who have good food/bad food divisions in their minds, and the pattern needs to be modified with behavior education. If you believe you will never be allowed to eat chocolate cake again, the likelihood of a binge on chocolate is greater. But when you realize you can eat chocolate cake again, but eat less of it, and find low-fat versions, the pressure of forced deprivation is released. While binge eating can be biochemical in origin or emotional in origin, it is an unhealthy eating practice that can escalate if it is not dealt with and moderated. The term *binge*, as used by dieters, is a borrowed word that comes from a more serious eating disorder and should not be confused with the binge common to bulimia. *See* Break.

BINGE/PURGE SYNDROME

Eating and then vomiting or taking laxatives, or both. *See* Bulimia.

● BLAME

Finding fault, usually in yourself. A self-critical habit pattern. *See* Relaxation, to let it go.

BLOOD PRESSURE

The cardiac output of your heart—stroke and volume. Good blood pressure is systolic below 140, and diastolic below 90, or below 140/90. To reduce your blood pressure, reduce your sodium and fat, eat more fiber, exercise, and don't smoke.

BODY COMPOSITION

The nutrient structure of your body. A healthy body at ideal weight has approximately the follow composition:

Water	55 percent
Protein (body muscle tissue)	20 percent
Fat	15-20 percent
Carbohydrates	2 percent
Minerals	2 percent
Vitamins	Less than 1 percent

If you have more fat, you have less muscle. The rest should remain stable. You have to replace your water, vitamins, minerals, carbohydrates, and protein daily. But if you have extra fat, you don't need to include much fat in your diet.

BODY IMAGE

How you see yourself. *See* Mirror Images and Imagery, for a healthy body image.

BODY TYPE

Your genetic shape, form, and composition; physique.

There are three primary body types that can be determined by clear, observable features. These types were identified from classification of athletes for sports participation: *Ectomorph*, linear, symbolized by column; *Mesomorph*, broad shouldered, symbolized by inverse triange; *Endomorph*, round all over, symbolized by circle.

One of the biggest mistakes people make is moving out of their body type for their weight-loss goal. This causes two basic problems: you can't reach your goal so remain dissatisfied, and you don't take advantage of the potential within your body type. When you learn to appreciate your own unique body type and work within its limits and capacities, you gain a better body image and have more realistic goals for fitness.

How to Optimize Your Body Type

Ectomorphic men and women who want more upper body differentiation can build upper body muscles with weight lifting or swimming.

Mesomorphic men and women have the best results with weight loss, because of their innately high muscular content. However, women who don't want to appear too broad shouldered and muscular should avoid weight lifting, or do it with low weights and lots of reps, rather than high weights, since mesomorphs have a tendency to build up fast. This must be combined with a low-fat diet that is carbohydrate rich and balanced in protein, so that muscles aren't pumped up under a layer of fat. Stretching and limbering exercises are excellent for mesomorphs, especially men,

---

▲ Food Skills　　● Behavior Skills　　◆ Exercise Skills

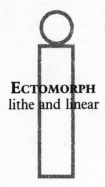

ECTOMORPH
lithe and linear

Small boned
Long arms, legs
Shoulder to hip line is similar
Low muscle, low fat
Lithe bodies
Can eat more without
    gaining weight

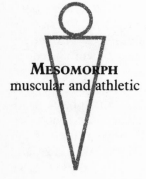

MESOMORPH
muscular and athletic

Denser boned
Average length arms, legs
Shoulder to hip line narrows
    in at hips
High muscle, medium fat
Athletic bodies
Lose weight and gain
    muscle easier

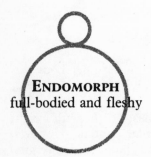

ENDOMORPH
full-bodied and fleshy

Medium boned
Short arms, legs
Shoulder to hip line is similar
    from wider hips
Low muscle, high fat
Round large bodies
Have the most difficulty
    with weight loss

⫸ How-to Skills   ❤ Good for Heart

to avoid that bulky, nonflexible look that can develop with weight lifting.

Endomorphic men and women have the most trouble losing weight, because of their innately high body-fat content. However, endomorphic women are known for their hourglass figures and can carry more fat without it making their bodies look off balance. (Example: Marilyn Monroe.) Endomorphic people should guard their fat intake on a regular basis to avoid excess fat. Rapid weight-loss diets are the least preferred method for endomorphs who can regain more rapidly than ectomorphs or mesomorphs (who have more body muscle). Full-body aerobic workouts are most beneficial to endomorphs, along with stretches for muscle lengthening, so the overall appearance is longer, rather than rounder. This body type is best served by staying on a diet a little longer, to insure that the ideal weight you reach is stablilized by higher body-muscle content inside. This is also the body type that needs regular exercise to keep weight gain away, but the results are worth it. Your efforts are more noticeable, since fat loss really shows, and this incentive can outweigh the fact that it's more difficult for you to lose weight.

Most people fall midway on the line between body types, and all types can share common fat distribution tendencies. *See* Fat Distribution.

BODY WEIGHT
Water, muscle, and fat. *See* Weight.

▲ BREADS
Grains; a food in the grain group for essential nutrition. The processed breads with white flour and added sugar and fat don't really qualify as real grains. They're fats in grain suits. The whole-grain breads are the better sources, as low in sugar and fat as you can find them. *See* Grains in The Problem Solver Diet section.

● BREAK
A lapse in dieting; a guilt state for hard-core dieters. Fear of breaking your diet is more common on rapid weight-loss diets that presume you have to lose weight by a certain date and you won't

---

▲ Food Skills   ● Behavior Skills   ◆ Exercise Skills

lose it if you eat foods that are not on the program. If you are on a natural diet plan, where you are eating leaner foods with a wide variety of options, a break doesn't mean disaster or doom.

Guilt comes into play when you have abnormal food views built into the diet—you have your foods, and the other foods aren't good for you. When you see food from this perspective of bad and good, can't have and can, then the odds are greater that you'll long for the ones you aren't allowed.

This doesn't mean that you can lose weight if you eat anything you want. It means you understand the challenge you are undertaking with food moderation and weight loss. You don't need to spend energy on guilt and self-recrimination. They aren't feelings that move you forward. They can set you back. In fact, they can make you eat. Often people break diets for very substantial reasons:

1. The diet is too restrictive. Regimented eating and narrowly focused eating plans can create diet stress and head-wars about food. After a few weeks of feeling ostracized from the real world, you might need a break.
2. Your nutritional needs aren't being met. If you are on a diet that does not provide your essential nutrients, you will be hungry constantly, and you will break your diet. In this case, it is beneficial. Getting nutrients through a lapse in your diet is your body's way of protecting itself.

Of course, most dieters don't go for nutrition when they break a diet. They go for sugar or fat. This is part of the reward/ punishment principle that is inherent in rigid diets. After you spend three weeks without a sweet on a rigid plan, you feel punished for having a weight problem. To reward yourself, you eat something it won't allow, a food that made you feel good in the past. It's the double-edged sword of deprived diets. You can spend most of your time on a deprived diet feeling like a child who was sent to your room without dessert because you were bad. Some programs even use childish language that enhances your sense of guilt: "You didn't lose weight this week. You were a bad girl/boy."

Some dieters like this kind of feedback and feel it keeps them on track. But it doesn't mix well with the rest of your life. That same guilty child, who was bad for not losing weight this week, has to go to the office and lock up a big business deal, then go home and feel he or she can't be trusted to make decisions about food. Does that sound familiar to you? Does it sound logical or self-supportive?

If you're tired of guilt and don't need more, try a healthy food plan where you make your own choices. Realize that you will make a few good decisions and you'll make a few bad ones, and keep retraining yourself to make the good ones. That's personal power.

➠   *How to Manage a Diet Break*

If you are on a diet and you have a piece of cake or eat half the contents of the refrigerator, handle it logically.

1. Write down what you ate and tally the fat, sugar, and calories.
2. Decide which energy you wanted, the fat or the sugar, or maybe the salt. Jot down your feelings about what you ate.
3. Go for a walk or do a relaxation exercise to ease your stress.
4. Identify nonfattening foods you can substitute for the foods you ate and have them on hand in case you feel yourself wanting to break again.
5. Begin again the next day.

If you break your diet again, follow the same plan. As long as you keep the majority of your week intact with lean choices and regular exercise, you won't put on a pound of fat from a break. Keep trying to resolve your food issues, without guilt or blame. That's the nature of healthy eating, and healthy weight loss.

▲ BREAKFAST

The first source of energy in your day. This is one of the most important meals for a dieter. If you skip it, you miss the metabolic benefits, since your metabolism comes out of sleep burning at a lower rate. The introduction of food in the morning starts the production of heat and kicks off an active metabolism early in the day. This keeps you on an even keel all day, burning fat at a steady pace. The less fat you eat in the morning, the better off you will be, and there are many breakfast fares that are high carbohydrate and low fat: cereal, milk, and fruit; a whole-wheat waffle with strawberries; a toasted bagel with jelly and a piece of fruit. Breakfast is also important to ensure that you get your calcium. Don't skip it thinking you'll lose weight faster. You'll burn fat better when you eat breakfast.

▲ Food Skills　　　● Behavior Skills　　　◆ Exercise Skills

● BREATHING

A gas-exchange process where oxygen is supplied to your blood on inhaling, and carbon-dioxide wastes are released by exhaling. Since oxygen is mandatory to all life processes, breathing is often synonymous with life and your oxygen uptake a barometer of that life. Better oxygen uptake means better health, heart circulation, digestion, metabolsim, cell regeneration, and repair. Dieters should note that oxygen is needed for fat burn, and to enhance that, you need to improve your breathing capacity.

The two basic types of breathing are chest breathing (shallow breathing) and diaphragm breathing (deep breathing). Babies breathe from their diaphragms as nature intended, while adults tend to fall into the habit of chest breathing and need breathing retraining to take up more oxygen.

The goals of breathing exercises are:

1. To increase your breathing awareness—how you are currently breathing as opposed to how you should be breathing.
2. To expand your breath capacity, in order to increase your oxygen uptake. This will energize your body, relax your mind, and improve your overall health.
3. To provide an instant relaxation technique you can use in times of stress.

The benefits of proper breathing are immediate, and you don't need special equipment, clothing, or location. You can do it without interrupting other work. At first, you should practice at home alone to learn the techniques, then you carry them over to other activities and sports. An especially good combination is walking while using deep breathing techniques.

BREATHING AWARENESS

⫘   *How to Improve Your Breathing*

Sit in a comfortable chair and breathe normally. Notice whether you breathe from your upper chest or deeply into your abdomen. In chest breathing, you would be inhaling from your upper lungs and your shoulders would tend to rise up. In diaphragm breathing, you would be inhaling from your lower lungs, and your abdomen would balloon out, then your ribs would rise up, then your lungs

---

⫘   How-to Skills   ❤   Good for Heart

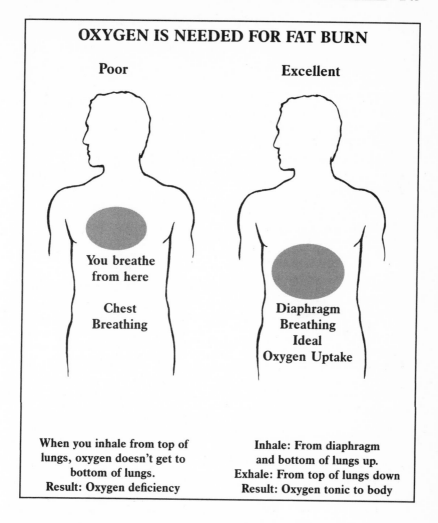

OXYGEN IS NEEDED FOR FAT BURN

Poor   Excellent

You breathe
from here

Chest   Diaphragm
Breathing   Breathing
                            Ideal
                            Oxygen Uptake

When you inhale from top of   Inhale: From diaphragm
lungs, oxygen doesn't get to   and bottom of lungs up.
bottom of lungs.   Exhale: From top of lungs down
Result: Oxygen deficiency   Result: Oxygen tonic to body

would fill with air. Practice deep breathing and compare the two experiences.

Deep Breathing. Sit in a comfortable chair with your feet flat on the floor and your back straight, to free up your diaphragm. Regulate your breathing process for ten minutes. Breathe in and out through your nostrils down to your abdomen to the following count:

Inhale while counting slowly to three.

Exhale while counting slowly to three.

Your goal is to make the inhale and exhale match. You can increase your breathing capacity by increasing the count, as it becomes more comfortable. If you find yourself getting dizzy or hyperventilating, you can prevent this by alternating your breaths between shallow and deep. Practice diaphragm breathing until it becomes like second nature.

Breathing Expertise. Sit in a comfortable chair with your feet flat on the floor and your back straight. Regulate your diaphragm breathing to this count:

Inhale while counting slowly to three.

Exhale while counting slowly to six.

Many experts feel that this style of breathing creates the best benefits. The exhale length is double the time for inhaling. You will feel the difference immediately.

BREATHING HINTS:

- Never strain. Never try to force air into your lungs.
- Keep your mind blank by concentrating on the breathing itself.
- Keep your mouth closed. It helps if you keep your tongue on the roof of your mouth.
- You can place your fingers lightly on your abdomen to insure that it is ballooning out, to show that you are breathing from your diaphragm.
- Keep your jaw relaxed.
- Wear loose, comfortable clothes that don't restrain your diaphragm.
- You can mildy contract your abdomen at the end of breathing to expel the last stale air.
- You can vary your breathing with a holding count of three, between inhaling and exhaling. This retains oxygen and enhances its pickup.

➠ *How to Use Your Breathing Expertise*

Stressed and about to eat? Consciously switch to a pattern of deep breathing from your diaphragm. You will relax and feel in control.

Combine your breathing exercises with assertive statements, such as "In with health, out with fat," or "In with positive, out with negative." It will strengthen your inner resources.

Combine your breathing exercises with mental rehearsals for success, by creating stressful situations which can cause you to eat and resolving them in your imagination. *See* Relaxation.

CHEST BREATHING	DIAPHRAGM BREATHING
half-breathing	whole breathing ♥ deep breathing
Decreases oxygen uptake by limiting the amount of air that reaches your lower lungs	Increases your oxygen uptake by pulling air into lower portion of your lungs where most of your blood circulates. This makes more oxygen available to your blood.
Puts strain on your heart, making it pump more blood. Blood has to circulate faster to carry available oxygen. This means higher blood pressure.	Lowers blood pressure Reduces heart rate Reduces stress on heart
Associated with anxiety Related to stress breathing and its accompanying symptoms	Associated with calmness Increases production of endorphines—natural opiates

BROWN FAT

A type of fat in your body that is viewed as "fat that keeps you lean." The primary site of brown fat is the upper back (identified in animals). It is more metabolically active than the standard white fat that is found in your adipose tissue. It is usually activated in cold climates to keep you from freezing. Only 1 percent of your fat is brown fat, as opposed to white fat which can be 20 to 30 percent of your body weight. Since brown fat is active fat, and very little is stored in your body, it's not fat that you need to lose.

● **BUDDY SYSTEM**

A next best friend for a dieter; an individual, group, or network of friends to support your weight-loss efforts and be there when you need help. An ideal buddy would be a former dieter who succeeded, because no one understands the struggle to lose weight better than someone who has been through it. If your buddy is a current dieter, be sure you don't support each other's desire to let go and fall back into old habits. If you choose a buddy who is overweight and settled into it, what might that indicate about you? (A secret desire to stay overweight? Fear of failure?) If your buddy is a slim person who never had a weight problem, be sure that person has a genuine appreciation for health and fitness, not just image or appearance.

Try not to think of a diet counselor or program representative as your buddy, because their role is an overseer, and their professional obligations to their own programs make it hard for them to be objective. Also, when you use your counselor as a buddy, it's like handing your control over to someone else, and you want to avoid that. Many dieters find buddies in their families, but it's not the usual choice because of the emotional connections. It can put too much stress on family members and thwart your efforts. Part of taking control of your weight and health is getting independent. It's difficult to get independent from a family member. Your diet buddy should not be someone who intimidates you, pressures you, or makes you feel uncomfortable in crisis. He or she should be someone who reinforces you, relaxes you, reminds you of your achievements, and guides you to make the right decisions, *not someone who makes decisions for you*. The reason your diet buddy isn't your best friend is simple. That role is waiting to be claimed by you.

You might say, "I don't know anyone who can be my buddy. I have no one to turn to." That's a very common problem, or we wouldn't have the weight problems we see today. Be creative about finding your buddy system. You can rely on your spiritual beliefs as a buddy system or you can acquire audio and video tapes for support. In a pinch, you can call Overeater's Anonymous. They're there for everyone.

BULIMIA

An eating disorder characterized by bouts of overeating followed by self-induced vomiting, abuse of laxatives, diuretics, or excessive exercise—for the purpose of weight control; also called binge/purge syndrome. Literal meaning: "ox hunger." High-carbohydrate (refined) foods are common binge choices. Often, no outward signs of the disorder seem observable, since most bulimics stay within normal weight ranges and binge/purge secretly. Bulimia is a serious eating disturbance which requires professional evaluation and treatment with individual or group therapy combined with other disciplines such as behavior modification, nutritional counseling, and medications.

The problem is of special concern to dieters because mild eating disorders can spiral out of control and become major eating disorders, particularly after bouts of bad dieting. Bulimia frequently occurs in adolescents after rigid dieting. This raises concern for teenagers and college students who have been known to experiment with purging and laxatives as forms of weight control.

The following list of problems common to bulimia is alarming because it reads like a profile of an average dieter.

1. Good food/bad food syndrome—seeing diet foods as good foods and most other foods as bad foods.
2. Obsessive concern with slimness.
3. Distorted eating patterns.
4. Food preoccupation.
5. The need for rigid diet rules, often self-imposed.
6. Body image disturbances—seeing yourself fatter than you are.
7. Shame, guilt, excessive anxiety.
8. Private binging, often with fear of being unable to stop.
9. Difficulty accepting feelings—tendency to transfer feelings to food.
10. Distorted thinking—eating meals which result in full feeling or distended stomach, equated with losing control over body weight.

The bulimic's problems are chronic versions of some of the issues that concern dieters. In the beginning stages of the disorder, purging and laxative use is voluntary, but as the disorder progresses, purging and laxative use become automatic, involuntary. A dieter may binge and feel guilty after eating 800–1000 calories, while a bulimic can eat 5,000–10,000 calories in one eating episode. This makes it even more important to educate younger people on the dangers of excessive eating and unrealistic weight control practices, and to act as role models for healthy behavior

▲ Food Skills   ● Behavior Skills   ◆ Exercise Skills

and nutrition habits. With social pressures for slimness and expectations for perfection mounting in our society, it's not difficult to see why eating disorders are escalating.

In its severe phases, bulimia can create electrolyte imbalances, irregular menstrual cycles, irregular heart rate and blood pressure, enlarged salivary glands, constipation, diarrhea, and more dangerous symptoms such as cardiac rhythm abnormalities. If you are struggling with this disorder, please seek help from a registered dietitian, psychologist, your doctor, or a hospital clinic. You deserve a healthy life.

C

▲ **CAFFEINE**

A central nervous system stimulant. Caffeine excess is similar to stress symptoms: increased respiration, pulse rate, and blood pressure. You feel all revved up with no place to run, like the fight or flight response. When you are on a diet, it's best to limit your caffeine intake, since the effects will be more pronounced when you are eating fewer calories.

The maximum dosage should be no more than 400 mg/day, but watch out for decaffeinated coffee as a substitute. The decaf that is water processed is the safest kind. The other variety contains formaldehyde. Your best bet is to substitute water or juices for coffee or tea, instead of using decaf.

One of the benefits of caffeine is for asthmatics, since it speeds respiration, letting air in.

COMMON SOURCES OF CAFFEINE

Chocolate (dark)	26 mg/bar		Coffee, drip	85 mg/cup
Chocolate (milk)	10 mg/bar		Coffee, instant	60 mg/cup
			Coffee, decaf	3 mg/cup
Aspirin	32 mg/pill	Cola		
Cold		32–65 mg	Tea, brewed	50 mg/cup
Preparations	30/mg dose	per can	Tea, instant	30 mg/cup
Stimulants	100 mg/tablet		Cocoa	6–14 mg/cup
Antacids	32 mg/tablet			
Pain relievers	32–66 mg/pill			

▲ **CALCIUM**

An essential mineral. The most important fact about calcium that you need to consider is the issue of absorption. Only about 20–30 percent of your daily intake is absorbed. This is one of the reasons you should pay particular attention to your calcium intake, keep-

---

▲ Food Skills   ● Behavior Skills   ◆ Exercise Skills

CALCIUM AT A GLANCE	
	Recommended dose—800 MG/DAY Women over thirty—1000–2000 MG/DAY
AVOID	**RELY ON**
Steroids	Skim milk 300 mg
	Cottage cheese 160 mg
Chocolate	Low-fat yogurt 360 mg
	Green leafy vegetables
Smoking	Beans
	Whole grains
Fat and fatty proteins	Vitamins and minerals
	Bonemeal supplement ½ Tsp.
	Daily exercise

ing at the maximum daily level in the lean choices. Lack of calcium can cause an increase in cholesterol, leading to calcium deposits in the arteries (arteriosclerosis). Lack of calcium can also lead to osteoporosis, particularly in women, who are a higher risk group because of hormonal changes in menopause which also accelerate calcium losses. When calcium levels are low in your bloodstream, and calcium is not provided in the daily food you eat, your body takes calcium from your bones and teeth. Bones usually store enough calcium to meet your body's needs, but when it doesn't come in through your diet, the losses are never restored to your bones. They lose density and become brittle, resulting in pain, loss of height, spinal deformities, and easy fractures (osteoporosis).

Lack of calcium shows up in loose teeth, receding gums, infected gums, gingivitis, spasms in your muscles, severe menstrual cramps, and constant headaches.

The good news is, when you get 1200–1500/mg of calcium each day, you can restore a good part of your bone density, have lower blood pressure, and gum problems will ease. It takes about six months, so today is the day to start ensuring your calcium needs.

The latest news in exercise is about calcium and strength training. It seems that strength training can help to restore the calcium in your bones. One more reason to exercise!

The best sources for absorption are low-fat dairy products and low-fat protein, along with foods that contain phosphorous. The reason you want your calcium in a low-fat format is because calcium combines with fat in your intestines and it can be excreted instead of absorbed. The best way to take your calcium would be between meals, when you are not eating fat. Many experts recommend that you take 30 percent of your daily calcium before bed to ensure absorption and get the added benefit of a good night's sleep, since calcium is a sleep aid. It also protects against sunburn, prevents depression, regulates your heartbeat, and activates enzymes in metabolism.

Calcium metabolism occurs in the presence of vitamins A, C, D and B complex, along with the minerals phosphorous and potassium. If you are a chocolate eater, the oxalic acid can prevent calcium absorption. Smoking or taking steroids can also lead to calcium deficiencies.

♦ CALISTHENICS
Nonaerobic, rhythmic exercises for strength and endurance.

♦ CALLANETICS
A stretching exercise routine that combines relaxation, breathing, and stretching in one program. In addition to being an excellent form of muscle and spine elongation, the exercises tone, shape, and benefit well-being.

♦ CALORIE EXPENDITURE
Output. *See* Exercise.

▲ CALORIE INTAKE
Input. *See* Food Groups.

▲ CALORIES

Units of energy derived from food. Foods are grouped according to the nutrient energy (calories) they yield. There are only three nutrients that provide calories:

1 gram protein	4 calories
1 gram carbohydrates	4 calories
1 gram fat	9 calories

These three nutrients are essential to your body for its growth, maintenance, and repair. A healthy diet provides these nutrients in the proper proportions to meet your body's needs, without adding extra fat. Those proportions are:

Protein: 20 percent of total calories
Carbohydrates: 55 to 60 percent of total calories
Fat: 20 to 25 percent of total calories

➠ *How to Estimate Your Daily Calorie Needs*

To estimate your daily calorie needs, use the following formula, which is a weight maintenance formula, the amount of calories needed to maintain your *current* weight.

Active Women	12–14 calories per pound of body weight
Inactive Women	10–12 calories per pound of body weight

Smaller-framed women use the lower number. Larger-framed women use the higher number.

Active Men	14–16 calories per pound of body weight
Inactive Men	12–14 calories per pound of body weight

Smaller-framed men use the lower number. Larger-framed men use the higher number.

➠ *How to Determine Daily Calorie Needs for Dieting*

Use the same formula as above, except you will use your *ideal body weight* (the weight you should be) for the weight. For instance, if you currently weigh 160 and should weigh 130, use the weight of 130, and multiply the calories/per pound of body weight to that number. In addition, *use the inactive calorie number* to tally your diet calories, not the active one.

This will put you in the lean range of calories for dieting. Example: Our 160-pound woman wants to weigh 130. She uses the inactive level of calories (10–12) to multiply with her ideal body weight (130). She comes up with a calorie range for her diet:

1300–1560 calories per day.

If her ideal body weight should be 120, her calorie range would be:

1200–1440 calories per day.

If she wanted to diet very seriously, she would use the lower number of calories for her daily calorie maximum. If she wanted to diet moderately, she would use the higher number of calories for her daily maximum.

▲ CANDY

A source of sugar. *See* Sugar.

▲ CARBOHYDRATES

The nutrient source of primary energy for your muscles and brain. Carbohydrates are your body's preferred source of energy and primary brain food. They are divided into two groups—simple (sugar) and complex (starches). Complex carbohydrates are long-chain simple sugars that are linked when you eat them and then split into simple sugars when your body digests and absorbs them. Why, then, are complex carbohydrates considered good and simple carbohydrates considered bad? The reason is found in the nutritional quality of the foods that contain these carbohydrates and your body's response to them.

First, complex carbohydrates are less-refined foods, and therefore are good sources of many naturally occurring nutrients. Simple carbohydrates, or sugars, are usually very refined foods that have been stripped of their naturally occurring nutrients. Second, your body has a slower, more natural response to eating

_____

complex carbohydrates, gradually breaking down the longer chain to use for energy over prolonged periods—a longer energy boost.

Complex carbohydrates start to be broken down earlier in digestion, with an enzyme in your saliva. They go through a longer process of digestion, and many experts feel that few carbohydrate calories ever get to fat storage. One aerobic workout can deplete your body's carbohydrate stores. The beneficial effects of carbohydrates doesn't apply to the highly processed versions, because they usually have added fats and sugars and very little fiber. The fresh, natural sources are the best.

Sugars exist in a very simple form, which stimulates a very rapid insulin response. They are absorbed easily and leave you feeling hungry sooner than if you ate a complex carbohydrate. People who eat high-sugar diets get short bursts of energy and big, tired letdowns. The energy is not first quality, and for fat loss, the simple sugars are self-defeating, since they usually occur in foods that also contain a lot of fat.

The starch group of complex carbohydrates includes grains and grain products as well as starchy vegetables such as corn. They are excellent sources of B vitamins and fiber, especially when whole-grain varieties are eaten.

Vegetables and fruits are often mentioned together because they have similar nutrient compositions. While fruit contains natural simple sugar that makes it sweet and higher in calories than vegetables, both fruits and vegetables provide healthy supplies of fiber and essential nutrients such as vitamins A and C. In fact, one fresh grapefruit and one medium carrot will satisfy your total daily requirements for vitamins A and C.

See Sugar for a comparison between natural complex carbohydrates and processed carbohydrates.

♦ **CARDIOVASCULAR CONDITIONING**

Using exercise to reach maximum oxygen uptake and target heart rate for best heart health.

Aerobic exercise improves the power of your heart and circulation. When activity is performed regularly and for sufficient periods of time, it can produce beneficial physiological changes. Your body becomes a better machine. It can take in, transport, and use oxygen at an increased rate. Your heart becomes a better pump, pushing more blood out with each stroke, and it rests longer between beats. Distribution and blood flow in your lungs and working muscles are enhanced, and slowing of your heart rate (pulse) occurs both at rest and at any given level of activity. As a result, your cardiovascular system operates more efficiently.

To achieve cardiovascular conditioning, certain conditions must be met:

- Duration: the exercise must be performed at a suitable level of intensity for twenty to thirty minutes (not counting warm-ups or cool-downs).
- Frequency: the exercise should be performed at least three times per week, preferably on alternate days.
- Intensity: the exercise must be strenuous enough for you to reach a level of exertion that is about 70–85 percent of your maximum heart rate.

The most suitable sports for cardiovascular conditioning are the ones that require repeated and continuous movement: running, swimming, cycling, brisk walking, rowing, rope skipping, running in place, stationary cycling, basketball, handball, racquetball, squash, skating, hockey, cross-country skiing, soccer, and hiking.

Other sports might not be adequate for cardiovascular conditioning if they allow long pauses between action or the movement takes place in brief spurts. In the same way that you want to keep the heat constant in your eating style, you need to keep the heat steady with your exercise. Low-heat exercises include baseball, softball, golf, and bowling.

Calisthenics that emphasize slow bending, stretching, and graceful movement will not provide cardiovascular benefits as well as continuous, rhythmic calisthenics that are performed at a higher level of intensity, such as the active *step* programs. *See* Exercise.

CAUSES (of overweight and obesity)
Factors that influence weight gain.

Diet. What you eat. What you *don't* eat. Both must be taken into account because you can eat a low-calorie diet and fail to lose fat, if your calories don't provide proper levels of protein, carbohydrates (fiber), and nutrition in the low-fat format needed for fat burn. The *source* of your calories has a greater effect on weight gain and weight loss than the *number* of your calories.

▲ Food Skills   ● Behavior Skills   ♦ Exercise Skills

Exercise (including daily activity). The more sedentary you are, the greater your tendency for weight gain. The more fat you have to lose, the greater your need for exercise. You must burn more calories than you eat in order to lose fat, and there is a limit to the number of calories you can cut back. If you only cut calories, and do it indiscriminately, you can lose body muscle, which will in turn cause you to burn fewer calories. Increasing your exercise and daily activity level is the only known way to burn enough calories while protecting your body muscle. This ensures healthy weight loss and safeguards your weight maintenance.

Eating Patterns and Lifestyle (adult and childhood). Your eating habits are learned behaviors that you gain over a lifetime and ingrain by repetition. Many eating problems carry over from your formative years and shape your lifestyle without your conscious awareness. Since poor eating habits reinforce what you eat, why, how, when, and where you eat, they are weight promoting and can remain weight promoting even after you've lost weight and think you are safe from fat. Changing these habits is the only known way to make your weight loss last.

Personality and Attitudes. Who you are and how you feel about yourself are both a reflection of weight and an indicator of your potential success or failure. Low self-esteem and lack of assertiveness have been linked to excess weight. While no studies exist to identify specific personality profiles for *future* weight gainers, a wealth of data shows that self-strengthening is crucial to successful weight loss.

Aging. Your metabolic rate decreases with age, and this reduces your ability to burn calories as efficiently. While it is common for people to gain weight with age, it is not mandatory. With increased exercise and improved diet, you can remain slim in spite of the averages. You can raise your metabolic rate and lose weight at any age.

Genetics. This is the elusive territory you have no control over. It involves fat metabolism, fat cells, body heat, and body type, along with a host of weight-gaining factors that may not be identified yet. For instance, many scientists are studying brown fat, thinking that may provide a link to why certain people gain weight and others lose it successfully. Others are studying genes and hormones and little trigger mechanisms in cells, looking for genetic causes of overweight and obesity. The wisest course is to leave genetics to researchers and concentrate on improving the factors that you can change, since they account for approximately 90 percent of the causes of overweight and obesity. A small minority of people (less than 1 percent) show genetic problems in relation to weight gain, and many can override their genetic tendencies with improvements in diet, exercise, and behavior.

CELLULITE

Lumpy fat, commonly found on hips, thighs, and buttocks in women, and in the abdomen in men.

Fat leaves proportionately from your body and, unfortunately, you can't change fat. But you can change your diet and exercise patterns and that will take care of all of your fat, including the lumpy variety. But beware! Your diet has to protect your muscle (body protein) and be low-fat, and it must include all the food groups, otherwise you might wind up thinner, with lumpy bags. The combination of healthy diet and regular exercise builds your body muscle while it is removing fat. This gives you a firmer look all over at the end of your diet.

If you are over forty, or if you've had excess fat since childhood, it will take a little longer for the lumpy look to improve. Be patient and disciplined in your exercise. As your muscles strengthen and build up, the problem areas will become firmer. And don't forget, the places that have the most fat will be the last places to get thinner and firmer.

Cellulite and Liposuction

Forget about liposuction, unless you intend to stay on a very low-fat diet after it. New fat will form in areas that didn't have fat before. Then you have lumpy fat somewhere else.

Cellulite Myths and Reality

There are two versions for the causes of cellulite—fad and fact. The fad version is short and clever and the treatment list is long and expensive. The fact version is complex and not selling any-thing, so the treatment is simple and inexpensive.

▲ CELLULOSE

A type of fiber found in carbohydrate foods. Excellent weight-loss food. *See* Fiber.

▲ Food Skills   ● Behavior Skills   ♦ Exercise Skills

FAD DESCRIPTION

Cellulite is a special kind of fat created by waste products (toxins) and water trapped in fat cells and the tissues around fat cells.

FAD TREATMENTS

AT HOME: $10–40 each item: loofas, special sponges, creams, cactus cloths, vitamin/mineral supplements, herbs, waffle-topped massagers, bath tonics, rubber suits, rollers, toners, electric muscle stimulators, spot reducing exercises. There's even a cream with hot pepper that makes skin red and tingly.

AT THE SPA: $25–50 per treatment: muscle stimulators, vibrating machines, whirlpools, air-streams, inflatable leggings, massages, thermal treatments, hormone injections, enzyme injections, wax treatments, heat.

FACT DESCRIPTION

All fat is the same. But fat distribution sites are different in men and women. Women tend to be lower-body fat distributors, depositing more fat in hips, thighs, and buttocks. Men tend to be upper-body fat distributors, depositing more fat in abdomen and chest.

Cell sizes differ. Hypertropic cells swell with fat and can increase to 5 times their size. Hyperplastic cells are smaller and more numerous—more cells store less fat over a great cell area, giving a more level appearance.

One half of your body fat is deposited directly under your skin, and women's outer layer of skin is thinner then men's. Therefore, women's fat, concentrated in the lower body in hypertrophic cells, can appear lumpier than men's fat in the same area.

FACT TREATMENT

Diet from the food groups, low-fat

Exercise to burn fat and build muscle

Drink water to flush out wastes

▲ CEREALS

Grains; one of the required food groups. Grains are needed to round out your complete daily nutritional profile. But be cautious! Commercial cereals can be rich sources of sugar and fat in the over-processed versions. Whole-grain cereals are the preferred ones, especially with the bran and germ of the grain intact. They are the best nutrient and fiber sources, but check the labels to insure that they are low in fat and sugar. *See* Grains in The Problem Solver Diet section.

● CHEWING

A factor in digestion; also called rate of eating. Chewing your food slowly is an important aid to digestion, weight control, and hunger control. Carbohydrate digestion begins in your mouth with the help of enzymes from your salivary glands. When you eat too fast and swallow too fast, carbohydrate digestion is limited in its first stage. What you eat is equally important, since processed carbohydrates have no fiber or texture; and lacking this consistency, chewing becomes minimal. Hunger takes approximately twenty minutes to abate from the time you begin eating, and chewing helps slow the eating process, so hunger ceases earlier in your meal. When you don't chew sufficiently and slow down the process, you can eat more calories without feeling satisfied, because hunger is still in full swing.

Eating faster doesn't mean speeding up your digestion, rather it's a form of bypassing the natural process of digestion. This can alter the whole cycle of digestion. Food arrives in your stomach in bulk and digestion is prolonged there. Enzymes in the stomach only break down protein. Carbohydrates that bypassed your mouth too quickly may have to wait to get broken down in your intestines along with fats. This prolongs digestion in your small intestines. All of these factors contribute to calories being stored. The result of a faster rate of eating is weight gain.

CHILDHOOD EATING PATTERNS

Food and weight-related habits that were learned in childhood. These carry over to adulthood to form adult eating habits and lifestyle. They are part of the causes of overweight and obesity. *See* Causes; Habits.

▲ CHOCOLATE

A derivative of the cacao bean. Chocolate contains the stimulants caffeine and theobromine, which speed up your central nervous

---

▲ Food Skills   ● Behavior Skills   ◆ Exercise Skills

system and heartbeat. It also contains oxalic acid, which can interfere with your calcium absorption. So why do dieters love chocolate so much? Usually because of the added sugar and fat. Chocolate by itself is quite bitter, not a tempting food at all. If you have a real chocolate desire and want to lose weight, try carob instead. It's lower in fat, rich in B vitamins, minerals, and is similar in flavor to chocolate. It has no caffeine and is non-allergenic.

You should limit your use of chocolate on a diet, but should you try to use willpower and deprivation to cut it out entirely? That will only send you straight to chocolate for a snack. A small mint patty can satisfy your chocolate desire with only 1 gram of fat. Cocoa can be substituted for a candy bar. The skillful dieter can still have chocolate and lose fat. If you believe the diets that say you can never have chocolate again, you're buying lack of trust in yourself and an attitude that you have no control over food. When you believe that, you lose your control.

You can learn to make wise diet decisions that allow you variety and pleasure without adding fat. A decade of dieting based on depriving oneself only proved it didn't work, because weight regain has become a major problem as a result. A good start is to get your baseline nutrition daily. That alone prevents a number of urges and desires that occur in a nutrient deficient state. With nutrition as your basis, you're healthier, and you're in a better frame of mind to make good choices and stick to them.

CHOLESTEROL
A fatty substance produced in your liver and found in some foods.

Body Cholesterol
There are two kinds of cholesterol found in your body:
1. LDL (Low Density Lipoprotein). Called bad cholesterol, it carries cholesterol to your arteries where it can form deposits on the artery walls.
2. HDL (High Density Lipoprotein). Called good cholesterol, it picks up bad cholesterol and carries it back to your liver for excretion.

Lipoprotein literally means "fat" (*lipid*) plus "protein." These fat/protein substances carry cholesterol through your bloodstream. When you have too much LDL (carrying cholesterol), the excess can be deposited in your arteries and build up to form

---

⯈ How-to Skills   ♥ Good for Heart

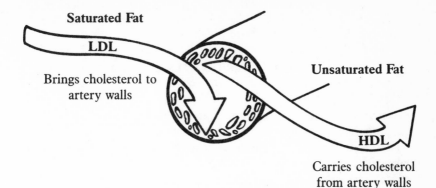

Saturated Fat

LDL

Brings cholesterol to
artery walls

Unsaturated Fat

HDL

Carries cholesterol
from artery walls

plaque. It is believed that the deposits occur in arteries that have
been predamaged or stressed. The artery wall thickens with these
deposits and becomes less flexible, less capable of handling the
blood flow. It's like water trying to pass through a clogged hose.
The passage narrows from the deposits, and the blood backs up,
causing more pressure to push the blood through a smaller opening. Eventually an artery can completely close.

In an artery to the brain, this causes stroke: no blood to the
brain.

In an artery to the heart, this causes heart attack: no blood to
the heart.

In an artery elsewhere, this causes damage to tissues that require blood.

Food Cholesterol.

Two types of food fat are associated with LDL and HDL:
saturated fats and unsaturated fats.

1. Saturated fats. Fats from animal sources, but also coconut oil
   and palm oil. These fats are solid at room temperature, such
   as a stick of butter. If you equate this fat with your LDL, or
   bad cholesterol, it will make it easier to sort out fats. (This is
   the fat that leads to plaque deposits in arteries.)
2. Unsaturated fats. Fats from vegetable sources: corn oil,
   cottonseed oil, olive, soy. These fats are liquid at room
   temperature, such as bottled oils. If you equate this fat with
   your HDL, or good cholesterol, you'll know what you're
   looking for on labels. There are two kinds of unsaturated
   fats: polyunsaturates, which actually raise the level of good
   cholesterol in your body; and monounsaturates, which were

▲ Food Skills   ● Behavior Skills   ◆ Exercise Skills

thought to have no effect either way, but that opinion is beginning to change. The unsaturates, then, whether mono- or poly- are the best bets in fats.

SAT FATS—fats to limit   UNSAT FATS—OK fats

Here's the tricky part. To get an *unsaturated fat* oil to appear like butter and be useful as a spread, it has to be hardened. This is accomplished by a process called *hydrogenation*. The more hydrogenated a margarine is, the worse it is for you. The best choice of margarine, therefore, is the *softer* one, because it is less hydrogenated. The softer margarines come in tubs. If you make the mistake of leaving one out on the counter, you'll see the oils separate. The stick margarines are more hydrogenated and remain hard at room temperature.

Regardless of which type of margarine you buy, check the lables. After the total fat content, you'll see the numbers for *saturated fat* and *unsaturated fat*. The first fat, and the most grams, should be unsaturated. It might read unsaturated 5 and saturated 2. That means you get 5 grams of unsaturated fat (OK fat) for every 2 grams of saturated fat (bad fat). That's considered a healthy ratio. If it's reversed, pass it by. If it says corn oil margarine and the highest fat content says saturated or hydrogenated, pass it by. Look for the lowest grams of a saturated or hydrogenated fat you can find on a margarine. If it doesn't tell you what kind of fat it contains, pass it by.

Because of this fat fandango, the best course would be to switch to apple butter and jams or jellies on your toast or muffin. They have no cholesterol. Cook exclusively with unsaturated oils. If you can't give up margarine on your toast or roll, at least switch to a tub margarine instead of a stick which is more hydrogenated.

➠   *How to Lower Your Cholesterol*

Many people who have tried to lower their cholesterol have been disappointed in the results. Cutting fat isn't enough. Increasing your fiber has been shown to have a more dramatic effect on cholesterol levels. Also studies on lecithin show that it has the interesting ability to hold cholesterol in solution, so it doesn't deposit.

You can get lecithin from soy products, which are excellent protein foods. Also niacin has been found to help reduce cho-

---

lesterol, and you can find that in poultry and grains. If you add exercise as a booster, you'll see your cholesterol level come down, since exercise raises the level of HDL (good cholesterol).

The guidelines for cholesterol reduction are:

Reduce total fat intake.
Reduce saturated fat intake.
Increase unsaturated fat intake.
Eat less cholesterol in your diet.
Eat more complex carbohydrates (for fiber, lecithin, niacin).
Exercise.
If you smoke, stop.

The above list sounds complicated to someone who doesn't study fat for an occupation, but you can turn to Cholesterol at a Glance, which combines all of these factors into a quick view of where your cholesterol is coming from and how to get the better variety of fats.

Cholesterol Tests
Your cholesterol level can change at different times. In fact, you can have it done twice in the same day at different places and get different readings, depending on how accurate the measurement was. Naturally, you'd like to go home with the lower number in mind and have a double cheese pizza with cholesterol in the cheese. But for your health's sake, you should get regular tests at your physician's office to get your cholesterol *range*. If your cholesterol remains high, that's cause for concern. In the meantime, you can make the adjustments in your diet and exercise, and you will be accomplishing what the doctor will tell you to do. Some people need medication, so it's best to check your level at every annual physical.

When you have your body cholesterol checked, it is a reading of both your good cholesterol (HDL) and bad cholesterol (LDL). You can have a borderline LDL level, and a high HDL level, and it is not as risky as a high LDL level and low HDL level. The key is in the ratio between the cholesterols.

The recommended level is:

LDL level: less than 130 mg/dl. (DL means deciliter of blood.)
HDL level: more than 35 mg/dl.

▲ Food Skills ● Behavior Skills ♦ Exercise Skills

The total cholesterol level ratings are:

Desirable   199 mg/dl or lower
Borderline   200–239 mg/dl
Too high   240 mg/dl or higher

Cholesterol Medications
Even when you have a high cholesterol level, the first course of action is to try diet and exercise improvements. If that fails, medications are recommended. However, these medications still require that you change your diet and exercise, so it's best to change first. Recent evidence shows that the medications combined with diet and exercise actually remove the plaque buildup. If plaque buildup continues unabated, balloon surgery—angeoplasty—or heart surgery may be required.

The medications for cholesterol reduction are called antihyperlipidemics, meaning they reduce the excess lipid concentration. The most commonly used medications are:

1. Clofibrate. This medication is not considered as safe as others because of increased deaths from noncoronary causes (36 percent higher).
2. Cholestramine, Colestipol. These work in the stomach, and are therefore considered safer. They can cause constipation, nausea, vomiting, flatulence, and diarrhea, but the symptoms often abate as use continues.
3. Niacin. This can create gastric distress, more frequent cardiac arrhythmias, and possible liver dysfunction.
4. Neomycin, Probucol. These can cause mild diarrhea. Often a combination of these medications is used.
5. Mevacor. A newer medication that selectively lowers LDL cholesterol.

➠   *How to Avoid Cholesterol Confusion*

Best Sources of Food: Low cholesterol foods, with little saturated fat—vegetables, grains, fruits. Eat hearty!

Cholesterol and saturated fats are justified in lean meats and poultry, because the other nutrients are essential. Don't be afraid of meats because of their cholesterol content. When you eliminate the main sources—eggs, butter, fatty dairy products, and cheese—lean meats are moderate sources of cholesterol, and the saturated fat content is not way out of proportion to the unsaturated fat.

Worst Offenders: Cholesterol content is high for the portion size, despite nutrient composition. Most cheeses, butter, lard, creams, ice cream, and desserts that contain these ingredients are high in cholesterol. When you eliminate two or three of your main sources, you'd be surprised how much you take out of your diet.

Easiest Solution: Avoid or limit the highest cholesterol foods and switch to vegetable oils for cooking. Get fiber in your diet and exercise. Check the next two lists for the highest source of cholesterol in regular food and desserts.

Recommended maximum of cholesterol is *300* mg/day.

Twelve Cholesterol Elevators

Egg yolk (1)	312 mg
*8 clams	240 mg
*4 oz. lobster	225 mg
4 oz. bacon	249 mg
4 oz. liver (CKN)	629 mg
*4 oz. crab	113 mg
1 hot dog	74 mg
4 oz. dark turkey	114 mg
1 cup sour cream	102 mg
4 pats of butter	140 mg
1 cup ricotta	124 mg
2 slices most cheese	54 mg

A bacon double cheeseburger will top your daily cholesterol maximum.

Eight top cholesterol desserts

1 piece of cheesecake	163 mg
1 piece of apple pie	156 mg
1 piece of sponge cake	123 mg
1 piece of lemon meringue pie	130 mg
1 serving bread pudding	170 mg
1 eclair	145 mg
1 piece of custard pie	278 mg
1 piece of pumpkin pie	91 mg

*Shellfish are being reevaluated in terms of cholesterol, because of omega 3 oils. However, these are still high fat compared to other fish, and two of them are often dipped in butter for eating.

_____

▲ Food Skills   ● Behavior Skills   ◆ Exercise Skills

Remember that sweets or pastries with cheese, custard, eggs, cream, or butter will be naturally high cholesterol.

For the exact count of cholesterol, saturated and unsaturated, see the Easy Cholesterol Counter on the following pages.

EASY CHOLESTEROL COUNTER

The primary sources of cholesterol are high-fat dairy products, high-fat meats, and processed desserts with added fats. When you moderate these sources of cholesterol, it really makes a difference.

The complex carbohydrates are cholesterol-beaters, since they are high in fiber and low in fat. You don't need to count them, just increase them to reduce your LDL and raise your HDL.

Recommended cholesterol maximum—300 mg per day
Dairy, 1 cup

	Total Fat	Cholesterol	Saturated	Unsaturated
Buttermilk	2	9	1	.7
Chocolate milk	8	30	5	3
Condensed	27	114	17	8
Dried whole	34	124	21	11
Dried nonfat	.9	24	.6	T
Evaporated whole	19	74	12	7
Evaporated skim	.5	10	.3	.2
Goat milk	10	28	7	3
Human milk	1	4	6	6
Low-fat milk	5	18	3	2
Malted milk	10	37	6	3
Skim milk	T	4	T	T
Whole milk	8	33	5	3

Creams, 1 cup

Half & Half	28	89	17	9
Heavy cream	88	326	55	29
Sour cream	49	102	30	16

T = trace (next to no fat)
— = not available

———————————————————————————————————————

⇒ How-to Skills   ♥ Good for Heart

Milk desserts, 1 cup

Ice cream	14	59	9	5
Ice milk	6	18	4	2
Sherbet	4	14	2	1
Yogurt	7	29	5	2
Yogurt, low-fat	3	14	2	1
Yogurt, low-fat, fruit	3	12	2	1

Eggs, 1

Egg, large	5	312★	2	2
Egg, small	4	219	1	2
Egg, whites	0	0	0	0
Eggnog	19	149	11	7

★One large egg has more cholesterol than the recommended daily maximum

Oils and Fats, 1 Teaspoon

	Total Fat	Choles- terol	Satur- ated	Unsat- urated
Bacon fat	14	—	6	4
Butter	12	35	101	66
Chicken fat	14	—	—	—
Lard	13	12	5	7
Margarine, stick	14	0	2	9★
Margarine, tub	7	0	1	6★
Cod liver oil	14	119	0	0
Corn oil	14	T	1	11
Cottonseed	14	0	3	9
Olive	14	T	1	11
Peanut	14	T	2	10
Safflower	14	T	1	12
Soybean	14	T	2	10
Sesame	14	T	2	11
Sunflower	14	T	2	12
Wheat germ oil	14	T	2	9
Vegetable shortening	12	—	3	9

★Margarines differ in saturated and unsaturated content. The best choice is tub margarine, because it requires less hydrogenation (is softer at room temperature). However, even tub levels can differ. Check the label to be sure.

▲ Food Skills ● Behavior Skills ♦ Exercise Skills

Cheeses, 1 Ounce or 1 Slice

	Total Fat	Choles- terol	Satur- ated	Unsat- urated
American cheddar	9	27	6	3
Blue	8	21	5	2
Brick	8	27	5	3
Brie	8	28	0	0
Camembert	7	20	4	2
Cheddar	9	30	6	3
Cheese spread	6	16	4	2
Colby	9	27	6	3
Cream cheese	11	31	6	4
Edam	8	25	5	2
Gouda	8	32	5	2
Gruyere	9	31	5	3
Limburger	8	26	5	3
Monterey	9	—	—	—
Mozzarella	6	22	4	2
Mozzarella, skim	5	15	3	2
Muenster	9	27	5	3
Parmesan, hard	7	19	5	2
Parmesan, grated (1 Tbsp)	1	4	1.5	—
Port du Salut	8	35	5	3
Provolone	8	20	5	2
Roquefort	9	26	5	3
Swiss	8	26	5	2
Swiss, pasteurized	7	24	5	2
Softer cheeses, 1 cup				
Cottage cheese	9	31	6	3
2% cottage cheese	4	19	3	1
Ricotta	32	124	20	10
Ricotta, skim	19	9	12	6
Cheese soufflé	16	159	9	7

Desserts, Sweets

	Total Fat	Choles- terol	Satur- ated	Unsat- urated
Brownies	9	25	1	6
1 piece of sponge cake	2	123	1	1
Custard	14	278	7	6
Apple pie	17	156	5	12
Lemon meringue	14	130	4	8
Pumpkin pie	16	91	5	9

➠ How-to Skills   ❤ Good for Heart

Pudding (Bread)	16	170	8	5
Cheesecake	26	163	6	6
Eclair	13	145	4	6

Meats, Poultry, 4 oz.

These are listed in 4-ounce serving sizes, the total daily allowance. Note that the recommended *serving* size for a meat selection is 2 ounces. The average person tends to eat larger portion sizes, so keep an eye on your meats.

	Total Fat	Choles- terol	Satur- ated	Unsat- urated
Bacon	80	249	25	45
Beef				
Chuck roast	19	67	9	8
Ground, lean	11	74	5	5
Ground, reg	24	77	12	11
Rib roast	39	65	18	18
Rump roast	24	65	19	19
Bologna	33	208	13	17
Braunschweiger	31	—	11	16
Canadian bacon	16	100	6	8
Chicken				
Back	10	92	3	6
Breast	4	60	1	3
Drumstick	7	60	2	4
Liver	5	629	2	2
Neck	5	92	0	0
Thigh	8	92	2	5
Wing	13	92	4	8
Chili w/beans	15	0	7	7
Club steak	33	65	16	15
Duck	32	80	8	20
Flank steak	6	65	3	3
Frankfurters	32	74	12	18
Goose	38	—	10	22
Ham, cured	34	80	12	17
Knockwurst	36	84	14	17
Lamb				
Leg	15	66	8	6
Chops	24	68	13	9
Shoulder	23	68	13	9
Pheasant	13	—	4	7
Polish sausage	29	0	10	16

▲ Food Skills   ● Behavior Skills   ◆ Exercise Skills

Pork chops	22	65	8	11
Pork link sausage	57	0	20	29
Rabbit	7	73	3	3
Sausage,				
Blood	41	0	0	0
Country-style	35	0	12	18
Salami	38	0	13	22
Vienna (7)	22	0	0	0
Steaks				
Flank steak	6	65	3	3
Porterhouse steak	37	65	18	17
Round steak	13	65	6	6
Sirloin steak	28	65	13	12
T-Bone steak	42	65	17	22
Turkey				
Dark	9	114	2	6
Light	4	87	1	2
Canned	6	0	2	4
Veal				
Breast	15	63	7	7
Chuck	9	80	4	4
Cutlet	10	63	5	4
Rib roast	12	63	6	5
Rump	8	63	3	3
Venison	4	0	3	4

Seafood

	Total Fat	Choles- terol	Satur- ated	Unsat- urated
Abalone	T	—	0	0
Anchovy	T	5	0	0
Bass	2	—	T	T
Bluefish	3	—	0	0
Carp	5	—	T	3
Catfish	3	—	1	2
Caviar (1 tsp)	T	7	—	—
Clams (4)	2	120	—	—
Clams, canned	T	240	—	—
Cod	T	57	T	T
Crab, steamed	2	113	—	—
Crab, canned	4	161	—	—
Eel	21	57	5	7
Flounder	1	57	T	T
Frog legs	T	10	—	—

⟶ How-to Skills ❤ Good for Heart

SOURCES OF EXCESS CHOLESTEROL

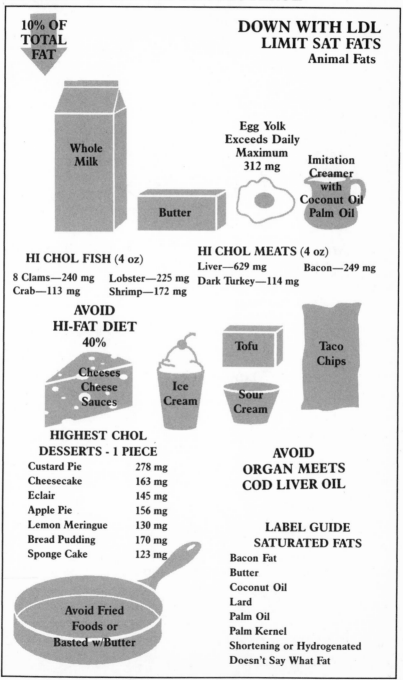

10% OF TOTAL FAT

DOWN WITH LDL
LIMIT SAT FATS
Animal Fats

Whole Milk

Butter

Egg Yolk Exceeds Daily Maximum 312 mg

Imitation Creamer with Coconut Oil Palm Oil

HI CHOL FISH (4 oz)

8 Clams—240 mg   Lobster—225 mg
Crab—113 mg   Shrimp—172 mg

HI CHOL MEATS (4 oz)
Liver—629 mg   Bacon—249 mg
Dark Turkey—114 mg

AVOID HI-FAT DIET
40%

Cheeses Cheese Sauces

Ice Cream

Tofu

Sour Cream

Taco Chips

HIGHEST CHOL DESSERTS - 1 PIECE

Custard Pie	278 mg
Cheesecake	163 mg
Eclair	145 mg
Apple Pie	156 mg
Lemon Meringue	130 mg
Bread Pudding	170 mg
Sponge Cake	123 mg

AVOID ORGAN MEETS COD LIVER OIL

LABEL GUIDE SATURATED FATS
Bacon Fat
Butter
Coconut Oil
Lard
Palm Oil
Palm Kernel
Shortening or Hydrogenated
Doesn't Say What Fat

Avoid Fried Foods or Basted w/Butter

▲ Food Skills   ● Behavior Skills   ◆ Exercise Skills

SOURCES FOR CHOLESTEROL CONTROL

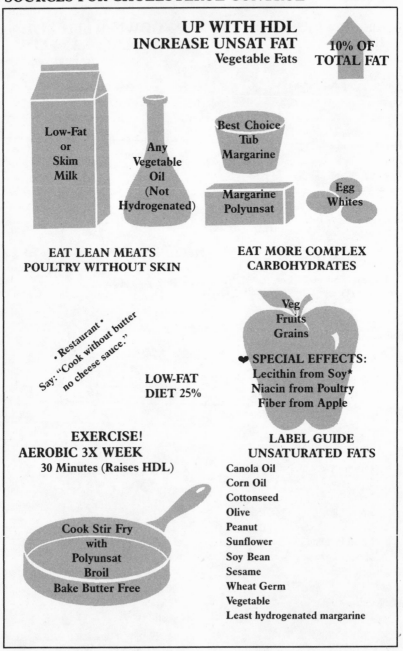

UP WITH HDL
INCREASE UNSAT FAT
Vegetable Fats   10% OF TOTAL FAT

Low-Fat or Skim Milk

Any Vegetable Oil (Not Hydrogenated)

Best Choice Tub Margarine

Margarine Polyunsat

Egg Whites

EAT LEAN MEATS POULTRY WITHOUT SKIN

EAT MORE COMPLEX CARBOHYDRATES

• Restaurant • Say: "Cook without butter no cheese sauce."

LOW-FAT DIET 25%

Veg Fruits Grains

♥ SPECIAL EFFECTS:
Lecithin from Soy★
Niacin from Poultry
Fiber from Apple

**EXERCISE!
AEROBIC 3X WEEK**
30 Minutes (Raises HDL)

**LABEL GUIDE
UNSATURATED FATS**
Canola Oil
Corn Oil
Cottonseed
Olive
Peanut
Sunflower
Soy Bean
Sesame
Wheat Germ
Vegetable
Least hydrogenated margarine

Cook Stir Fry with Polyunsat Broil Bake Butter Free

★Keeps LDL in suspension. Prevents deposits.

⇒   How-to Skills   ♥   Good for Heart

	Total Fat	Choles- terol	Satur- ated	Unsat- urated
Haddock	7	68	T	T
Halibut	1	56	T	T
Herring	7	96	2	4
Lobster	2	225	—	—
Mackerel	11	107	3	7
Oysters	2	56	—	—
Oysters, canned	1	27	T	T
Perch, ocean	2	—	T	T
Perch, yellow	1	80	—	—
Pike	1	—	T	T
Pollock	1	—	T	T
Salmon, fresh	15	68	T	T
Salmon, canned	3	19	1	T
Sardines, oil drained	12	80	—	—
Scallops	T	39	—	—
Shad	11	—	—	—
Shrimp, fresh		172	—	—
Shrimp, canned	T	48	—	—
Smelt	2	—	—	—
Snails	T	—	—	—
Snapper	1	—	T	T
Swordfish	4	—	—	—
Trout	12	62	2	3
Tuna, oil drained	13	104	5	6
Tuna, water-packed	1	126	—	—
Whitefish	9	—	T	4

CIRCULATION

Blood movement through arteries and veins to deliver oxygen to tissues and take away waste products and carbon dioxide. Your rate of circulation has an indirect effect on weight gain, but the effect can be significant. Blood circulation facilitates many processes that are central to fat burn. It carries oxygen to your muscles, where fat burn occurs; it carries nutrients from your intestines to your cells for metabolism; it carries vitamins and minerals to your cells, which is essential for the chemical reactions of metabolism; it carries wastes away from your cells after metabolism; it carries salt to your kidneys which aids in their elimination. All of these processes are part of your internal calorie regulating cycle that better circulation can enhance. You can improve your

▲ Food Skills ● Behavior Skills ◆ Exercise Skills

circulation with regular exercise and diaphragm breathing, earning double benefits. The exercise burns calories and breathing exercises help you stay calm when stressed.

▲ **COLAS**

Drinks with 100 percent sugar. *See* Sugar.

● **COMMITMENT**

The deal you make with yourself; the amount of energy, time, and effort you make to make your diet succeed; the trust you place in yourself; the pledge you keep.

Commitment is a very critical factor in successful dieting. It's important to understand that you're not making a commitment to a particular diet plan, a contract to a clinic, or a pledge to your favorite counselor or nurse who weighs you, even though these people are there to help you keep your commitment. The only pledge that works is the one you make to yourself. That way, if there's a snowstorm one day and the roads are closed, you won't stop dieting because you can't check in to get weighed.

To help you make the best pledge you can make to yourself, try not to jump into a diet on an impulse—because a wedding or a reunion is coming up—unless you plan to go the distance to ideal body weight. The more you start and stop diets, the harder it will be to believe the commitment you make to yourself. Choose a diet carefully, and don't begin it if you have any doubts about your ability to comply with it. Ask questions, and if you are unsatisfied with the answers, find another program. Try to find a diet that doesn't feel like punishment, and there are many around. Avoid gimmicks and extra purchases if you can, since real, fresh food is the best fuel for energy and fat burn. Don't hesitate to call other people who have been on the diet and ask their opinions. Use every resource at your disposal to make your decision, and take your time making it. It's better to wait and make your commitment real than to start too quickly, without being ready to make the changes you will need in your lifestyle. Once you make your decision, stick to it! You'll prove to yourself that you can succeed at other things.

───
⟶ How-to Skills   ♥   Good for Heart

● COMPLIANCE

Adhering to a diet program, following the rules and regulations.
Many dieters have problems with compliance for a variety of
reasons.

1. The diet you choose doesn't fit into your lifestyle. The plan
   you use for weight loss should be one that is comfortable to
   do, or you won't continue doing it for long. When a diet
   causes too much disruption of your normal routines, it becomes stressful and a chore, and you find yourself getting
   angry at a hundred little things. Eventually, these emotions
   lead to a break from the plan. Diets that are too far out of
   line with everyday life aren't much use to you over the long
   term; they can create new problems instead of resolving your
   old ones. One of the reasons dieters choose unfitting plans is
   because they see a diet as a form of short-term punishment
   that has to be endured for the purpose of weight loss. This
   doesn't have to be you, if you close the gap in your mind
   between diet and everyday life, and select a program that
   makes you feel positive about working toward health on a
   daily basis.

2. The diet you choose is too regimented and repetitive. A diet
   doesn't have to be a robotlike routine where you do everything someone else tells you to do, blindly following rules
   and feeling that if you don't you'll gain weight. On diets like
   this, when you find yourself breaking the rules, you don't
   tell anyone, because you feel guilty, like a kid with your hand
   in the cookie jar. While diets involve discipline, weight loss is
   not an either/or situation—their way or no way, the one and
   only solution. Before entering a program, ask to see the
   menus and rules. Be sure you have a clear picture of what's in
   store for you, so you won't be disappointed later. Don't sign
   on to a program because the woman at the front desk is fun
   to talk to. Sign on because it offers what you want and shows
   you what you're getting. If they tell you that their rules and
   food lists are private information that can only be divulged to
   a client, go someplace where weight loss isn't treated like a
   big secret.

3. You are half-hearted about dieting. This can be because you
   see dieting as an unpleasant experience, when it doesn't have
   to be. Or you can be afraid to go through the process and
   face another failure. Or you may have convinced yourself
   that you were born to be fat. There are as many reasons for

▲ Food Skills   ● Behavior Skills   ◆ Exercise Skills

this as there are dieters. Before you take on the project, make sure you're ready to make a change in your eating habits and lifestyle. If you're not quite ready, don't make the investment. Losing and gaining can be worse for you in the long run. Explore the reasons you might feel reluctant to diet, and make an effort to resolve these conflicts before you start dieting. Give yourself time to get ready to make a commitment. That way you'll be setting yourself up for success.

4. You jumped into the plan too quickly. Don't buy into a diet because a wedding is coming up in two weeks. Do it because you want to lose your excess weight for life. Don't let the immediate stress of weight cause you to sign with the first program you find. The faster you jump in, the faster you will jump out. Each time you do that, you lose a little belief that you can work out your weight problems. If a wedding is coming up in two weeks and you want to lose weight, go for a brisk walk and think about the marriage of low-fat eating and regular exercise and what it can do for you. Then just start doing it.

5. You want instant results. This is the biggest reason people quit diets: false expectations of rapid weight loss. It's also the reason people regain weight so fast. The faster you lose, the faster you regain. You didn't gain your excess weight overnight, and you're only hurting yourself if you plan to lose it within a week or two. If this was the only change you made in your weight-loss perspective, it would be the best one you could do. When you want instant results, you choose plans that promise instant results, and you get what you ask for. So ask for something else. Ask for lasting weight loss and enjoy seeing the slow, steady changes in your weight and well-being on a weekly basis. These diets are the ones that comply with a lean life.

● **CONFIDENCE**
The surety that you will succeed with your goals, based on support skills (not willpower). *See* Control.

CONSTIPATION
Intestinal slowdown. This can be caused by a variety of factors:
  You're not drinking enough water.

You're not eating enough fiber, or you increased your fiber intake too fast and didn't drink water simultaneously. If you drink water when you increase your fiber, you will not have problems with fiber. Fiber binds with water in your intestines and speeds up your food transit time. But it's got to have water to do it.

You're eating too rapidly, swallowing too fast, and not chewing sufficiently. This throws off the natural process of digestion at the outset.

You're too stressed or anxious while eating. This can tighten your diaphragm and stomach muscles and interfere with digestion. Before you eat, five minutes of deep breathing will let go of the stress and tension.

You're eating too late at night, particularly heavy proteins. Late night eating doesn't give your food time to digest. Your metabolism slows down dramatically when you sleep, and you aren't digesting the food properly.

Your diet is imbalanced on a regular basis. This makes everything work less efficiently.

You're not getting enough exercise. Exercise increases your food transit time and keeps food from lingering in your intestines where it can stagnate.

Constipation may also be due to other medical conditions. If it is severe or prolonged, see your doctor.

● **CONTINGENCY PLAN**

A coping skill to use for emergency situations; a problem-solving technique. During weight loss, contingency plans center around food and eating problems, such as meal planning, developing strategies for eating out at parties, restaurants, vacations, and planning behavior substitutes like exercise, breathing exercise, and relaxation to replace your usual emergency eating habits.

In maintenance, your contingency plans are more geared to relapse prevention or weight regain. This means taking action *before* you regain ten pounds so you don't have to get caught in the cycle of losing and regaining excessive amounts of weight. Most dieters never take the time to develop successful coping skills and contingency plans during their diet routine. They see weight loss as their *only* diet goal, and even if they achieve it, they are stranded at ideal weight without the skills to keep it. Gradually, they fall back into old habits because they have not developed controls to prevent this. Coping skills act as *controls*, habits you can use on a

---

▲ Food Skills   ● Behavior Skills   ◆ Exercise Skills

regular basis for fitness insurance. Without these skills, weight loss is seldom permanent. *See* ● topics for coping skills, especially Lifestyle.

● CONTROL

Taking charge of, or authority over; to direct.

Anyone who has ever been on a diet has heard the word *control*. It's the byword of most commercial programs. Control your appetite. Control your portions. Control your will. Control yourself.

Weight gain is seen as loss of control, and weight loss is seen as taking control.

The problem is, control is the like the two-headed monster. When you start to take control, you feel great and in control. Then the other face turns and you feel the overwhelming tension of having to be in control all the time. Control starts to control you, and you feel like you're going to break. The easiest way to get out of control is to think you can control everything in your life at the same time.

Control isn't what you really need on a diet. What you really need is to *own* your decisions, actions, habits, and lifestyle. You need to feel part of it—in charge, but flexible, able to go with the flow without losing your sense of self-support. That's very different from control.

Take stress, as an example. If you tell someone to take control over stress, it can make them feel more stressed. First, it assumes they have no control and are deficient. Working from a feeling of deficiency isn't a positive mindset, directed to positive goals. Second, it puts the blame on the person, who seemingly lost control. Working from a feeling of blame and guilt isn't self-supporting or productive. Third, it's a paradox. More people get stressed from needing too much control and not getting it, than people who let go of the need for control and rely on step-by-step decisions about health.

Willpower is an example of a control technique. You're supposed to exercise your "no" power over foods you think you want. The more you try to resist the food, the greater the hold of that food. You think about it all the time. In supermarkets you stare at it, saying no. You dream about it at night. Finally, one day, when no one's looking (not even you), you go out and get that food. You eat it until you satisfy the three-week obsession you had while saying no.

Skill power is an *owning* technique: You own your desire for that food. What are you going to do about it? Know the food inside out, what it does and does not provide in nutrition and fat burn. Study your reactions and desires for the food. How does it get to you, when, and why? How does it make you feel after you eat it? Guilty? Temporarily satisfied? Happy? Admit what you really feel and deal with it. Make reasonable choices. Gradually limit your dependence on that food by replacing it with healthier alternatives. If you're going to faint without a slice of cake, have a sliver, then go back to limiting it in your life. When something owns you, no matter how small (even a truffle), it is something worth dealing with. It won't go away by itself. You own it, and you have to let it go.

As adults, most of us have a number of different factors in our lives that we control, and we do reasonably well at it. To believe that you are out of control because you are overweight is neither helpful nor particularly accurate. Thin people can be out of control in areas of their life that you are skilled at handling. The best way to view your weight and food problems is as an issue you want to deal with. List the issue as a priority and think about the choices you can make and want to make. Step by step, change one unhealthy food habit into a healthy one. One day you'll turn around and find that your efforts have dominoed; one healthy habit has led to another and another. One day, you'll own your new habits and health. *See* Eating Habits.

▲ COOKING

How you treat what you eat. To create a healthy, low-fat lifestyle, you need to set up a kitchen that will promote easy cooking, while you give yourself a whole new view of eating and cooking without fats, sugars, and sodium. This means that you don't want a kitchen that looks deprived or depressed, stripped of food and pleasure. You want a kitchen that is alive with pleasure and energy, so that cooking low-fat becomes a gourmet delight.

Try to enjoy the pleasure of cooking while you are on a diet. If you only rely on microwave dinners or oven entrées in a box, you deny yourself the smell of food and the sensual pleasure that comes from preparing a good meal, with hot and cold fares.

⮕ *How to Design Your Diet Kitchen*

1. Start by adding a spice rack full of herbs and spices, free of the ingredients that give you too much sodium. You might even consider taking up pottery as a hobby (to substitute for eating), and you can make your own herb and spice jars. Make your herb and spice rack a real eye catcher with fresh cinnamon sticks and perhaps a planter of fresh basil, so the sight and smell can permeate your kitchen, giving you a new feeling about cooking with low-fat pleasure. Use herbs and spices for flavoring in sauces and sautés. Lemon, garlic, and basil are excellent for fish. Orange, basil, and whole-wheat flour make a delicious, creamlike sauce for chicken. Use your imagination to create your own herb and spice combinations to replace the butter you may have used in the past.
2. Set up a rack of unsaturated oils to use instead of butter or margarine. There are many, including peanut oil, cottonseed oil, and olive oil. You can find a collection of bottles that will show off the oils, and you might think of painting designs on the bottles yourself. If you keep a rack of the varieties of unsaturated oils that are available, you won't feel so limited when you're cooking low-fat. Different oils have subtle taste differences, and you can experiment with herbs and spice mixes to make your own oil mixes. Keep a selection of wine vinegars on your rack of oils. There are many varieties, and the colors will be pleasing to your eye.
3. Keep jars of colored pastas in plain sight instead of cakes, candies, and fattening snacks. Pastas are complex carbohydrates—fat burning foods.
4. Keep fruits under your glass cake saver. It's artistic and a clear message to snack on fruit instead of sugar and fat.
5. Hang pictures of fresh fruits and vegetables to remind yourself that these are the foods that will lighten up your life.
6. Keep sugar free candies and menthol throat drops in a glass bowl to soothe a sudden desire for something sweet.
7. Set a beautiful glass by the sink to remind yourself to make water drinking a habit. Put a lemon or lime next to it, to remind yourself that fruit spritzers are better than sodas.
8. Keep a selection of fruit nectars in sight. They make excellent bastes for lean meats.

This is a kitchen that will make you feel healthy and inspire you to cook and eat low-fat.

⮕ How-to Skills   ❤ Good for Heart

◆ COOL DOWNS

A mild exercise or stretch for a minimum of five minutes after a vigorous exercise. This prevents that after-exercise ache or soreness in your muscles by breaking down lactic acid which can build up if oxygen supply to your muscles is limited (as in anaerobic exercise). In addition, it allows you to bring your heart rate down gradually, instead of abruptly. The cooling effect occurs as your body heat is reduced and your temperature returns to normal. You can use a brief easy walk for a cool-down exercise, or repeat the full body stretch or yoga you used as a warm up. *See* Stretching; Warm Ups.

◆ CROSS-COUNTRY SKIING (MACHINE)

Skill sport aerobic exercise. *See* Nordic Track.

◆ CROSS TRAINING

A combination of exercises that includes endurance, strength, flexibility, and aerobic conditioning; a method for exercise versatility and best effect. An example of cross training might be: on Monday, you power walk; on Tuesday, you do stretching exercises; on Wednesday, you walk, and so on through the week. The next week you might want to develop more upper body strength, so on Monday, you lift weights, on Tuesday you stretch, on Wednesday you power walk, on Thursday, you stretch. The goal is to combine weight-bearing exercises with flexibility exercises to gain strength along with grace. It also combats boredom with exercise for high achievers. For the ideal cross training, see The Problem Solver Calendar.

⎯⎯⎯⎯⎯⎯⎯⎯⎯⎯⎯⎯⎯⎯⎯⎯⎯⎯⎯⎯⎯⎯⎯⎯⎯⎯⎯⎯⎯⎯⎯

D

♦ **DAILY ACTIVITY**

Routine motion that produces heat and burns calories. The more active you are on a daily basis, the greater your metabolic rate. Activity levels can be responsible for burning 25 percent of your calories. It doesn't take a great deal of effort to activate your daily life. If you have a desk job, get up and move around on breaks. Walk to the store sometimes, instead of taking your car. Use more stairs than elevators, and park farther away from your destination. Use the seasonal opportunities to get outside: rake leaves, shovel snow, landscape around the house. If you live in an apartment, you might find a trampoline easy for exercise, since there's no impact on the floor. You can walk on it, run, or bounce. Take up an outdoor sport, preferably not one that lets you stand around a great deal, like golf. The little activities add up, even though you might think they don't mean much. They help you become a more active person overall, then it's easier to think about starting an aerobic program for real fat burn. *See* Exercise.

▲ **DAIRY PRODUCTS**

One of the daily essential food groups; animal sources of protein, calcium, riboflavin, vitamins, and minerals. The recommended servings daily are: two servings for adults, four servings for teens, three servings for children, four servings for pregnant and lactating women. The best source is the low-fat version. Dieters often forego their calcium, thinking that milk and milk products are fattening. This is a harmful habit, since lack of calcium can lead to osteoporosis—dry and brittle bones—and it can upset your protein balance, leading to muscle losses. Less muscle means more fat gain. *See* Calcium.

♦ **DANCING**

A daily activity exercise, nonaerobic (unless it's break-dancing for thirty minutes sustained). *See* Exercise.

◆ DANCE AEROBICS

Aerobic exercise to music.

Benefits:
- Full-body workout;
- Easily accessible—from health spas and community centers to home use with video and audio tapes and instructional guides;
- Entertaining, incorporating high-energy music.

Guidelines:
- Check the credentials of the instructor; he or she should have formal training or certification in physcial fitness rather than just "liking to dance."
- Assess the facility: type of floor surface (wood preferred); amount of ventilation; average number in class.
- Find out about the levels of classes offered: how they differ in length of class, degree of difficulty and supervision, length of warmup and cool-down periods, frequency of supervised heart-rate monitoring.
- Join the best program that offers low- to high-level classes and take responsibility for yourself. Use target heart rate to avoid overexertion; forcing yourself to keep up is more harmful than not dancing at all.
- Always warm up. Never just jump into a class late. If you arrive late, take time to do your own warm-up first.
- Wear good, supportive shoes. *See* Exercise.

DEFICIENCY

Lack of one or more essential nutrients needed for body growth, repair, and maintenance. Nutrient deficiences can occur for a variety of reasons.

1. Improper eating. You can overeat and be deficient in your daily nutrients if you are not eating a balanced diet from the daily food groups. Or you can be eating certain energy to excess, such as sugar, which will deplete other nutrient sources. Taking one vitamin to excess will throw off the others. Excess protein can deplete calcium from your bones. That's why it's so vital to be sure you get balanced nutrition, regardless of the amount of food you eat. Your metabolism requires all of the daily nutrients in the food groups to function properly, and that also means burning fat better.

▲ Food Skills ● Behavior Skills ◆ Exercise Skills

2. Metabolic disorder. You can have deficiencies if you have an inability to digest or metabolize certain nutrients, as in diabetes, where carbohydrates cannot be metabolized, or you can have a problem with lactose metabolism, which can cause nutrient deficiencies to occur.
3. Prolonged stress. The stress response speeds up your body processes, including your heart rate and metabolism. This causes your nutrients to be burned off faster and can result in deficiencies.
4. Illnesses, injuries, or surgery can cause nutrient deficiencies, since the body needs more energy for repair.
5. Weight-loss diets are a common source of nutrient deficiency, since many dieters feel that anything is acceptable if it gets rid of fat. But beware! Nutrient-deficient diets don't get rid of much fat at all. They get rid of your body muscle and water, and that adds more fat.
6. Obesity. You can have major nutrient deficiencies if you have obesity. Your fat mass steals your nutrition and keeps your nutrients out of balance on a regular basis. That's why obesity is considered a disease of *malnutrition,* instead of a disease caused by overeating. You can eat the same calories as a normal-weight person, but you gain weight because nutritional deficiencies keep you in a fat-gaining cycle. For nutrient needs, *See* Food Groups.

DEHYDRATION

An excess loss of body fluids and water. This condition should not be confused with mild fluid loss and needs medical attention if the condition persists. However, dehydration can occur if you exercise in a hot, dry climate without taking water breaks to replace lost fluids, or it can occur on severely imbalanced diets that allow water losses. The immediate solution is to drink plenty of water on a steady, regular basis, not all in one gulp. Also cut back on your salt intake. If the condition does not improve in a day or two, see your doctor.

DESIRABLE BODY WEIGHT

The best weight you can be for your height, frame size, and sex. *See* Ideal Weight for height/weight tables.

DIABETES/MELLITUS

A disease of the pancreas, known as sweet urine because of the increased concentration of sugar excreted in the urine.

There are two types of diabetes.

Type I Insulin Dependent: The pancreas produces no insulin, or low insulin. This results in an inability to metabolize carbohydrates, since insulin is needed to convert glucose to energy for metabolism. The unmetabolized glucose remains in the blood and accumulates. This can lead to coma or death. Ten percent of all diabetes is the insulin-dependent type, requiring insulin injections.

Type II Noninsulin Dependent: The pancreas produces insulin, but excess fat prevents the body from using insulin, creating an insulin resistance. As a result, the pancreas has to make larger amounts of insulin to metabolize carbohydrates. Ninety percent of all diabetes is the insulin-resistant type. It can be brought on by excessive intake of sugar, and obesity. This type can be treated by weight loss and proper nutrition.

- Upper body fat distributors have a greater risk of developing diabetes.
- People who are obese have three times the risk of diabetes, while people who have upper body fat and obesity have ten times the risk.
- Since men are primarily upper body fat distributors, obesity in men presents a greater risk of diabetes.

Symptoms of diabetes include loss of weight, increased appetite, excessive thirst, frequent urination, vision problems, skin itches, and poor healing. It must be treated by a physician.

◆ DIARY, EXERCISE

A daybook of activity; the story of you and your energy output. The exercise diary should be tacked on to your food diary for the best effect, but many people have a difficult time with food. While food is becoming more controllable, it might be best to keep your exercise diary separate. Its goal is to get you moving and to keep you moving on a regular basis.

Since most overweight people have a tendency to resist exercise, your exercise diary is both a record of your aerobic activity and your feelings before, during, and after it. This will give you feedback you can use to develop an effective program for yourself. You can record the exercise you did, the amount of time you did it, where you did it, and how you felt about it. You can use this as a gauge to find a comfortable place to exercise, to choose exercises that please you (so you'll keep doing them), and to release your resistance on paper. Also include your average daily activity level, since this burns calories too.

The Ideal Dieter's Diary

Both diaries combined—food and exercise—make the ideal weight-loss record. If you keep a combined record from the first day of your diet, tracking your food, and ensuring that you exercise three times each week, you get four stars for successful dieting. Your diary will be your best diet ally and a fabulous support system. It provides diet, exercise, feelings, behavior, and self-monitoring in one easy system.

SAMPLE EXERCISE DIARY

Moods and Feelings Before Ex	Aerobic Choice	Minutes Performed	Other Daily Activity	Moods and Feelings Afterward	Total Cal Burned

➠ How-to Skills ❤ Good for Heart

Notice the column on the far right of your diaries. When you keep a combined diary and add up the calories you ate each day and the calories you burned with exercise, you can track your progress like an athlete.

▲ DIARY, FOOD

A daybook of eating habits; the story of you and food. The dieter's diary is a four-star aid for behavior modification. Its goal is to teach you to become master of your eating habits, but to do that you first must know what those habits are.

The ideal food diary is both an *eating* record and a *feeling* record. You list what you eat, the time you eat, with whom, and how you feel about what you eat—on a daily basis. This will give you a wealth of information about yourself that you can use for a wide range of personal fitness goals.

What Your Food Diary Can Do for You:

1. It makes you aware of what you're actually eating, not what you think you're eating. Everyone makes mistakes when they try to remember their day's intake, even undereaters. Your diary provides an accurate record to use for a variety of problem-solving issues.
2. It takes the guilt out of your personal evaluation. The simple act of recording your daily food intake objectifies the situation. You don't have to keep that neon sign "I ate cake" in your head all day. It's on paper, where you can see it more objectively, like a scientist viewing food.
3. It's a personalized dietary analysis, and a bargain at that! It shows you the quality of food you eat. You can use this to compare with the quality of food you should be eating in the food groups.
4. It records your eating patterns:
   • Your preference for certain foods;
   • Times of day or days of the week you eat most often;
   • Food cues that get to you.
5. It shows you your weak points and strong points. You can use these for habit change.
6. It reveals the emotions and feelings that you equate with food. You can use this to understand more about yourself and to find substitutes to feed your emotional needs.

▲ Food Skills   ● Behavior Skills   ◆ Exercise Skills

7. It's a personal weight control monitor. You can use your diary for feedback to adjust your food intake when you find yourself gaining weight.

Many people lose weight simply by keeping a diary and using it to improve their food intake and eating habits. But keep in mind that a diary isn't a menu or meal plan. A diary is what you actually eat, even with a menu or meal plan in front of you. Be completely honest in your record keeping. It's your record for you. The better your record, the better your progress and self-evaluation.

SAMPLE DIETER'S FOOD DIARY

Food	Amount Servings	Who I Ate With	Time	My Moods & Feelings	Calorie Total

How to Use Your Diary

Prediet Diary

This diary is used to target problem areas. You list your regular food intake when you are acting normally. You write down everything you eat—no cheating—including the fluids you drink. It's best to keep this diary for one week before a diet, since that will give you a realistic picture of your average intake and eating patterns on week days and weekends. Using the Problem Solver pyramid recommendations for dieters, you can compare what you've been eating to what you should be eating and plug in the gaps to create a balanced, slenderizing food plan. You can study your eating patterns, moods, and feelings to use as guides to problem areas that need resolution.

During Diet Diary

This diary can be used to track your progress, to keep you in line, and as a tool to monitor yourself. Keep this diary for the first four weeks of your diet, then one day a week as a checkpoint. Every so often, keep a weekly record again to see if fat foods are creeping in, your protein is up to par, and you're getting enough fiber, calcium, and water. In addition, you can see how your eating habits are improving.

Fail-safe Maintenance

This diary can be used to keep you at ideal weight for life. If you see yourself gaining more than five pounds (five pounds can be water weight), keep a diary for a week and evaluate what happened. By maintenance, you will be so knowledgeable about your intake and eating habits, you'll be able to take action in a snap. *See* Maintenance.

● DIETARY ANALYSIS

A review and rating of your average food intake. There are four steps to making a dietary analysis:

1. Recording what you actually eat;
2. Adding up the nutrient value of what you eat;
3. Comparing your nutrient intake with recommended daily nutrient intake (RDAs);
4. Filling in the missing gaps in your diet. This might mean adding some foods, while subtracting others, not simply adding in the missing nutrients.

Dietary analyses are best when prepared by a registered dietitian, because they have all the information for nutrient calculations in their heads or on floppy disks. This makes an extremely complicated process seem easy. In addition, they can make on-the-

---

▲ Food Skills ● Behavior Skills ◆ Exercise Skills

spot evaluations and personal recommendations from speaking with you and reviewing the outward signs of your physical health. In a sense, in a one-half-hour dietary analysis with an R.D., you are getting ten years and one-half hour's worth of education, and you're only paying for the half-hour.

Standard dietary analyses don't include behaviors and moods, which is a big part of your eating idiosyncrasies. What you eat is often contingent on how you feel and how you react when you face situations like stress. If you change what you eat, without changing your headset about eating, old habits creep in and one day you find you're eating for weight gain again.

⦿   *How to Make a Dietary Analysis*

Record what you eat for one week. Compare your servings of meats, dairy, fruits, vegetables and grains to the recommended servings in the Problem Solver pyramid. Plug in the servings in food groups that you are not eating, and take out the servings in food groups you are overeating. You have an excellent analysis and solution in a snap.

▲ DIETARY GUIDELINES

A fundamental set of standards for nutrition and health from the U.S. Department of Agriculture and the U.S. Department of Health and Human Services. First issued in 1980, these guidelines cite six areas for concern in your daily diet, and one major health concern as the second point: "Maintain your ideal weight." If you're a part of the population (more than one-fourth) who has to get to ideal weight before you can think about maintaining it, you might not think these guidelines apply to you. Look again! The other six guidelines set the example for a very healthy diet for weight loss and maintenance.

The seven standards are:

1. Eat a variety of foods (from the basic food groups).
2. Maintain ideal weight.
3. Avoid too much fat, saturated fat, and cholesterol.
4. Eat foods with adequate starch and fiber (carbohydrates).
5. Avoid too much sugar.
6. Avoid too much sodium.
7. If you drink alcohol, do so in moderation.

⦿   How-to Skills   ♥   Good for Heart

If you use the six food guidelines as the basis of your daily diet, you'll gradually lose weight and be in good shape to maintain it. Many people say the guidelines are too general, but they were intended to be that way. Every year, researchers come closer to finding more exact information that explains what "too much" or "adequate" means for weight loss, maintenance, and health. The government simply weighed in on the safe side, confining itself to guidelines that adhered to the Hippocratic Oath: First do no harm. If more commercial diets followed that principle, we'd be seeing less weight regain. You might add two extras to the list of standards to boost your fitness results: (8) Exercise regularly, and (9) Drink plenty of water daily. *See* Food Groups for more specific guidelines. And ▲ topics.

DIETS, WEIGHT LOSS

Calorie-restricted diets that result in weight loss. The key point to remember with calorie-restricted diets is what kind of weight loss? All weight loss is not created equal. The weight you want to lose is fat. The weight you do *not* want to lose is muscle. The weight you want to balance is water.

When you lose muscle, you regain your weight after your diet phase is over. Why diet if you are going to gain your weight back because of the kind of diet you chose?

There is a simple rule you can use to determine if a diet is going to provide fat loss or muscle losses:

Balanced diets provide fat loss.

Unbalanced diets provide muscle loss (and fat loss), especially very low calorie diets (VLCDs) for rapid weight loss.

How can you determine if a diet is not balanced? Compare the foods used in the diet to the foods required daily in the Problem Solver food pyramid for dieting. This will give you a very easy way to rate commercial diets to ensure that you are paying for a proper program. If the diet does not include all of the food groups, it is not balanced.

There are certain circumstances that require unbalanced diets, such as diabetes, since the person cannot metabolize carbohydrates. But this condition is a metabolic disorder that requires the care of a physician; therefore, it is a different issue than the ones facing average dieters.

▲ Food Skills   ● Behavior Skills   ◆ Exercise Skills

Guide to Dieting

If you are obese and have no other medical complications, your doctor would most likely recommend a food-group plan as the diet of first choice. Anything less will not be the best for you.

If you are overweight, your diet of first choice should not be one that provides less than 1,000 calories per day (women) and less than 1,400 calories per day (men). They allow you to lose muscle.

If you go on a very low-calorie diet for rapid weight loss or an imbalanced diet, you can wind up fatter than you started and have greater hunger after the diet is over—hunger that wasn't present before the diet. Your weight gain will be rounder all over. You can face bouts of binge eating that were not part of your life before the diet.

The diet you choose for weight loss is one of the most important choices of your life. You are investing your body, time, energy, health, money, and emotions. You are not just investing your extra weight.

The *best and most lasting* form of weight loss is achieved with the following diet components:

- Real food
- Balanced food groups—Lean version—Low-fat, high complex carbohydrates, optimum protein and calcium.
- Healthy calorie levels:
  Women   1,000–1,500
  Men   1,400–1,800
- Exercise
- 8 Glasses of water
- Behavior modification for a healthy lifestyle
- A vitamin/mineral supplement daily

Believe it or not, dieting is not as complicated as you've been told. Learning how to eat a healthy, balanced diet is the complicated part, especially for dieters who have been trained to eat oddly by unbalanced diets. But once you make the shift, you have it as a healthy skill for life. Make the next diet you choose a healthy, balanced one. That way, you build yourself up on a diet, rather than break down. See The Problem Solver Diet (pages 69–85) for everything rolled into one.

Types of Diets

Fads *See* Fads.
Fasts *See* Fasting; Undereating.
Fruit *See* Fruit Diet.
High Protein *See* Liquid Protein Diets; Protein.
Ketogenic *See* Ketones; Ketogenic Diets.
Low- or No-Carbohydrate *See* Ketogenic Diets.
Modified Fast *See* Ketogenic Diets.
Powdered Protein *See* Supplements.
Protein-Sparing Modified Fast *See* PSMF.
Rapid Weight Loss *See* Rapid Weight Loss.
Starvation *See* Starvation.
Vegetarian *See* Protein.
Very Low-Calorie Diet *See* VLCD.

DIGESTION

The process that breaks down food into smaller and smaller nutrients until they take the form that can be absorbed by your blood.

Foods contain nutrients, but these nutrients do not occur in a form your body can use for energy, repair, or maintenance. For instance, meats, fish, poultry, eggs, and dairy products are sources of the nutrient protein, but the protein in these foods has a different molecular structure than the protein in your body needs for making muscle. To turn food protein into body protein, the bonds of the food protein are broken during the long process of digestion, yielding amino acids that your blood can pick up and deliver to the areas of your body that require protein (such as cells for building muscle tissue).

In the same way, fats are broken down to form fatty acids and glycerol, which can be used for energy or stored for later use. Fruits, vegetables, and grains are broken down into glucose, your body's preferred source of energy and primary brain fuel.

Digestion and Your Diet

If you take a look at the digestive process, you'll notice that *the order* in which nutrients are digested is the pattern for healthy eating and healthy dieting. Carbohydrates start digesting first, and

▲ Food Skills   ● Behavior Skills   ◆ Exercise Skills

these are the foods that should make up more than half of your diet. Protein begins to digest next, and it should make up one-quarter of your diet. Fats, the foods you should eat the least of for the best results, are digested last.

Now you know why science is the best source for fitness and health. No fad can match that magic formula.

1. Mouth. Chewing breaks your food into smaller pieces for swallowing.

○ *Salivary Glands.* Saliva is produced to moisten your food. Saliva also contains the enzyme amylase that begins to break down carbohydrates.

2. Pharynx. The food goes to your pharynx by your voluntary motion. After this point, peristalsis takes over. Peristalsis is a slow, wavelike motion that moves food through your entire digestive tract.

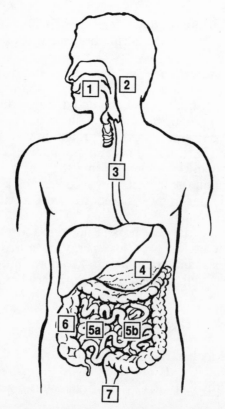

⟩ How-to Skills   ♥ Good for Heart

3. Esophagus. Peristalsis pushes food through your esophagus into your stomach.

4. Stomach (mid-section) one to four hours. Food mixes with gastric juices in your stomach. They include water, hydrochloric acid, and the enzyme that begins to break down protein. A semiliquid mass called chyme is formed. Peristalsis pushes the chyme out of your stomach into your small intestines.

5a. Small Intestines. When chyme enters your small intestines, your pancreas secretes digestive juices that include acid neutralizers. If fats are present, bile is secreted from your gallbladder. Bile separates fats into droplets to prepare them for reaction with pancreatic enzymes. These chemical reactions convert food into nutrients that can be absorbed by your blood. The remainder of the chyme goes into your large intestine.

○ Your *liver* produces bile acids that store in your gallbladder for use in fat breakdown in small intestines.

○ Your *pancreas* produces digestive juices and enzymes for additional carbohydrate and protein breakdown in small intestines.

5b. Absorption (from small intestines). Nutrients pass into your bloodstream from your small intestines.
   Glucose (from carbohydrates)
   Fatty acids and glycerol (from fats)
   Amino acids (from proteins)
   Vitamin and minerals (water and fat soluble)
   Chyme with lymph (and other substances)

6. Large intestines. Undigested chyme (plus fiber) enters your large intestine where it absorbs water. Your large intestines have no enzymes, so no further digestion takes place.

7. Rectum. After chyme passes through your large intestine, it is excreted as waste.

DISEASES, WEIGHT RELATED
See Risks.

▲ Food Skills   ● Behavior Skills   ◆ Exercise Skills

DIURETIC

A medication that increases urine output, such as lasix or diazide. Diuretics are used for serious conditions and should not be confused with laxatives, which increase overall bowel excretion. Mild diuretics are often called water pills, but even these should not be used casually. Loss of body water can cause serious fluid imbalance and major disorders if prolonged. *Diuretics should not be used without medical supervision.*

DRUGS

Prescription or nonprescription medications or aids. The excessive use of any drug causes depletion of essential nutrients from your body. Absorption is hampered, excretion of nutrients is increased, and appetite can be decreased, which adds to nutrient depletion since you are not replacing them in your daily diet. A dangerous combination is sleeping pills with use of stimulants and alcohol. It can start gradually, by taking stimulants as a diet aid, leading to sleeplessness and the need for sleep aids. Add alcohol to the mix and it can be deadly, since your system is constantly swinging up and down, and your perceptions and responses are altered. It's best to avoid over-the-counter drugs or diet aids, since they can often be a catalyst for use of other medications. Recommended therapy is to discontinue all nonprescription drugs and adhere to a balanced diet and exercise program, drinking plenty of water. If use is excessive, see your physician.

E

● **EATING**

The process of acquiring energy you need for metabolism. In its ideal state, eating is a physiological process, but it can also be influenced by emotions, psychology, and environment. *See* Appetite; Digestion; Hunger; Metabolism.

● **EATING HABITS**

Your eating style; how you eat, as opposed to what you eat; patterns of eating. Your eating habits may play a greater role in weight gain than any other factor. They include your adult eating patterns and habits carried over from childhood, where you first learned about food. Often food is used for rewards or punishments in childhood, with desserts being withheld for punishment or proffered as rewards. No one can recall hearing, "I'm so proud of you. Here's a cup of fruit." It's more like, "You can have a double scoop of ice cream tonight." This is how sweets and fats come to be regarded as the foods that give comfort or pleasure.

Eating habits are also cultural and ethnic, and many of your food cravings (emotional) center around family gatherings where people bring their favorite recipes and talk about old times. Food also has peer links. The foods your teenage friends perceived as "cool" are foods you can equate with being popular or fun; therefore *not* eating them makes you think you're dull or uncool.

The primary eating habits that lead to weight gain are:

Emotional eating: using food to satisfy other needs you may have.

Stress eating: using food to soothe you when you are tense.

Eating on the run: eating too fast, which means you can eat more without being aware of it.

Late night eating: your metabolism is slower in the evening and it gets even slower in sleep. Late night food doesn't digest easily and more calories can store.

Not eating breakfast: this is the first meal of the day to give you energy and fire up your metabolism. When you don't eat breakfast, your metabolism can be sluggish until noon.

▲ Food Skills   ● Behavior Skills   ◆ Exercise Skills

Social eating: feeling obligated to eat because everyone else is doing it.

Relying on sugar for energy boosts: sugar is empty calories and usually comes along with excess fat. This keeps you in a sugar/fat cycle that tends to take precedence over healthy foods.

The key to resolving your fat-promoting eating habits is to find rewards for yourself that are not food. You can substitute pleasurable nonfood activities for your most common habit problems. A good way to keep yourself from falling into poor eating habits is to practice a regular program of relaxation or meditation every day. *See* Meditation; Relaxation.

ECTOMORPH

A body type that is characterized by a long, thin, linear look, symbolized by the column. *See* Body Type.

ENDOMORPH

A body type that is characterized by roundness all over, symbolized by the circle. *See* Body Type.

ENERGY

The heat of living and being active. Every process in your body generates heat. When you eat, it produces heat; when your body takes up the nutrients from food, it generates heat. The nutrients give you the energy you need to be alive and active, and the process of using that energy generates heat. This heat is measured in units, or calories. From this heat measurement, scientists were able to measure the nutrient density of foods and the energy effects of exercise, along with thousands of other substances and processes in the universe.

When you eat, the heat you produce should match the heat you give off. Eating is *input* (taking in the nutrients). Movement and activity, including exercise, is *output* (using those nutrients).

When your *input* matches your *output*, you are at ideal weight. Overweight (obesity) and dieting are not balanced energy states. In overweight and obesity, your *output* is less than your *input;* and in dieting, it's intentionally reversed—your *output* exceeds your *input*. We put this in the food pyramid for you in each of these states. *See* Obesity, for energy and the food pyramid.

⇒ How-to Skills   ❤ Good for Heart

♦ ENERGY EXPENDITURE

Output. The amount of calories you burn daily. *See* Exercise.

ENZYMES

Chemicals that can break down other chemicals without being changed themselves. There are dozens of enzymes involved in digestion and metabolism of your food. Each one can only act on a specific nutrient, and no other. In digestion alone, there are three enzymes for carbohydrates, six for protein, and one for fat. During digestion, these enzymes split the molecules of carbohydrates, proteins, and fats into smaller molecules in each part of digestion from your mouth through your small intestines, where absorption finally takes place. Gastric juices in your stomach stimulate the release of hormones, which in turn stimulate the release of enzymes. It's a chain reaction that keeps on splitting molecules into smaller and smaller forms, until they wind up in the form that can be absorbed by your blood. Carbohydrates become glucose, proteins become amino acids, and fats become fatty acids and glycerol. From your blood, they go to your cells where a whole new series of enzymes activates the chemical reactions of metabolism.

This entire process starts all over again with each meal. This is known as enzyme-catalyzed reactions. Diets that claim that they catalyze important enzyme reactions that burn fat are only talking about the natural process of digestion and metabolism that your body does automatically. So you're paying for what you've already got. *See* Digestion; Metabolism.

EPINEPHRINE

A hormone produced by your adrenal glands that reduces hunger by stimulating the release of glucose from your liver. When your blood glucose levels rise, hunger is abated (in your brain). Exercise increases the production of epinephrine, which is one of the reasons it decreases your appetite.

The Epinephrine Effect

Have you ever had a shaky feeling, where you can literally feel tremors inside and feel weak even though you just ate? That's the epinephrine effect.

▲ Food Skills ● Behavior Skills ♦ Exercise Skills

It's caused by eating too much sugar.

If you wake in the morning and have orange juice, pancakes, and sugary syrup, and the pancake mix has added sugar, you can experience the epinephrine effect. Your sugar intake causes your blood glucose to shoot up. Insulin is secreted to metabolize the glucose, and your blood sugar starts to drop quickly. Epinephrine is released, which reacts on your liver to release glucose, and the shakes start. Rapid heartbeat, cold sweats, a feeling of sudden fear or dread—your body literally quakes inside.

To stop the effect, you need protein and sugar back to back— one-half cup of orange juice and one-half cup of milk. The orange juice will stop the quick sugar drop and the protein will prolong digestion, stabilizing the effect.

If you had protein with a high carbohydrate breakfast in the first place, you wouldn't have the effect, and you'd be in great shape for weight loss.

● EUSTRESS

Good stress, specifically the good stress of exercise. Exercise is stress, but it's a beneficial stress, meeting a challenge and over-coming it. The benefits are the opposite of negative stress, *after* you complete the exercise. You see a lower heart rate, lower blood pressure, soothed respiration. That's why it's important to do the required twenty to thirty minutes of an aerobic exercise. It's the time needed to create those after-exercise effects. If you break earlier, you can be in the midpoint of stress and feel tenser as a result. The part that is not computed is the feeling of well-being that you get from meeting that challenge and mastering it. It gives you a sense of confidence and pride that shines from within.

EXCHANGE LISTS

Energy equivalents. Exchange lists are a system that allows foods in one food group to be substituted for foods in another group for therapeutic use, such as diets for diabetes (since the diabetic has trouble metabolizing carbohydrates) or in lactose-allergy diets, where the person has trouble digesting milk. The exchange list indicates the other sources of energy that can replace those foods, while still providing equal nutritional value.

The term *exchange list* is sometimes used in weight-loss diets to refer to foods in the same group that can be used in place of another food in that group to achieve similar energy, but lower in fat or for preference. Or it can cross groups, as in a vegetarian's diet for weight loss, which would have to provide alternate sources of protein, instead of animal sources.

● EXCUSES

Reasons why you think you can't accomplish something. They're simply attitudes, and you can change them. *See* Rationalizations.

◆ EXERCISE

Motion; dynamic action. The motion in exercise sets off chemical reactions in your body that use nutrients and produce heat as a by-product.

There are two forms of exercise—aerobic and anaerobic—named after the type of energy that is used for each form.

First, it is important to know that the chemical in your body that acts as the energy carrier for all processes is called ATP—adenosine triphosphate. It's made by a chemical called ADP—adenosine diphosphate. When you eat food, the molecules are broken down into smaller forms. When the bonds of your food molecules are broken, energy escapes and some is captured by the bonds of ADP and stored in the bonds of ATP. ATP travels around your body bringing energy to every part. When your heart beats, it means that a bond of ATP has been broken to provide energy. If you run down the stairs, bonds of ATP are being broken to provide the needed energy. When you exercise, the source of your energy is ATP. To break the bonds of ATP, oxygen is necessary.

Aerobic exercise
The source of energy for aerobic exercise is ATP and oxygen. The bonds of ATP break with oxygen and supply glucose and fatty acids for fuel. This is your muscles' *preferred* form of energy. The suppy of ATP must be increased for aerobic exercise, and at first your circulation can't keep up with your activity if you burst into aerobic exercise too quickly. If you are a jogger, for instance, you walk first before you run, so that your circulation can pick up and supply more ATP, which will be needed for your aerobic workout. The entire aerobic workout is sustained on ATP and oxygen (providing fuel).

Anaerobic exercise

The source of energy for anaerobic exercise is different. It's ATP without oxygen to break the bonds. Since you burst into action without warming up and increasing your circulation, your body has to make ATP without sufficient oxygen. This is called the glycolytic method, meaning that your body uses glucose and glycogen to make ATP. This process produces lactic acid along with the ATP. Lactic levels that accumulate to critical levels result in fatigue. There is a limit to the amount of ATP that your body can make anaerobically. If you burst into a run with your muscles tensed up, and you aren't breathing deeply, you can use up your anaerobic ATP and not get enough oxygen to produce aerobic ATP; you can collapse from exhaustion. Lactic acid levels to excess (ketones) can be toxic.

Sudden, spontaneous motion that is sustained is not the way to start exercising aerobically. Under ordinary circumstances, if you burst into exercise with anaerobic ATP, part of the way into your activity your aerobic ATP will catch up and start being manufactured with the necessary oxygen. But dieters' circumstances aren't ordinary; they are restricting their calories. And if you're on a diet that is restricting its carbohydrates (the primary muscle fuel), you're producing a high level of ketones to begin with. Sudden, spontaneous exercise on a no- or low-carbohydrate diet could be dangerous.

This is one more reason you should think seven times before you go on an imbalanced diet.

Anaerobic energy use is something that trained athletes deal with as a part of training. Mile runners, for instance, start with a sudden anaerobic burst, and the speed of the run is so stressful that the aerobic ATP never gets a chance to catch up. They learn to gauge their point of exhaustion; and using this, they have to meter their anaerobic ATP, or they could collapse from fatigue. But athletes eat sound, balanced diets to achieve this ability.

You should too. Eat plenty of carbohydrates daily, in case you need sudden and sustained energy in a crisis situation. It's your body's best protection.

Why You Need to Exercise

To fine-tune your metabolism. Calorie restriction can reduce your calorie-burning power by causing your metabolic rate to drop as much as 10 to 15 percent. You can burn fewer calories, even

---

though you cut them to burn more. This could cause you to stop losing weight or to lose very slowly. Exercise raises your metabolic rate by 10 to 15 percent to offset this loss of burning power.

To preserve your muscle. Fat is the only loss you can afford on a diet. Muscle losses undermine your metabolism and reduce your burning power. Exercise preserves muscle during a diet to ensure that you burn only fat.

To balance your body composition. At the end of your diet, your fat-to-muscle status is of primary concern. It will determine how many calories you can eat at maintenance without gaining weight. Studies showed that two people of the same height, weight, and sex can eat the same number of calories at the end of a diet, and one will gain while the other will not. Why? The one who won't gain has a low-fat/high-muscle body.

To gain oxygen for fat burn. When you exercise, you use more oxygen. For fat to be burned, oxygen is necessary. With aerobic exercise, you can expect greater burn of stored fat.

To increase intestinal motility. Food passes through your intestines better when exercise is a regular routine. An average nonexerciser can take twenty-four hours to complete one digestive cycle; an obese nonexerciser can take up to forty-eight hours, which is too slow. Food that lingers in your intestines can stagnate and lead to digestive disorders or increase your risk of bowel cancer. Exercise speeds food transit time through your intestines. Athletes show intestinal motility of four to six hours to complete digestion.

To regulate your appetite. Loss of appetite follows a good workout. When activity levels are low, studies show that people increase their calorie intake.

To fight anxiety and depression. Endorphins are opiatelike chemicals produced in your brain that modulate pain and moods. Exercise increases their production, leaving you with a euphoric feeling. Your circulation is improved and this creates a sense of well-being. Therapists are beginning to prescribe aerobic exercise and dance as therapy against anxiety and depression, with one study boasting an 82 percent success rate in hard-to-treat patients.

To reduce stress. From 50 to 75 percent of all organic illnesses are aggravated by or related to stress. Stress stimulates your sympathetic nervous sytem, speeding your heart rate, increasing your blood pressure, and contributing to cardiovascular disease. Exercise reverses the stress response by reducing your heart rate, lowering your blood pressure, and improving your sense of control.

▲ Food Skills ● Behavior Skills ◆ Exercise Skills

HEALTH BENEFITS OF EXERCISE

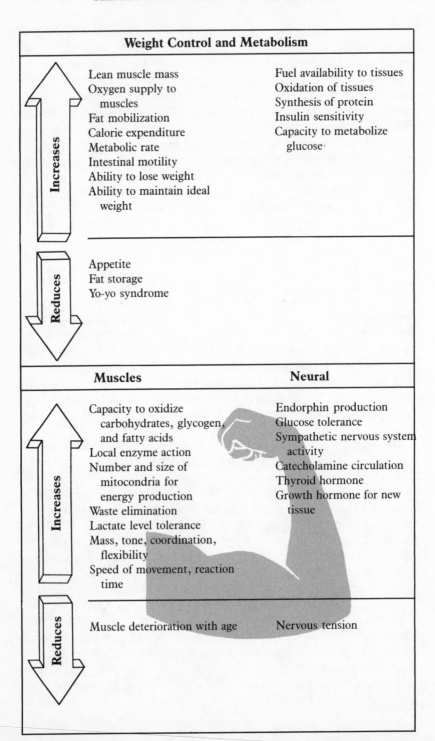

Weight Control and Metabolism

Increases

Lean muscle mass
Oxygen supply to
   muscles
Fat mobilization
Calorie expenditure
Metabolic rate
Intestinal motility
Ability to lose weight
Ability to maintain ideal
   weight

Fuel availability to tissues
Oxidation of tissues
Synthesis of protein
Insulin sensitivity
Capacity to metabolize
   glucose

Reduces

Appetite
Fat storage
Yo-yo syndrome

Muscles   Neural

Increases

Capacity to oxidize
   carbohydrates, glycogen,
   and fatty acids
Local enzyme action
Number and size of
   mitocondria for
   energy production
Waste elimination
Lactate level tolerance
Mass, tone, coordination,
   flexibility
Speed of movement, reaction
   time

Endorphin production
Glucose tolerance
Sympathetic nervous system
   activity
Catecholamine circulation
Thyroid hormone
Growth hormone for new
   tissue

Reduces

Muscle deterioration with age   Nervous tension

RECOMMENDED DOSE   **AEROBIC (LOW IMPACT)**
                         3 x per week, 30 min. session

❤ Heart & Blood

Cardiac output	HDL—good cholesterol
Stroke volume	Number of capillaries
Heart rate recovery	Size of arteries
Strength of heart muscle	Collateral circulation to with-
contraction	stand heart attack
Blood volume	Elasticity of blood vessels
Circulation	Oxygen content of arteries
Oxygen carrying capacity	Ease of blood movement
Number of red blood cells	
Hemoglobin content	

Increases

Resting heart rate	Risk of hardening of arteries
Vulnerability to arrythmias	Clotting time
EKG abnormalities	Lipid, triglyceride, and
Blood pressure	cholesterol levels

Reduces

Brain   ### Bones

Mental alertness	Density
Glucose and oxygen	Tensile strength
supply to brain	Joint stability
	Strength of connective tissue

Increases

Depression	Incidence of osteoporosis
Anxiety	Compression in vertebral
Perception of effort	column

Reduces

Lungs   ### General

Volume and capacity	Immunity to disease
Gas exchange ability	Rate of healing
Strength of respiratory	Stress tolerance
muscles	Quality of sleep
Ventilation and breathing	Ability to relax
efficiency	Sense of accomplishment
Oxygen uptake	

Increases

To lose fat for disease prevention. High body fat has been linked to most of our major lifestyle diseases, including hypertension, heart disease, diabetes, and cancer—specifically colon cancer in men and breast cancer in women. Since exercise reduces body fat, you reduce the risk of acquiring these diseases by exercising. Recent studies show that exercise can significantly reduce the risk of heart attack by improving heart and lung function and increasing the concentration of HDL (good cholesterol).

To increase your energy output. Movement requires energy. The more you move, the more energy you use, which means more calories burned.

In addition to its metabolic benefits, exercise is the best behavior substitute for eating.

See Skill Sports, Cardiovascular Conditioning. Also see all topics with ♦ for a complete exercise guide. For the *ideal* exercise program to use while dieting, see The Problem Solver Calendar (pages 107–112).

CALORIE BURN FOR EXERCISE AND ACTIVITIES

The average calorie burn for exercise and activities is based on 150-pound adults. If you weigh less than that, you will burn a little less than the levels shown here. If you weigh more, you will burn a little more.

Activity	Calories per hour	Activity	Calories per hour
Aerobic dance	445	Cooking	100
Badminton	350	Cross-country skiing	700
Baseball	280	Dancing	250
Basketball	750	Desk work	100
Bed making	210	Dishwashing	135
Bicycling	415	Downhill skiing	595
Bowling	190	Driving	100
Calisthenics	415	Eating	90
Canoeing	300	Floor washing	250
Car washing	230	Football	600
Carpentry	305	Gardening	390

➡ How-to Skills   ❤ Good for Heart

Activity	Calories per hour	Activity	Calories per hour
Hiking hills	600	Sleeping	65
Ice hockey	900	Snow shoveling	610
Jogging	655	Soccer	600
Lacrosse	900	Square dancing	420
Martial arts	790	Squash	775
Mowing lawn (reg)	460	Swimming	300
Mowing (power)	270	Swimming (power)	600
Painting (walls)	165	Table tennis	300
Reading	90	Tennis	425
Riding a horse	415	Volleyball	350
Rowing	648	Walking (brisk)	255
Running in place	510	Walking (power)	345
Running (power)	800	Watching TV	80
Sailing	155	Weight lifting	300
Shopping	165	Window washing	250
Skating	350	Writing	90
Skipping rope	510	Yoga	230

F

FAD

A diet or diet-related aid that is popular for a brief time, even though it may not be healthy, safe, or do what it promises. Fad diets play on your vulnerability as a person with weight problems, luring you with claims that equal your secret desires: Fat Melts Like Magic! Miracle Food Removes Fat! Secret Formula Makes You Slim Overnight! Some fads, like liquid protein diets, were downright dangerous, and others, like patches, were harmless as pet rocks. But even a harmless fad isn't worth the price of emotional setbacks. You want to believe it will work; you try it believing; and your spirit takes a beating when weight loss fails again. The best way to combat the lure of fad diets is to consider the investment you're making—your body, health, money, pride, self-esteem—then get all the facts you can about dieting safely and compare the risks. You'll probably find that safe dieting is the secret formula you've been looking for all along. *See* The Problem Solver Diet.

FAMILY TENDENCIES

Your predisposition for obesity based on genetic and trained factors. Scientists have not been able to determine what part of overweight or obesity is exclusively a matter of genes and how much is a matter of conditioning or childhood training. Childhood eating patterns carry over into adulthood as part of the family tendency picture. Therefore, the following figures represent both aspects:

If you have one overweight parent, you are 30 percent more likely to be overweight.

If you have two overweight parents, you are 70 percent more likely to be overweight.

Studies of adopted children support the "learned" aspects of obesity as a major factor. Adopted children tend to display the same incidence of obesity as their unrelated brothers and sisters.

⟹ How-to Skills   ❤ Good for Heart

However, the older the child was when adopted, the less likely these tendencies become, which suggests that overweight habits are learned at a very early age. On the plus side of the picture, learned behaviors can be unlearned or changed. Changing your eating patterns carried over from childhood is one of the purposes of behavior modification. *See* Eating Habits.

▲ FAST FOOD

Food you can buy quickly and eat quickly, usually processed and nonnutritious. And fattening.

You don't have to give up fast foods on a diet. Make your own variety in low-fat stews, casseroles, pasta salads, and soups that you freeze and reheat or microwave in a snap.

With a little detective work, you can find healthy fast foods in the neighborhood near your job, so you're not caught in the drive-through window of a processed food palace because you need a quick lunch. Many restaurants and supermarkets have salad bars with light dressings, and most delis have barbecued chickens (you can remove the skin). Make eating out an adventure rather than an exercise in denial. Have fun finding slim foods in local eateries and keep your own restaurant guide. But change one feature about fast foods: don't eat them fast! People who have a slower rate of eating stay slimmer.

FASTING

Going without food. *See* Starvation.

FAT, BODY

Lipid stores. There are two types of fat in your body, white fat and brown fat. White fat is the most prevalent form of fat, but the least active body tissue. Brown fat is a small percentage of your total body fat (usually 1 percent), but it is metabolic active, meaning it is more related to burning energy than storing. *See* Brown Fat.

▲ FAT, FOOD

Concentrated energy. One gram of fat gives you 9 calories, twice the amount in protein or carbohydrates. You need some fat in your

---

▲ Food Skills   ● Behavior Skills   ◆ Exercise Skills

body for insulation, support, and protection of your organs, and to act as a carrier for the fat-soluble vitamins A, D, E, and K, aiding in their absorption.

Fat supplies essential fatty acids, including linoleic acid, which is needed for proper growth in children, to maintain cell membranes and regulate cholesterol metabolism, and to prevent drying and flaking of the skin. But how much fat do you need?

Studies show that one tablespoon of corn oil—rich in linoleic acid—provides all the essential fat needed by most people. The rest is extra fat, and it arrives in a form that stores easily in your body.

The average American derives 40 to 50 percent of his or her calories from fat. In fat intake studies of thirty-five- to forty-year olds, only 13 percent of the males and 17 percent of the females had a fat intake of less than 36 percent of their total calories. Over a third had a fat intake providing 45 percent or more of their total calories.

Dietary trends over the last decade indicate that our total intake of calories is down, so why are we still fat? Our fat consumption is up. We are eating more fat packed into fewer calories.

When you keep your diet low in fat, the results are dynamic. You feel a cleaner, lighter system in the absence of excess fat. You begin to notice the flavor and subtle tastes of other foods that you may not have appreciated before, because your taste buds were blunted by your desire for the taste and texture of fat.

FAT CELLS

Storehouses for fat. Also called adipose tissue.
There are two kinds of fat cells in your body:

Hypertrophic: oversized cells filled with fat
Hyperplastic: normal-sized cells in greater numbers

The nutrients left over after metabolism which were not needed for body maintenance and repair, and not burned off with activity and exercise, store in your fat cells as lipids. When you accumulate a higher-than-normal level of lipid storage, you have obesity.

In infancy, your fat cells grow primarily by increasing their number, not their size. The number of cells you produce can range from two to five times the normal number. At some undetermined point in adolescence, the production of new cells slows down, and weight gain increases the size of cells. Cell size can range from two to five times the normal size.

Adult-onset obesity is associated with hypertrophic cells—fatter fat cells.

Infant- or adolescent-onset obesity is associated with hyperplastic cells—more normal-sized cells.

Both types of cells exist in most people, but more hypertrophic cells exist in obese people or people who have been obese and have lost weight. It is assumed that excess weight gain in infancy and childhood causes overproduction of these fatter fat cells, and prevention of childhood weight gain will limit their production. The thinner you are younger, the fewer fat cells you will have in adulthood, making it easier to stay slim.

Losing weight can shrink the size of cells, but not their number. Until liposuction surgery, there was no known way to change the number of fat cells in your body. By removing fat cells, liposuction alters this phenomenon. However, it does not change the fact that remaining cells can increase in size. This means that weight gain after liposuction will appear in isolated areas, swelling existing fat cells to a greater size. The result is unevenly distributed fat, or pockets of fat in formerly nonfat areas. Men have been found to deposit fat in the breast area after liposuction for midriff and abdominal fat. Women can deposit fat in their upper bodies, when they were formerly lower-body fat distributors. Existing cells don't change their location or spread out over a larger area after removal of some cells. They stay where they are and fat goes to the areas where cells are. Losses of blood can be extensive in fat-cell removal. As a result, cell removal isn't recommended as weight-loss therapy. Shrinking the size of the cells by shrinking the fat content of the diet is the best fat-cell therapy to date.

FAT DISTRIBUTION

Where fat predominates; primary fat sites. Where you deposit your fat is an important issue to consider, since fat sites influence health risks. Two types of fat distribution have been classified as the primary ways you deposit fat.

Either sex can deposit fat in the upper or lower body, but the crossover is more common in women. Upper-body fat distributors are the ones who should be more concerned about losing weight, since it increases your risk of heart disease and diabetes. For example, obese people in general have three times the risk of

Upper-Body Fat	Lower-Body Fat
The common sites are neck, back, abdomen, waist, upper hips	The common sites are hips, thighs, stomach, calves to ankles
Predominates in men Predominates in men with diabetes	Predominates in women More common after menopause
Also seen in women with diabetes	Not linked to disease
More common in smokers	Harder to lose
Linked to heart disease	
Easier to lose	

acquiring diabetes, but obese people who are upper-body fat distributors have ten times the risk of diabetes.

Since liposuction surgery can lead to fat distribution in areas of the body where fat didn't predominate before, it is an issue for women who think it is harmless to remove fat cells from their hips and thighs. If it changes you from a lower-body fat distributor to an upper-body depositor, it will make the fat that you carry more risky.

● **FAT EYES**

A behavioral term for seeing yourself fatter than you are after losing weight.

Many people who have carried weight for a long time have difficulty seeing themselves without that weight around them. In a sense, they wear a shadow of their old fat. This can cause a diet relapse, and steps must be taken to own your new, leaner self. Weight is often seen as strength or power to a person who has carried it, and thin can seem weak or vulnerable. Often, diets that cause rapid weight loss can foster this image problem, because the physical changes occur too fast and there isn't time for adjustment to the new, slim image. This is one of the reasons why thin/within imagery is so vital during a diet. Your thinner self is claimed in your mind, and you are more familiar with the sight and feeling of being slimmer when you arrive there. Any change in your outer appearance should be accompanied by supportive work on your inner view of yourself, since that makes the change ring true. *See* Imagery; Mirror Exercises.

FAT TOOTH
Desire for fats; the shadow behind your sweet tooth. The phenomenon of fat tooth emerged from studies on taste-preference at Rockefeller University. Normal-weight college students were given a variety of mixtures of sugar and fat and asked to rate them. Their findings showed:
  • Heavy cream solutions (37 percent fat) and 8 percent sugar were rated as pleasant.
  • When the sugar content was increased to 10 percent, the rating was *not* pleasant.
  • When the fat content was increased to 52 percent with 9 percent sugar, the mixture got the *highest* rating.

These studies suggest that a preference for fat may be hiding behind the desire for sugar. A higher fat mixture can increase your tolerance for sweets. On the reverse side of the coin, decreasing your fats can lead to a decrease in your tolerance of sugar. That means two problems can be solved for the price of one.

FAT-TO-MUSCLE RATIO
Body composition; the proper proportion of body fat and muscle. *See* Scale.

FATIGUE
Exhaustion. This can be brought on by nutrient deficiency on an imbalanced diet, or it can be the result of anaerobic exercise. Prolonged fatigue can be caused by a medical disorder and needs your doctor's care.

▲ Food Skills ● Behavior Skills ◆ Exercise Skills

FATTY ACIDS

The nutrients derived from fats, used by your body for energy. *See* Digestion.

● FEAR OF FAILURE

An obstacle course of feelings. Fear is an emotion that sets barriers in front of you, whether those barriers are real or emotional. It is natural to feel fear about change, and weight loss is change, especially for a person who carries a great deal of weight. It is also natural to fear failure if you have a history of rapid weight-loss dieting, which led to rapid weight regain. Or you can fear the person who might emerge from the process, because you aren't familiar with that person; you're familiar with weight. You may have a spouse who would feel threatened by changes in your attitude and lifestyle, and this can generate fear. Or you may have unrealistic expectations.

Setting unrealistic expectations is one of the biggest reasons for failure with weight loss. For instance, you've been overweight for several years, but you want to lose your weight in four weeks. That's an unrealistic expectation, especially if you are more than 20 percent over your ideal weight and have used very low-calorie diets in the past. However, this expectation—or desire—will send you to a diet that says, "Lose thirty pounds in one month." That diet might be able to provide what it promises, but it will starve you and deprive you to do it. If you hang in for the duration and lose your weight, you'll gain it back because you lost too much muscle tissue. You will think you're a failure, when it was the diet that failed you. You're left with the residue. The next time around, you fear what you're trying to do.

To deal with these issues, first you have to redefine failure. Then you have to plan how to deal with fear.

When you set a goal and try to achieve it, that's a success-minded attitude. If you fail to achieve it, that isn't failure; the effort is the achievement. Failure is an illusion, or imaginary monster. It will remain in front of you like an obstacle, until you kick it out of the room.

⟱   *How to Combat Fear of Failure*

An excellent technique you can use is imagery to identify failure and decide how to get rid of it. This form of imagery is best done with paper and pencil, instead of your mind, because you don't need any more pictures of failure in your mind. They can frighten you.

Take a notebook and write FAILURE in big letters on the top of the page. Then draw something that comes to your mind to represent failure. It can be a stick figure, a cartoon monster, or anything. Once you have your picture of failure, you want to think of something that will remove it. For instance, if failure is a stick figure of some kind, draw yourself as a bigger stick figure with a broom sweeping failure out of the picture. Or failure can be a black cloud, and you can cross it out and draw a sun overhead. Draw as many pictures as you want, until you find the one that makes you laugh or feel better. Every time you think of failure, draw another picture of it and resolve the image.

Fear can be managed with relaxation exercises, especially the ones for meditation. In addition, you can change how you feel about fear by using the same formula as the one used for failure. You can use this process for most of your obstacle-emotions and feelings. Back this up with positive self-talk to replace negative self-talk, and you'll find you don't feel as much anxiety about trying again.

When you decide to try again, set healthy expectations. The way to prevent big gaps in your emotions from here to there—from overweight to ideal weight—is to use a step-goal approach. First lose five pounds, then accept yourself at that place and with that thinner image. Then lose ten more pounds and stabilize yourself. Use this approach to get to ideal weight.

▲ FIBER

The undigestible part of plants; also called roughage. The fact that fiber is undigestible means it doesn't get absorbed or stored as fat. Most foods are broken down by digestive enzymes by the time they reach your intestines, but not fiber. It binds with water in your intestines, smoothing out bowel movements and preventing constipation and many digestive disorders. Where is fiber found? In complex carbohydrates.

▲   Food Skills   ●   Behavior Skills   ◆   Exercise Skills

FIBER AT A GLANCE

Recommended Diet Dose
25–35 grams/day
from the 5 fibers

➠ **2 FIBERS AT EACH MEAL, INCLUDE ALL GROUPS**

1 **CELLULOSE**			
Bran	Whole-Wheat Flour	Cabbage Young Peas	Wax Beans Green Beans Brussels Sprouts
Apples	Broccoli Peppers	Cuke Skins	Carrots
2 **HEMI-CELLULOSE**			
Bran	Cereals	Whole Grains	Beet Root
	Mustard Greens		Brussels Sprouts
3 **GUMS**			
Oatmeal	Rolled Oat Products		Dried Beans
4 **PECTIN**			
Apples	Squash	Citrus Fruits	Cauliflower
	Cabbage	Carrots	Green Beans
5 **LIGNIN**			
Bran	Cereals Eggplant	Older Veggies Strawberries Potatoes	Green Beans Pears Radishes

CARBOHYDRATES

➠ 6 Servings Fiber Daily

Average Serving
Veg, Fruit, Cereal ½ Cup
Whole Fruit 1 small
Bread 1 Slice

Vitamin
Mineral

Water
2 Qts
Daily

Fiber binds with water. Drinking water keeps fiber from blocking.
Fiber binds w/trace minerals and can be excreted. Vit/min supplement recommended.
➠ Increase fiber intake gradually over 2-8 weeks to prevent gas.

FIBER'S BENEFITS FOR DIETERS

Bonuses to Dieters:
- Fiber expands with water to fill your stomach, and fullness terminates hunger. Fullness also means a sense of satisfaction, and that's important when you're on a limited-calorie program.
- Since fiber doesn't store as fat, you can use fiber foods to fill out a diet, so you don't feel deprived.
- Fiber-rich foods are lower in overall calories than nonfiber foods.
- Increased fiber intake leads to decreased intake of more fatty, sugary foods.
- Fiber foods take longer to chew, a very important habit to use to say slim.
- Fiber increases your food transit time—the time it takes food to pass through your intestines. Faster transit time means less chance of food stagnation and calorie absorption. The longer food stays in your intestines, the more calories can be absorbed.
- Fiber lowers your levels of bad cholesterol (LDL) without reducing good cholesterol (HDL).
- It stimulates bile flow from your liver and prevents bile absorption, which keeps gallstones from forming.
- It reduces intestinal pressure and allows food to be cleared from pouches that cause diverticulosis.
- It can help to prevent colon cancer by reducing bacteria that interact with fat and bile acids to create carcinogens. By moving stool more quickly, it prevents carcinogens from coming into contact with intestines.
- Gums in fibers are thought to delay emptying of the stomach and absorption of glucose, resulting in lower insulin levels in diabetics. It smoothes sugar surges.

● **FIGHT OR FLIGHT**
The stress response. *See* Stress.

● FOOD CUE

Something that triggers you to eat (other than mealtime). This can be a person, place, situation, event, or stimulus that causes you to reach for food on automatic pilot. Some of the most common food cues are:

- People in your family, or people who remind you of your family (where early eating patterns developed).
- Places other than the kitchen or dining room where eating has been an accepted activity—eating in bed, in front of the TV, at movie theaters, at your desk in the office during breaks.
- Situations that are emotionally charged, such as vacations, parties, family gatherings, weddings.
- Events that cause stress, anxiety, fear, or any strong emotion such as moving, a family illness, a job change.
- Stimulus about food, such as pictures of food, food commercials, the refrigerator, kitchen, bakeries, supermarkets.

Here's how it happens:

1. You get the cue: You're making out your taxes. You owe more than you thought.
2. You feel an emotion (anxiety, frustration, depression).
3. To assuage that emotion, you eat.

➠ *How to Control Food Cues*

Food cue control is a study of action/reaction. Notice the typical actions that cause you to eat, then devise strategies that change your reaction to a nonfood response, such as taking a walk, reading, working on a hobby, meditating. Your nonfood reactions are called substitution behaviors, because you are replacing a bad habit with a good one. It helps to make a list of habits you find pleasurable and easy to do in a pinch, so you can arm yourself in advance with alternatives to food. The longer your list, the better equipped you'll be to conquer eating on cue.

▲ FOOD GROUPS

The scientific system that sorts foods into groups according to the nutrients they yield (calories). The nutrients that provide calories are proteins, carbohydrates, and fats; and these calories are essential to your body for its growth, repair, maintenance, and metabolism.

Eating for health means eating what the food groups recommend for essential energy. Eating less is not better for you; it leaves you deficient in your daily needs. When you are deficient, every body process is slightly altered to make up for these absences in nutrients. Over time, the mild alterations can turn into major imbalances. If you only make one change in your life, the best change you could make is to _eat everything in the food groups on a daily basis_. The food group recommendations for minimum daily nutrition are the following:

6–11 servings from the grain group
5–9 servings from the fruit-vegetable group
2–3 servings from the meat group
2–3 servings from the dairy group

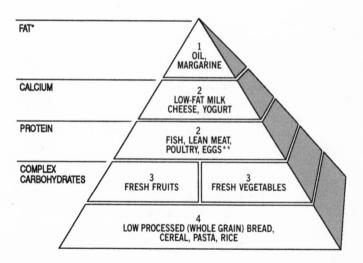

For a diet using the food groups, see The Problem Solver Diet on pages 69–85.

● FOOD SCALE

A weight-measuring device for portion control. _See_ Scale, Food.

_____

▲ Food Skills   ● Behavior Skills   ◆ Exercise Skills

FOOD TRANSIT TIME

The time it takes for food to pass through your intestines. Also called intestinal motility. This is a very important factor in weight gain. The longer food stays in your intestines, the more calories you can absorb and store as fat. Athletes have food transit times of six hours, while obese people can have food transit times as long as forty-eight hours. The worst thing you can do is take laxatives to speed up your food transit time, because you lose valuable minerals and nutrients. The best steps to take are to increase your fiber intake, and increase your exercise and daily activity. Both increase your food transit time. *See* Exercise; Fiber.

FORMULA DIET

A program that relies on powders, drinks, or shake-and-pour supplements to replace average meals. *See* Supplements.

FORTIFIED

Resupplied with vitamins, minerals, or nutrients that are lost during processing of foods, particularly grains. Standard fortification includes three B vitamins, niacin, thiamine, and riboflavin, plus iron and vitamin C. Replacing lost vitamins and nutrients is no substitute for the original food. Fortified foods are also stripped of fiber, have added sugar, salt, and fat, which the real foods don't have. If you switch to the whole-grain varieties, you get ten times the nutrition at the outset. Whole-grain flour beats white flour by a lean mile for cooking and gravy-making. High-fiber cereals and breads made from whole grains keep your food moving through digestion and metabolism with real fat burning benefits. Many people find it difficult at first when they switch to whole-grain foods, after they've been used to the smooth, sugary version of cereals and breads that go down so quickly. Retrain yourself by using half-and-half mixes, half of the fortified kind, and half of the whole grain. Then gradually let the whole grains move the processed grains out. *See* Food Groups.

FRAME

Bone structure and density. People of the same height can have different bone structure and density. This accounts for a ten-

---

➠ How-to Skills ❤ Good for Heart

pound differential that is not body fat. For instance, a small-framed woman of five feet, four inches has a recommended ideal weight of 120 pounds, while a medium-framed woman of five feet, four inches can weigh 130 and a large-framed woman of the same height can weigh 140 and not be carrying excess fat. Bone weight can account for the extra pounds.

However, be careful that you don't use your frame as an excuse for extra pounds. Everyone likes to look at the height/weight tables and say, "I can weigh more because I have big bones." Then they take the highest weight on the tables and if they haven't exceeded it, they feel more comfortable about their weight. Your goal should be the *fittest* you can be, without using extreme or radical measures to achieve that fitness. That's why it's better to take the midpoint of the weight range indicated for your height, weight, and frame. That way, you are setting strong, realistic goals.

➠ *How to Find Your Frame Size*

1. Extend your arm forward, palm up. Bend your forearm upward to a 90-degree angle.
2. Keep your fingers straight and turn your wrist out, away from your body.
3. Place your thumb and index finger (other hand) on the two prominent bones on each side of your elbow. Measure the space between your fingers with a ruler or tape measure.
4. Compare the measurements to the following table.

This table gives you the measurements for *medium* frames. Anything below this measurement is a small frame, and above is a large frame.

Frame Size
Based on Height in 1-Inch Heels

WOMEN		MEN	
Height	Elbow Breadth	Height	Elbow Breadth
4'10" to 4'11"	2¼ to 2½"	5'2" to 5'3"	2½ to 2⅞"
5'0" to 5'3"	2¼ to 2½"	5'4" to 5'7"	2⅝ to 2⅞"
5'4" to 5'7"	2⅜ to 2⅝"	5'8" to 5'11"	2¾ to 3"
5'8" to 5'11"	2⅜ to 2⅝"	6'0" to 6'3"	2¾ to 3⅛"
6'0" to 6'3"	2½ to 2¾"	6'4" to 6'7"	2⅞ to 3¼"

▲ Food Skills ● Behavior Skills ◆ Exercise Skills

FRUIT DIET

A program that relies on fruits for primary calories, or a program that uses one fruit as a magic food, such as a grapefruit after each meal. While it is true that fruits are ideal diet foods, eating fruits without eating the other food groups can lead to nutrient deficiencies, dizziness, muscle losses, and a very inferior form of weight loss. Many diets use fruits as a focus, and are called fruit diets, when in actuality, they are calorie-cutting diets that highlight fruits. Most diets look for a handle or label to separate them from other diets, and isolating fruits is one way to get that handle. The problem is that these diets have led to confusion and misinformation about foods. Many dieters learned to dislike fruits after eating them exclusively for weeks and feeling the effects of solo fruit diets. Eating any food to excess, without the presence of the other food groups, is unhealthy, not only because of nutrient losses in the absence of other foods, but because this kind of eating creates distorted food habits and patterns. You can start out with a fat problem and wind up with major food problems after a bout with one of these extreme food diets.

▲ FRUITS

One of the essential food groups, sources of fiber, vitamins/minerals, and sugar; diet foods. *See* Fruits in the Problem Solver Diet section.

G

GALLSTONES

Hardened cholesterol/calcium deposits that are combined with bile. During digestion, your gallbladder secretes the bile needed to emulsify fats for metabolism. But bile can also be secreted by the liver. Deposits can form in the passage between your liver and gallbladder, in your gallbladder itself, or in the passage between your liver and intestines. The condition is more prevalent in people with diabetes, obesity, the elderly, and females. The recommended treatment is to avoid large meals and high-fat, high-cholesterol diets, and ensure that you are drinking plenty of water. The condition can require surgery and should be treated by a physician.

GASTRO-INTESTINAL

The parts of digestion that relate to your stomach and intestines, the two primary organs for breakdown of food into nutrients. *See* Digestion.

GENETIC

The inherited tendencies for disease or health. Many diseases, including obesity, have genetic tendencies. This doesn't mean that you *will* get them. Healthy diet and exercise can minimize your risk, and even prevent many diseases from occurring. *See* Causes; Risks.

GLUCOSE

The form of energy that carbohydrates take after they are digested and turned into nutrients that can be absorbed into your blood; a prime energy source for red blood cells; the simplest form of sugar. *See* Digestion.

▲ Food Skills   ● Behavior Skills   ◆ Exercise Skills

GLUCOSE HIGH

A sugar rush, usually accompanied by a dizzy feeling. It usually means your diet is too high in sugar. *See* Sugar; Epinepherine.

GLYCOGEN

The form carbohydrate nutrients take when they are stored in your body.

● GOALS

Expectations. The best way to achieve your diet goal is to take one day at a time, one pound at a time, using a healthy diet. This keeps you moving forward. Each step you take is an achievement, teaching you better eating and slimmer living. Over time, these habits will become natural—ingrained. This will keep you slim on a permanent basis.

GOUT

Inflammation of joints caused by uric acid salt deposts in joint tissues. This is a metabolic disturbance, where excess uric acid occurs in your blood. Protein is not metabolized properly, causing salt crystals to form around fingers, toes, heels, knees, or other joints. The deposits create bumps or growth that irritate your joints, and inflammation occurs. A gout attack begins in one joint and spreads to others before it abates. The pain is usually greatest in the morning, because your body processes have slowed down in sleep. An average attack can last five to ten days or more before abating. Reoccurrence is common. Gout is generally considered a hereditary disease that can be aggravated by obesity, aging, improper diet, overuse of alcohol, stress, and *rapid weight loss*. People with gout should avoid organ meats, since they contain purine, which can bring on an attack. The recommended treatment includes regular exercise, since that improves the circulatory system; good diet with moderate protein and low fat; and rest. The condition should be treated by a physician.

⇒ How-to Skills ♥ Good for Heart

▲ GRAINS

Seeds from grass such as wheat, rye, oats, rice, and barley; also called cereals, and used in flours, breads, and pastas. Known as the staff of life, grains can be viewed in two categories for easy references.

Whole grains: Grains that still contain the germ of the original grain.

Half grains: Grains that have been processed to remove the bran or germ or both. This is done to prolong the shelf life of grains, but all of the nutrients in the bran and germ are lost. These two parts are the most nutrient-rich components of the grain. The half grains are then fortified or enriched to replace some of the nutrients lost in milling, but it's not the same as the real thing.

The flours used in breads are ground and sifted grains. *Whole-grain flour* is the product of the first milling process. It contains the germ of the grain. The bran has been removed. Whole-grain flours still contain many nutrients. *Bleached flour* is refined flour, whitened to look good and is lowest in nutrients. *Enriched flour* can be a refined flour, or all-purpose flour, with added nutrients such as niacin, thiamine, riboflavin, and iron. *All-purpose flour* is a blend of different grains and can be mostly refined.

When you're choosing rices, the wild rices and whole-grain rices are the best. But check the labels of processed rice mixes or medleys, since they can contain fat and sodium. Look for the more natural ones.

White rice is dehulled and polished to look good. It has lost its B vitamins but can be enriched. *Converted rice* is the better of the white rices, slightly higher in vitamins. *Brown rice* is a rich source of B vitamins, calcium, phosphorous, and iron. *Wild rice* is the tops, containing twice the nutrients as white. *See* Grain varieties in the Problem Solver Diet section.

● GUILT

Self-criticism and blame, a useless emotion. *See* Relaxation to let it go.

H

▲ HABITS

Learned behaviors that are ingrained through repetition. How is a habit formed? Usually in childhood by watching other people or by responding to situations in your own unique way. You may still use yellow number nine pencils today because you used them in school during the year that you got A's. Or you may not like to use blue ink because that's the ink color on report cards when you got demerits. This generation's kids will use computers instead of pens or pencils when they're adults. Some may keep computers in their bedrooms, as they're doing now. Some may start working after midnight because they're night owls now.

You can reverse a habit you had as a child because it reminds you of something that felt uncomfortable then. For instance, you always walked to school, every day, rain or shine, while your neighbor rode in a red convertible her parents gave her when she was sixteen. You don't walk anywhere now—you drive. Your car may even be red.

Your moods and attitudes can also be habits. You may wake up every morning and dread getting out of bed. There doesn't seem to be a reason for it. It's a habit you picked up somewhere along the way in life. You may get up every day at dawn and run ten miles, after spending four years as a marine because the habit was trained into you. You may eat chocolate cream pie every time you feel depressed. Somewhere along the way, you ate chocolate cream pie and it cheered you up on a bad day.

Some habits help you gain weight, while others help you get lean. The art of behavior modification is to substitute good habits for poor ones. The more good habits you can gain to outweigh the poorer habits, the greater your chances of staying lean for life.

There are four areas to consider when you are reviewing your weight-gaining habits: eating habits, exercise habits, "diet"—specific eating habits—and overall daily habits. As you can see, these add up to the habits that make your lifestyle, or whole day. To see real results, you shouldn't expect to change all of these habits *at the same time*. That's too much change to introduce into your life at one time, and change causes stress. The best way to make positive

---

habit changes is to change one or two at a time, practicing the new habit until you do it naturally, on automatic pilot. Then you can change other habits in the same way. Slow, steady change is the best way to make a new habit last. If you try to shake up your whole life overnight for a diet, before long you'll be back to your old habits again.

⇒ *How to Change Weight-gaining Habits*

Eating habits
Change your irregular eating and low-nutrition plan to a regular food plan that ensures your daily nutrition.

Exercise habits
Change your no-action plan to a regular action plan three times per week, aerobic, thirty minutes a session.

Diet-related habits
Use skill power instead of willpower to get to ideal weight.

Daily habits
Change no-priority setting to regular priority review.
How do you do it all the easy way? *See* the Problem Solver Calendar.

❤ **HDL**
High Density Lipoprotein. Good Cholesterol in your body. *See* Cholesterol.

HEALTH
A state of well-being that is free of disease, and usually low-risk or risk-free for the major lifestyle diseases, such as hypertension, heart disease, diabetes, and cancer. This implies many things. First, you are at your ideal body weight and you got there in a healthy way. Second, you don't use addictive substances or sleeping aids. It also means that you adhere to the basic dietary guidelines for good health. To be considered healthy, you also have to use exercise on a regular basis. Most of the conditions of ill-health can be dramatically improved by a healthy diet for weight

▲ Food Skills   ● Behavior Skills   ◆ Exercise Skills

loss, since that automatically includes the factors needed for overall health. But is that all there is to health? It must include a good attitude, sense of purpose, stress control, self-respect, and even spiritual beliefs. The definition of health is an issue that can go on indefinitely, since health itself is never static. At any given moment, old cells are dying in your body while new ones are being created. At the same time, the environment is changing, creating new situations that will affect health.

In addition, you can have diabetes that is being controlled, and you can still be very healthy. The key to health, more than anything, is found in the efforts you make to achieve it. Seeking positive things and continuing to seek the positive are the foundation of a healthy life.

When it comes to weight loss, most people don't realize that the _process_ is far more important than a weight goal on the scale. When the process is positive, the results are positive, and the weight goal becomes secondary to the thrill of health. When you diet healthfully, everything else takes care of itself. This year, resolve to diet healthfully. It's the best thing you can do for your life.

HEALTH BENEFITS, OF EXERCISE
See Exercise.

HEALTH RISKS
Weight-related diseases or disorders. _See_ Risks.

HEIGHT/WEIGHT TABLES
Averages of people by weight and height, in relation to mortality statistics.

Height/weight tables are accurate indicators of height, but vague indicators of ideal body weight. The weights do not reflect body composition, simply overall weight. That's like weighing a one gallon container of water that is sealed, guessing that it's primarily water inside. The weight could be sugar and water, or it could be part water and part fat. In the case of your body, it has fat, muscle, and water. Your fat content is important, but your

---

⟹　How-to Skills　　　❤　Good for Heart

muscle content is far more important, because that determines how much fat you can keep gaining. The water content should remain stable at all times for proper metabolism and health, and water is 55 to 60 percent of your overall weight.

Dieters spend so much energy reading their weights on scales, unaware that those five-pound ups and downs can be water fluctuations, not fat loss or gain. A major part of the weight-loss seen in the first week or two on a rapid weight-loss diet is water, but you think you're losing fat because the scale says five pounds less. When you see your weight as a general indicator, and your body composition as the key to better weight loss, you'll be making a major step forward to ideal body weight in the right proportions.

Body weight is a personal and sensitive issue. Numbers on weight tables should never be read as judgments or rating systems for your sense of self-worth. They are simply numbers for ideal goals. You can be ideal at a higher weight if you're comfortable there and it isn't a weight-risk issue. Or you can go for the gold in fitness, which is reaching your desirable weight with a higher content of body muscle, just for the thrill of health and maintenance. If you change your scale-reading habit to a label-reading habit to get the weight out of your food, you'll reach the numbers on weight tables with a body composition to match. *See* Ideal Weight, for the height/weight tables. *See* Scale, to find the facts about your body composition, which is a better measure of fitness than weight alone.

▲ HERBS AND SPICES

Salt replacers, seasonings, and taste enhancers for dieters. Herbs and spices provide taste and pleasure, in addition to nutrition. You can use them in sauces and gravies to replace salt, fat, and sugar, without feeling deprived. They make excellent teas and garnishes for salads, soups, casseroles, and stews. They can spice up potato skins for low-fat snacks. Set up an herb and spice rack in your kitchen to take the place of all the salty condiments that lead to sodium excess, and eventually hypertension. Don't confuse the real herbs and spices with the herb or spice *salts* that are available in your supermarket. The salts contain sodium or MSG.

Choose the *powder* versions, but it might help to glance at the labels to be sure. There are a variety of spices to choose from, the fresher the better.

▲ Food Skills ● Behavior Skills ◆ Exercise Skills

Basil	Curry	Paprika
Bay leaf	Dill	Parsley
Caraway	Fennel	Peppers
Celery seed	Garlic	Poppy seeds
Chervil	Ginger	Pumpkin spice
Chili powder	Marjoram	Rosemary
Cinnamon	Mustard	Saffron
Cloves	Nutmeg	Sage
Coriander	Onion	Tarragon
Cumin	Oregano	Thyme

HORMONE

A chemical produced in one organ for a specific use in another organ during metabolism.

HUNGER, PHYSIOLOGICAL

The need for nutrients; biological hunger. It is controlled by your appetite center. *See* Appetite.

● HUNGER, PSYCHOLOGICAL

Desire for food (as opposed to a *need* for food.) Sometimes called "imaginary hunger," or conditioned hunger.

Hunger that follows feelings—such as anxiety, depression, boredom, fear, confusion.

Hunger based on habit—repeating a pattern of eating that was learned in the past, such as eating to ease stress. You can have a conditioned response to eat certain foods for reward, such as chocolate, ice cream, sweets. Often these foods were used for rewards in childhood, or withheld for punishment.

Hunger from food cues—such as seeing food, smelling food, or being in the presence of food. You can respond to the sight of food with an increase in salivation and blood insulin levels, as in biological hunger.

Psychological hunger is real, because you feel it, but it is not triggered by your body's need for nutrition. It is cued from a learning process. It's similar to an actor in a play, being *cued* to recite his lines after certain music, action, or gestures—and after constant rehearsals—except you are cued to eat. Eating will not satisfy the real need for emotional comfort, and in most cases eating will only increase the problems, creating guilt and feelings of helplessness after the eating is over. Something is needed instead of food. That's where behavior modification comes in. Using behavior skills, you learn to recognize your nonbiological hunger and deal with it. Once you identify the cues, habits, and moods that lead you to eat, you use your knowledge to change your responses and routines. In this sense, hunger becomes a catalyst to use for self-improvement. *See* Diary, Food to learn how to understand your hunger.

HYDROGENATED

A process used to turn a vegetable-oil fat into a harder fat, so it will be solid at room temperature for use as a spread. *See* Cholesterol.

HYPERPLASTIC

Fat cells that are normal size but occur in greater numbers. Common to adolescent-onset obesity. *See* Fat Cells.

HYPERTHYROIDISM

Hormone overproduction by your thyroid. Excessive thyroid hormones speed up your body processes, particularly your metabolism. This causes your nutrients to be used at a faster rate. The symptoms are sudden weight loss, rapid pulse, nervousness, fatigue, weakness, goiter. Since nutrient depletion can be extreme, muscle losses occur with hyperthyroidism. The recommended treatment is an increased nutrient diet with extra protein for muscle losses, and vitamin B complex for metabolism of extra protein and carbohydrates. This condition should be treated by a physician.

HYPERTROPHIC

Fat cells swollen with fat. Common to adult-onset obesity. *See* Fat Cells.

▲ Food Skills ● Behavior Skills ◆ Exercise Skills

HYPOGLYCEMIA

Low blood glucose, brought about by overproduction of insulin, which removes glucose from the blood. Hypoglycemia can be caused by several factors. Eating too much refined sugar can cause your blood sugar to rise rapidly. This, in turn, prompts your pancreas to secrete insulin. When too much insulin circulates regularly, too much glucose is removed. Underlying disorders can lead to hypoglycemia also, such as tumors in your pancreas that stimulate overproduction of insulin, or it can be caused by liver disorders. The symptoms are fatigue, constant hunger, weak legs, swollen feet, tight chest, headaches, eyeaches, pain, nervousness, insomnia, and often mental disorders. Reducing the consumption of refined sugars in your diet guards against the disease. A glucose tolerance test is recommended. The disease should be treated by a physician.

HYPOTHYROIDISM

Hormone underproduction by your thyroid. This is generally caused by heredity and includes an iron deficiency. Symptoms are decreased appetite, fatigue, insomnia, dry skin and hair, and constipation. This condition should be treated by a physician.

I

IDEAL BODY WEIGHT

The recommended weight for your height, sex, and frame, that gives you the best disease-prevention status. These weights as-

WOMEN			MEN		
Height		Weight	Height		Weight
FT	IN		FT	IN	
4	10	96-107	5	2	118-129
4	11	98-110	5	3	121-133
5	0	101-113	5	4	124-136
5	1	104-116	5	5	127-139
5	2	107-119	5	6	130-143
5	3	110-122	5	7	134-147
5	4	113-126	5	8	138-152
5	5	116-130	5	9	142-156
5	6	120-135	5	10	146-150
5	7	124-139	5	11	150-165
5	8	128-143	6	0	154-170
5	9	132-147	6	1	158-175
5	10	136-151	6	2	162-180
5	11	140-155	6	3	167-185
6	0	144-159	6	4	172-190

Small-framed women can weigh four to six pounds less than the lowest number. Large-framed women can weigh ten to twelve pounds more than the highest number.

Small-framed men can weigh six to eight pounds less than the lowest number. Large-framed men can weigh twelve to fourteen pounds more than the highest number.

These tables are based on lean versions of the Metropolitan Life Tables.

▲ Food Skills   ● Behavior Skills   ◆ Exercise Skills

sume that you have a high-muscle, low-fat body as your ideal. (*See* Scale for body-fat ratings.) If you are small framed, you should weigh less than these values at ideal. If you are large framed, you can weigh more. To find your frame size, *see* Frame.

● IMAGERY

The skill to imagine or visualize yourself successful with future goals. *Seeing* yourself slim and healthy. *Picturing* yourself successful. Imagery exercises are used in weight control to strengthen your mind's ability to claim or own what you want (a slimmer, healthy body), so that it will become more attainable and feel more real when you achieve it.

Imagery exercises are especially helpful if you have always been overweight, since the thinner image at the end of a diet can seem unrealistic or out of reach, because you've never felt it, never experienced it firsthand. The exercises allow you to experience the feelings of being slim, even when you are currently overweight. This lifts a great weight off your internal belief systems that keeps repeating that you are fat and keep you feeling fat. Combine the power of imagery with a healthy fat burning diet, and the weight can be lifted off for life.

How to Do Thin-within Imagery

The first step to thin-within imagery is to get a clear picture of yourself as a slimmer, healthy person. To do this, sit in a comfortable chair and let your entire body relax. (Close your eyes.) Let go of all distractions. Bring the picture into your mind of a slimmer you. Once you get your picture, let yourself experience what it feels like to be the slim you. Can you feel your muscles and a new sense of your body? Let yourself feel the movements of the slim you. Are they graceful, strong, confident? Feel the climate and the clothes you are wearing. Locate yourself in pleasant surroundings, feel the air on your skin. Feel yourself walking, running, swimming, or playing tennis with friends. Feel yourself breathing in and out. Now bring the image into the present and believe that you exist this way *now*. Talk to yourself, saying, "I feel strong and happy," or describe what you feel. Always use the present tense, such as "I am . . . ," not "I will be. . . ." This is *now*. You are slim and healthy. Suspend all doubt that enters your mind; forget

---

your present weight; and believe you are slim now. Let yourself feel this way for a few minutes, then open your eyes and go on with your day.

Try to use this technique each day for five minutes, when you wake in the morning, or before retiring in the evening. It's a powerful, exhilarating feeling to let go of your weight.

INCHES
Weight-loss measurements that are usually preferred to pounds on scales, since they don't fluctuate as regularly.

INNER SELF
The unique collection of attributes that make you distinct and different from everyone else. The inner self is often called the *real self* because it is not subject to superficial views of self-worth and self-value, such as appearance, physique, weight, or social opinions of worth such as money, clothes, popularity, or position in society. The inner self isn't rewarded by these things. It is rewarded by *feelings* of well-being and self-value, and often that means having spiritual beliefs as the source of strength. The inner self is the most valuable factor in weight loss, because you can change your outer self (get thinner) but still not satisfy your inner self.

▲ INPUT
Calories eaten, specifically on a daily basis. Input is one-half of the energy scale that determines your weight, or weight regulation. The balanced state is:
  • Input Equals Output
  • Calories Eaten Equal Calories Burned
Imbalances exist in the energy scale in overweight and the dieting phase. *See* Obesity, for the total picture.

INSULIN
A hormone produced by your pancreas to help metabolize glucose, the nutrient derived from carbohydrates in digestion. After a meal, insulin is secreted. This causes your system to go into a

---

▲ Food Skills   ● Behavior Skills   ◆ Exercise Skills

nutrient storage phase, to save part of the nutrients from digestion. Your liver stores glucose as glycogen; your adipose tissue
stores fatty acids as lipids. Other nutrients from digestion were
absorbed and are circulating in your blood. These nutrients are
delivered to the cells for energy for metabolism. A few hours after
your meal, when the blood supply of nutrients is depleted, insulin
decreases and your pancreas secretes another hormone—gluca-
gon. This causes nutrients to be released from storage for use as
energy. Your liver releases stored glucose, your adipose tissue releases fatty acids, and metabolism continues, this time from stored
nutrients. This process is repeated with each meal. It's your body's
way of conserving and metering out nutrients so that it can maintain itself throughout the day.

In diabetes, not enough insulin is produced, or none is produced. The process for metabolizing carbohydrates is not possible, and glucose metabolism is inhibited. *See* Diabetes.

♦ INTERVAL TRAINING

A method for gradually developing your aerobic potential without
stress or strain. Interval training is a fail-safe way for beginners to
build their fitness levels gradually. It lets you start at your own
pace and gradually increase your speed and build endurance. You
use timed bouts of exercise and follow with rest periods to enable
you to last the full exercise session. This is especially important for
beginners on exercise machines.

Your exercise sessions start off with short bouts and gradually
increase in duration, according to your progress. The exercise
bouts are continued until they total twenty to thirty minutes of
aerobic activity. Beginning exercisers finish with the satisfaction of
knowing they completed the same workout as a seasoned exerciser
would, but without jeopardizing their health or motivation.

How to Do Interval Training

- Start with three to five minutes on a machine at a slow pace, or
  as your target heart rate dictates.
- Take two to four minutes off, but keep moving—walk around
  the room until your heart rate slows down.
- *Never stop completely!* This would shock your system.

- Do another three- to five-minute session, then stop and walk around.
- Complete six sessions.

As your fitness level improves, the length of each session can be increased, but continue to monitor your heart rate. Do not wait until you get symptoms of overexertion such as dizziness or nausea—these are danger signals.

You should strive to increase the length of your exercise session every two to four weeks, but you will need to be faithful to your workout routine to attain this goal. This pace of advancement is not mandatory. Go at your own pace. An interval workout is the same as one long exercise session. *See* Exercise.

INTESTINAL MOTILITY
The speed at which your intestines digest and eliminate food. *See* Digestion; Food Transit Time.

◆ ISOMETRICS
An exercise technique based on tensing muscles, holding the tension, then relaxing, often against a stationary object; muscle resistance. It can be used to tone specific areas and is good for toning the skeletal muscles.

J

♦ JOGGING

An aerobic exercise.

Benefits:
- Excellent cardiovascular training
- Excellent calorie-burning activity
- Convenient: requires only the time to get dressed, warm up, and go
- Able to enjoy the fresh outdoors, altering your path for variety
- Easily transferred to an indoor track
- High degree of peer support

Guidelines:
- Jogging should not be an exercise choice if you are more than thirty pounds over your goal weight.
- A walk-jog pattern can be incorporated (walk five minutes, jog two minutes, for instance) as you gradually improve your level of fitness.
- Make sure you have very supportive running shoes and proper attire for the climate.
- Stop jogging (and walk) if you experience side cramps or any muscle or joint pains.
- Always warm up with stretching to avoid injury.

Some bodies are better structured for jogging then others. Yet, with any body type, there's a high risk of injury to knees, ankles, and calves because of pounding on hard surfaces.

▲ JUNK FOOD

A subjective view of food. To some people, junk foods are empty calorie food such as cola, jelly beans, taffy—100 percent sugar. To others, junk foods are ones with little nutrient value for the calories, such as refined and processed foods, vending machine foods, cinema snacks, candy. Many processed foods contain all of the requirements for junk foods—high sodium, high sugar, high fat, few vitamins and minerals, lots of additives, minimal fiber. To certain age groups, junk foods are preferred foods, such as burgers, fries, chips, franks, and shakes. To vegetarians, junk foods can be meats. To kids who don't like to eat spinach, that can be a junk food. To Popeye, it would be a power food.

The point is, seeing food as junk, regardless of the food, isn't good food sense. In areas of the world where there is no food, jelly beans would seem like manna, and they would provide a form of energy, even if it isn't the best. Extreme attitudes about food aren't healthy, because they can create food fears in your mind. When you tell yourself, "I can't have that," your first instinct is to want it. When you say "I can have it, but I don't want it," you're gaining control over food, instead of food controlling you.

The best way to handle your versions of junk foods is to learn the ingredients and make sensible decisions about those foods and you.

Ask yourself: How much nutrition am I getting for the calories? Does it replace other foods in my diet? Many people rely on low-nutrition foods for bursts of sugar energy, and they never get real nutrition on a daily basis.

The best plan for a dieter is to aim for the most nutritionally dense foods during the weight-loss phase to get the best fat burn. Later, in maintenance, you can reevaluate your junk foods, and see if they fit into your diet in a more restricted way, one that you can handle without gaining weight. Of course, by then, you may not want low-nutrition foods anymore. Somehow, they lose their magic when you realize what's in them and the price you paid in weight gain.

➡️ *How to Find the Low-nutrition Foods*

High-sugar foods. The foods that have large quantites of excess sugar are not the best for you. These include colas, many sodas, and fruit drinks, since they contain ten to twelve teaspoons of sugar in each can and provide empty calories.

High-sugar/fat foods. Usually the high-sugar foods are also high in fat, and it may be the fat that makes the sugar food so palatable. Check the labels on cereals to see if they are high in sugar and have added fats. Some cereals can have two to four teaspoons of sugar in one cup. Sweets and desserts are high-sugar and high-fat foods that provide little real nutrition because they are often over-

▲ Food Skills ● Behavior Skills ◆ Exercise Skills

processed. Cakes, pies, and ice cream fit in this category. That doesn't mean that you should never eat a slice of pie again. Select the ones with less sugar and fat, and if you make pies or cakes at home, modify your recipes to be less fattening. While you are dieting, it's best to avoid these foods, or learn to moderate your use of them by eating smaller portions less often. A piece of cake once a week will not add on a pound of fat, but cake every night will add up fast. Chocolate bars and candy bars provide a few carbohydrates, but the sugar and fat they contain are not worth the risk. If you rely on candy for quick boosts of energy, switch to fruit or grains instead.

High-sodium foods. You can find foods that are low in sugar and fat, but high in sodium, which is bad for your heart and overall health. Many canned foods are high sodium, so check the labels. Also be sure you're not adding extra sodium in cooking and at the table.

You will find that limiting sugar, fat, and sodium in your diet is the automatic way to lose your extra weight. Often, you can make the greatest impact on your diet by simply limiting the high-sugar foods, since they usually have those hidden fats that add so much weight.

If you have a particular food you eat to excess, and it's one that is not nutritious, slowly train yourself away from that food by cutting your portions in half, then to one-fourth, then to one-eighth. Also eat it less frequently and slowly decrease the frequency from eating it every day, to every other day, to once a week, then once a month. This is the best way to retrain yourself not to need this food.

K

KETOGENIC DIETS

Diets that produce excess ketones from carbohydrate restriction. Some experts feel that ketone-producing diets should be avoided, since they are associated with muscle tissue wasting. Others claim there is use for these diets in cases of severe or morbid obesity, where the overweight condition is life threatening. It is believed that muscle losses are acceptable in very obese people, since they have more muscle tissue, along with excess fat tissue. In these cases, measuring ketones with the use of a ketostick is seen as an aid in compliance, since dieters can see if they are adhering to the program by measuring their ketone output in daily urine. However, this is a subject of continued debate among scientists, since the risk/benefit ratio is unclear. *Ketone diets cannot be used by people with insulin dependent type I diabetes. Also, ketone diets should not be used without medical supervision.*

If you are *not* in your doctor's care for your diet, a ketone-producing diet is not a good choice. The primary source of energy for your muscles is glucose from carbohydrates. This is your body's preferred energy. If you have no carbohydrate energy in your body, your muscles can use ketones for metabolism, and your brain can use ketones, but this is a situation that is also associated with famine conditions. The best form of fat burn occurs with balanced diets that are high in carbohydrates, and you don't suffer muscle losses. Even if you are obese, this is the best way to burn fat and protect yourself against weight regain at maintenance.

KETONES

Byproducts of fat metabolism, specifically in low- or no-carbohydrate diets. Ketones are sometimes called incompletely burned fat. They are also produced during anaerobic exercise, when oxygen supply is limited. *See* Exercise, Anaerobic.

▲ Food Skills   ● Behavior Skills   ◆ Exercise Skills

KETOSIS
A metabolic state usually associated with no- or low-carbohydrate diets, where ketones are produced as byproducts of weight loss.

KILOGRAM
A weight measurement that equals 2.2 pounds.

● KITCHEN
A food cue; an environment that inspires you to eat.

There are two schools of thought about kitchen problems for dieters, and the diet you choose will dictate what skill you should use: approach or avoidance.

The problem with diets that are too different from everyday life is that they have no relationship to your real food issues. Therefore, they can't really solve them. And the feeling of being ostracized is associated with dieting, and that makes dieting seem like a negative thing. At their best, they can help you lose weight, but you've got to go through the entire approach phase to relearn how to relate to your real life. It's a lot to expect from a person with a weight/food problem. It drags out the diet process, and makes the whole business take so long.

The advantage of diets that are natural and lifestyle-related is that they are patterns for how to eat healthily and still lose weight. They don't disrupt your lifestyle, and they don't create a gap between dieting and maintaining. As a result, you are less likely to fall into the gap when you come off your diet and start maintaining your new weight. And they make kitchens places where you can feel safe. *See* Cooking.

➠ How-to Skills ❤ Good for Heart

Avoidance	Approach
Rationale: Since food cues make you eat, the best course is to minimize the food cues, stay away from food.	**Rationale:** Since you have to deal with food, and the problem isn't going to go away, learn how to take charge of it.
Theme: Don't deal with food decisions while on a diet. Use a follow-along plan. 　Save food decisions for maintenance.	**Theme:** Deal with food decisions while you're on a diet, and food problems will be solved by the time you reach maintenance.
Flaw: By maintenance, it's too late. You haven't learned the skills you need to avoid weight regain. 　Food still has all those old associations.	**Advantage:** You carry over the skills you learned, and adapt them to a higher calorie level. Food doesn't threaten you as it did. Weight regain is less likely.
Where it's most commonly used: In diets that are different from normal eating plans, such as diets with food replacement supplements, special foods, or eating styles that are not average.	**Where it's most commonly used:** In diets that are similar to normal eating plans, but are lower in overall calories, and based on nutrient density of foods.
Common avoidance techniques: Strip the kitchen of all nondiet foods.	**Common approach techniques:** Learn what's in the food you're eating so you can choose wisely.
Eat only certain foods.	Eat less fats and more carbohydrates. 　Moderate your food intake.
If you have a family, keep your food separate from their food.	If you have a family, your food isn't different from their food, you just eat better.

▲　Food Skills　　　●　Behavior Skills　　　◆　Exercise Skills

L

● LABEL READING

Food education made easy. Reading the labels on foods in the supermarket is a sure-fire way to wake you up quickly to the sources of your fat, sugar, and salt problems. First read the sections on sugar, sodium, and additives to get the information you need for expert label reading. Then take a day and investigate the labels of the most common foods you eat. Food is the fuel for your metabolism and the source of your health and energy. One day in the supermarket can make your future lean.

➡ *How to Read Labels*

Foods are listed on labels *in order of their weight* in the product. If you pick up a box of crackers or a pasta mix and sugar is listed first, that means sugar outweighs all the other ingredients in the box. You're eating sugar, not a grain product. You can pick up a pack of granola bars, a substitute for candy, isn't that right? Sugar can be the first ingredient on the label. You can pick up a cereal that has sugar listed first, grains listed about midpoint, and ten different additives—and the product is called a Natural Wheat Cereal, meaning that the wheat part, which is minimal by weight, is a natural wheat. What are you going to do? Pick the best products with the least fat, sugar, salt, and additives. Then make sure you fill in your diet with fresh vegetables for fiber that will be missing from these processed foods.

Label Guide to Diet Foods

Read the labels on diet foods, using the same technique as above. Diet foods are divided into three basic categories:

1. Light or Lite. The food inside contains no more than forty calories per ounce. The food must be similar in taste, smell, and texture to the food it is representing, but it must contain at least one-third fewer calories than an equal quantity of that food.

2. Low Calorie. The food inside contains no more than forty calories per ounce. As to what makes up those calories, you have to check the sugar and fat content.
3. Reduced Calories. The food inside must contain at least one-third fewer calories than an equal quantity of the same food. You have to check the fat and sugar calories.

At first you might feel defeated when you start reading the labels on foods in your supermarket, but don't give up. After you discover what's really in the foods you're eating and what is not, you'll be surprised at how quickly you pick up on the food game in packaging and advertising. The choices you make will automatically become better ones. Each choice is a big step toward better nutrition and fat burn. It will not only make you a better dieter, it's food education you can use for life.

The Label Game
The importance of label reading cannot be stressed too much. Think about a cola. Then think about taking the ingredients listed on a label and make a cola of your own, just to see what you're getting. Take ten teaspoons of sugar and put it in a glass. Add a touch of coloring. Take a teaspoon of salt (to represent all the additives), spray it with food coloring, and add it to the glass. Add water, shake, and add ice. Makes you think twice, doesn't it?

You can do this with an assortment of your favorite fattening foods. Be creative and show your friends. It will de-fat you. Take a piece of cake (find your favorite on the supermarket shelf and read the label). Go home and make a mix of white flour, sugar, liquid bacon fat, and salt to represent the additives. Think about baking it.

Reading labels can teach you everything you need to know about food. It's the quickest way to help you reduce the excesses in your diet. You don't have to cut these foods out forever. Limit them. Ration them. Put them in their proper place. Make a game out of them. When you don't buy them, the manufacturers snap into action and start producing better varieties. So everybody wins.

LACTOSE
Sugar in dairy products, naturally occurring, or refined and added to other foods. *See* Sugar.

▲ Food Skills   ● Behavior Skills   ◆ Exercise Skills

LBM

Lean body mass; also called body muscle, body protein, or muscle tissue. Lean body mass is usually a combination of muscle weight, water weight, and bones. It is generally assumed that everything that *is not fat* is your lean body mass, or fat-free mass. *See* Weight.

LDL

Low Density Lipoprotein; bad cholesterol in your body. *See* Cholesterol.

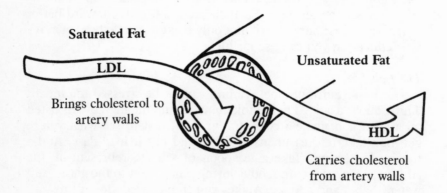

Saturated Fat

LDL

Unsaturated Fat

Brings cholesterol to
artery walls

HDL

Carries cholesterol
from artery walls

● LIFESTYLE

A series of habits that make your day. A single habit is a behavior that is learned and ingrained by repetition. For instance, what's the first thing you do in the morning when you get out of bed? Brush your teeth? Do a few stretching exercises? Head for the coffee pot? These are habits. How do you eat breakfast? At the table? On the run? In the car? None? Habits. How do you handle stress? Get angry? Take a tranquilizer? Eat? They're all habits.

Your lifestyle is the sum of habits you do each day from the time you wake to the time you reset the alarm at bedtime. Even your sleeping patterns fall into the lifestyle picture. Step by step, from morning to night, your habits create a pattern of life (your style) that can be healthy or harmful, that can add or subtract weight.

To create a lifestyle that leads to ideal weight and health; you need more than a food-restricted diet. You need to take conscious charge of your habits.

⇒ How-to Skills ❤ Good for Heart

MAKE A FEW COPIES OF OUR LIFESTYLE PIE

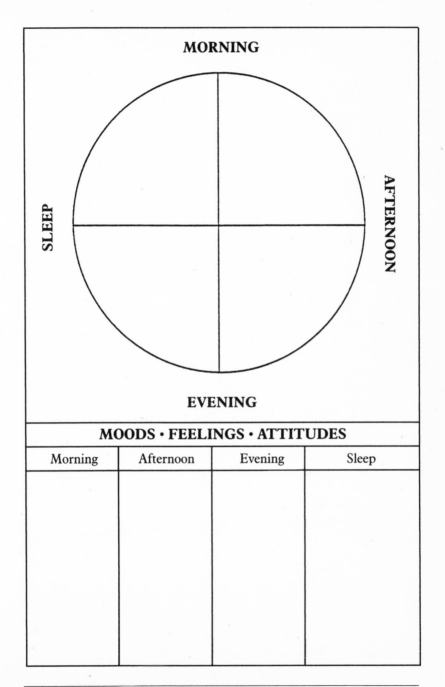

Morning	Afternoon	Evening	Sleep

▲ Food Skills   ● Behavior Skills   ♦ Exercise Skills

To do this, you need to know the patterns of your normal life-style and what you can do to make it work for you instead of against you.

The quickest way to get a complete picture of your lifestyle is to make a lifestyle pie. This is a behavior modification skill to make you aware of your current habits.

⟫ *How to Make a Lifestyle Pie*

Use the lifestyle pie design on the opposite page.

Fill in everything you do in one day as you do it, and include the time. Use the bottom of the page to make notes about your reactions to particular issues, your feelings, or comments you want to make. Use the back side of the page if you need more room.

Make a pie for at least four days, including two weekend days, to get an accurate picture of your lifestyle.

Review your lifestyle at the end of each day.

⟫ *How to Create a Slim Lifestyle*

What kind of lifestyle do you need to get lean and stay lean? You need to add the following as a routine part of your week.

1. Aerobic exercise every *other* day for thirty minutes. *See* Exercise.
2. Relaxation exercises for fifteen to twenty minutes every day. *See* Breathing; Meditation; Relaxation.
3. Food review daily for fifteen minutes. *See* the Problem Solver food pyramid.
4. Self time daily for fifteen minutes. For any self-strengthening exercise. *See* Behavior Topics ●; Imagery; Positive Self-Talk.

If you use this plan during your diet, you will reach ideal weight in the best physical and emotional shape to maintain your weight. The new you that emerges at the end of your diet phase will be an exhilarating experience.

Lifestyle checkup. Make a new lifestyle pie every four weeks to see how you are improving or if you are falling back into old habits and patterns that lead to weight gain. Adjust your pie regularly.

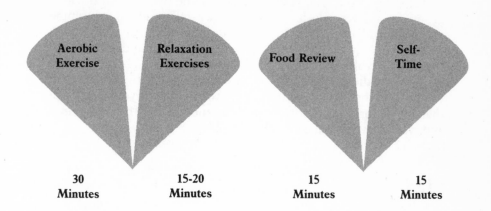

Aerobic Exercise	Relaxation Exercises	Food Review	Self-Time
30 Minutes	**15-20 Minutes**	**15 Minutes**	**15 Minutes**

Advanced lifestyle pie. Once you've added your slices of life to your pie and are comfortable with them, you can move on to advanced lifestyle study. Look at your other habits and see which ones need changing. The new strength you've gained from healthy eating, regular exercise, and positive self-support will give you confidence to achieve other goals.

● LIFESTYLE CHANGE

Substituting healthy habits for unhealthy ones to improve your style of life. If you see your lifestyle as a chain of habits that link together to make your day, then each habit is a link in the chain. When one link is weak, the chain is weakened. If three or four links are weak, the chain can break. To change your lifestyle, you take one habit at a time and strengthen it. Since the chain is interconnected, when you strengthen the weak links, you are strengthening the whole chain. The weakest links for dieters are exercise, food, and self-empowering techniques such as relaxation, meditation, and positive reinforcement on a regular basis. When you strengthen these links, you can reach ideal weight and maintain it. *See* Lifestyle, to find out how to do it.

● LIFESTYLE DIET

A program that uses exercise and behavior modification as part of its healthy diet program. The key here is healthy diet, because a program can use behavior modification and exercise, but the diet

▲ Food Skills   ● Behavior Skills   ◆ Exercise Skills

might not be up to par. A healthy diet is one that uses all the food groups in a lower calorie setting, so that you get all your essential nutrients and learn how to use food to accomplish your fitness goals. That way, you're set for life, because you can deal with real food in the real world where the problems began. When you settle for less in a diet, you lose. Learn to expect more from a diet than weight loss that doesn't last. You're worth it. And your body will thank you for it. You'll see the difference in health, well-being, and weight maintenance. *See* the Problem Solver Calendar (pages 107–112).

LIPIDS
Fat deposits in your cells or blood; also called triglycerides.

LIPOPROTEIN
A substance in your body that contains fat (lipid) and protein. It's the substance that carries cholesterol in your blood. *See* Cholesterol.

LIPOSUCTION
Surgery to remove fat cells. *See* Fat Cells; Cellulite.

LIQUID PROTEIN DIETS
Diets that were blamed for deaths from chronic muscle losses. These diets were a fad more than a decade ago and consisted of liquid drinks which were high in protein. It was found that the form of protein used in these formulas was a nonmetabolic variety, and this caused loss of muscle from vital organs such as the heart. Your body needs protein to rebuild its cells and muscle, including protein for hemoglobin in your blood. It must get the protein in the form of amino acids in the pattern needed to make a new protein. Eight of the amino acids can't be made by your body, and you must get them from food. The protein in these liquid diets did not provide the amino acids that the body could use. As a result, it was as if no protein was eaten, and the body had to take its protein from its own inner sources. *See* Amino Acids.

▲ LITE
A category for diet food labeling. *See* Label Reading.

M

♦ **MACHINES, EXERCISE**

Stationary aerobic exercise devices. Exercise equipment is a superior way to work out because of the intensity of the workout, but it is important that you gradually build up, so you prevent overexertion. This can be done with *interval training*. *See* Exercise; Interval Training. Look up machines by type of exercise, such as Rowing, Cross-Country Skiing.

MAGIC BULLET

A pill or pill-like formula that is seen as the cure for weight problems; a gimmick; fad. If you're the kind of dieter who looks for a magic pill for your weight problems, you're not alone. Most dieters have experimented with some form of fad, and it takes a lot of failure to cure the habit. Part of it has been created by our culture that promotes fast cures in TV and magazine ads, and it doesn't go away by pretending it doesn't exist. Even scientists are looking for magic pills to end our weight-loss problems once and forever, but they know the difference between realistic expectations and false one. So do you, and yet you still get lured by that magic pill idea. Consider this one: it's a pill-like part of grains—the center or *kernel*—filled with nutrition and a source of carbohydrates that are significant for weight loss. So there you are, it's the magic pill you've been looking for all along.

MAGIC FORMULA

A mix that is seen as the cure for weight loss. Everyone likes to believe in magic, and the entire staff of Walt Disney is there to prove that magic can be a positive part of life. It can be a positive part of weight loss too, if you look for the magic in the right place—your food and exercise.

The best formula for fat burn contains the following real food:

Complex carbs 60%
Lean protein 20%

▲ Food Skills   ● Behavior Skills   ♦ Exercise Skills

```
Low fat ............................. 20%
Water ............................... 2 Quarts
Vitamin/mineral tablet ............... 1
Exercise ............................ 3 x per week/
                                       30 minutes/session.
```

This formula would work on Prince Charming, Snow White, Rose Red, Bugs Bunny, Elmur Fudd, Mickey and Minnie Mouse, and you.

Who said science isn't filled with magic?

● MAINTENANCE, IDEAL WEIGHT

The energy eaten equals energy burned.

Maintenance Contingency Plan

Set a weight that you will not exceed, in the event that you start letting too much fat creep back into your diet.

```
Suggested signal:   Eight pounds
                    (Five pounds can be
                        water fluctuations)
      Pre-signal:   Five pounds
```

If you gain five pounds and stay there for two or three weeks, review your food pyramid and exercise and use them to evaluate where you're slacking off. Reduce your sodium intake and increase your water drinking, and if the weight stays there, begin to take action. Keep in mind that a five-pound gain can be muscle, if you are still eating soundly and exercising regularly. The best way to check is the fit of your clothes.

If your weight creeps up eight pounds, return to your diet phase for a few weeks. If you were carrying extra fat for a long time, it may be that you need a period of stabilization. Don't see this as a sign of failure! It's just another step to weight maintenance for life. Most people don't understand what maintenance really means. It doesn't mean staying at one precise weight for the rest of your life. It means staying within your weight range for healthy ideal weight.

When you learn to catch your weight before it exceeds eight pounds, your life becomes so much easier. The drama of dieting is diminished, and you are back in shape before it gets out of hand.

⟶ How-to Skills   ❤ Good for Heart

Women tend to get more of their fats from cream sauces and sugary foods, so keep an eye on them. Learn to continue your use of nonfattening sauces and gravies after your diet.

IDEAL WEIGHT MAINTENANCE

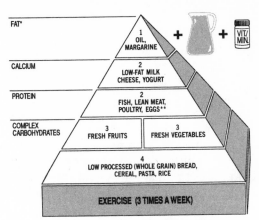

FAT*	1 OIL, MARGARINE
CALCIUM	2 LOW-FAT MILK CHEESE, YOGURT
PROTEIN	2 FISH, LEAN MEAT, POULTRY, EGGS**
COMPLEX CARBOHYDRATES	3 FRESH FRUITS / 3 FRESH VEGETABLES
	4 LOW PROCESSED (WHOLE GRAIN) BREAD, CEREAL, PASTA, RICE

EXERCISE (3 TIMES A WEEK)

**Your food stays powerful.
Your exercise stays constant.
They work together to keep you lean.**

Your food intake is ideal. This is the pattern to follow for life. It gives you fifty essential nutrients daily and is high-fiber and low-cholesterol.	**Exercise aerobically three times a week. This is the pattern you should use for life. It will keep you burning the food you eat, and it will continue to tone your body. It keeps you lean as you age.**

MAINTENANCE AFTER A DIET

YOUR GOAL: Stay balanced! To do that, you increase your calories in the complex carbohydrate group—vegetables, fruits, and grains. You can increase your fats, but you should ask yourself why you would want to. Every now and then you can eat something with more fat or sugar, but why do it on a regular basis? This is what you dreamed of. This is the power to stay lean. Use your ability to increase your fats within the group of high-yielding nutrient foods, not the low-yield processed ones. Keep up your water level. It will keep incoming fat going out. If you have a bowl of ice cream, choose the-low fat yogurt kind. Explore the world of food and nutrition that is now available to you. Always meet the minimum on the diet food pyramid daily. That will keep you stable.

▲ Food Skills ● Behavior Skills ◆ Exercise Skills

Men tend to get more of their fat from proteins—those big steak dinners. So keep an eye on your protein that contains hidden fats. A good plan is to stay with the leaner proteins on a regular basis, and only add the fatter ones now and then.

Maintenance mindset

Remember: You weren't born to be fat and to get fat even after you dieted to get lean. You were born to be lean. Babies are born with body compositions in the appropriate balance and with very little differentiation between male and female babies. Your life-style changes your body composition, and your lifestyle can change it back to its ideal state. Sure, it takes a little work, but that's part of the process of learning how to treat yourself right.

If your mind's eye is letting you gain eight extra pounds and you're letting it happen, take action against the picture of having your fat back. Each time you retrain yourself away from fat and away from seeing yourself fat, your inner power to stay lean gains more of a foothold. Your brain is a historical organ. It only remembers what you tell it about your needs, desires, and wants. If you tell it you are going to regain and your actions duplicate that feeling, you'll recreate the lifestyle that helped you gain weight. If you want to stop that cycle, you can.

If you see yourself gaining eight pounds, start eating according to the food pyramid again and regulate your exercise. The burnoff time will be faster.

What difference does it make if it takes two or three burnoff sessions to stabilize yourself? Does that make you feel less successful? It shouldn't. It should make you feel great. That's the strategy that normal-weight people use to keep their weight in line for life. That's successful maintenance.

▲ MARGARINE

A food that is more vegetable fat than animal fat (or should be); a butter substitute. *See* Cholesterol.

MEAL REPLACEMENT

A formula, usually protein, that is used instead of a regular meal in a diet plan. *See* Meal Replacement Diets; Supplements.

⟾ How-to Skills　　　❤ Good for Heart

MEAL REPLACEMENT DIETS

Plans that use formulas, usually protein, to substitute for meals. The reason protein is the standard formula for meal replacement diets is twofold. Meal replacement diets aim for the lowest calorie ceiling they can get. Fresh fruits, vegetables, and grains have minimal fat and calories, so it wouldn't make sense to replace them with a better variety. The protein foods are the ones that contain hidden fat, therefore making a protein with less fat reduces the overall calorie ceiling dramatically. Secondly, protein is mandatory on a diet to preserve your body muscle. A diet would be dangerous for your health without adequate protein. While this makes sense theoretically, in practice these diets don't pay off. It may be that the processed proteins don't have the same metabolic effect and benefits of real protein foods, but this has to be researched. It's also a calorie problem. When you go on very low-calorie diets, your metabolism slows down, and you burn fewer calories overall. Over time, as you continue to eat and burn fewer calories, your body adjusts to this lower calorie level, and your metabolism is burning at its low point. When you go off the diet, you aren't a good fat burner, and you gain weight fast. If you *must* use a meal replacement plan that is very low in calories, do it under a doctor's care where you can be supervised.

MEDICAL CHECKUP

A routine physical exam. Whenever you go on a diet, you should precede it with a visit to your doctor, who knows your medical history. You can use the results of your physical to take a look at your food input and energy output to see where you can make improvements. When you go on a diet that is 800 calories or less, it must be doctor-monitored. An 800-calorie diet (or less) is *serious* restriction and not usually preferred by doctors as the first, best course. The easiest and best way to diet is with a balanced food plan that meets your daily nutritional needs. That way, you avoid the risks and get double the benefits. And the next time you go for your physical, you'll be healthier as well as slimmer.

● MEDITATION

Mental stillness or calm, achieved through a specific method of relaxation; also known as transcendental meditation.

▲ Food Skills   ● Behavior Skills   ◆ Exercise Skills

Meditation is a process of relaxation that brings your mind and body into a deeply silent state. It's the ideal relaxation, easy to do, and richly rewarding. Advocates say it gives you a new lease on life. It deepens sleep, reduces insomnia and restlessness, and gets you in touch with your inner resources for strength, clarity, and self-appreciation.

Meditation Needs:
1. A quiet comfortable place.
2. A fixed time schedule for meditation. The same time every day. The best time is usually the first thing in the morning, since your mind is in a less frenzied state.
3. Uninterrupted time for ten to fifteen minutes to start.
4. No prescription drugs for twenty-four hours prior to meditation.
5. No food or beverages two hours before meditation.
6. Your own word or mantra sound, that you keep to yourself.
7. The right frame of mind. Don't see meditation as a duty or obligation. You are not being judged or graded on your progress. Trust the process, and don't concern yourself with results. Make it a gift you give yourself each day.

Meditation Goals:
1. Physical stillness. Find a posture where you can practice remaining still. The one suggested for beginners is sitting in a comfortable chair with your feet flat on the floor, hands resting loosely in your lap. You can also lie on the floor on a rug or mat, but for first-timers it's not recommended, since you can fall asleep. You want a position that will keep you from fidgeting, while allowing you to remain mentally alert.
2. Adjusting to stillness. Once you begin meditating, urges come over you to shift, itch, scratch, and cough, or be distracted by outside noises. Part of the process of meditation is to resist all of these urges calmly to achieve mental and physical stillness. Many meditators find that this takes time to learn and pass through. The point is to keep doing it.
3. Experiencing the sound vibrations. Sound is used in meditation for its tranquilizing effect. Since the mind's tendency is to be distracted, the sound also creates focus and the ability to concentrate. The sound that is required is very specific. It must be open and expansive to start, must have resonance and good vibrational power, and it must close at the end to keep the vibrations inside you. The sound *om* is the most

---

⇒ How-to Skills   ❤ Good for Heart

common mantra, and is considered the perfect sound for meditation. It is a word which combines three sounds— aaaa-oooo-mmmm, opening with the *a* sound and closing with the *m* sound. Many people like to use the word *home* or *calm* for the mantra. The sound or mantra is used with your breathing and should be used on exhaling, lasting the full length of the exhale.

⏵   *How to Meditate*

Assume your position and breathe in and out, using your mantra as you exhale. Repeat the process for ten minutes to start, and gradually extend the time to fifteen to twenty minutes each session. The more you repeat the meditation, the easier it becomes to go deeper into relaxation.

MEGAVITAMIN

Large doses of a particular vitamin or nutrient. Megavitamin therapy is usually used in the case of specific illnesses or conditions that are caused by chronic depletion of vitamins or nutrients. It should never be used as a dietary practice on an unsupervised basis. It can cause serious harm, since excessive intake of one vitamin can imbalance all the others. If you eat a balanced diet, your vitamins and minerals will be provided in your food. If you do not eat a balanced diet, and can't seem to get around to improving your food intake, you can take a balanced vitamin/mineral supplement, but you shouldn't view this as a solution to an inadequate diet.

Your system exists in delicate balance, using your vitamins, minerals, and nutrients in harmony. This is particularly true of the amino acids, which recently have been used as vitaminlike supplements on an isolated basis. Tryptophan, for instance, was promoted as a sleep aid and taken in handfuls by wired-up dieters. The unfortunate result is a rare blood disease, either brought on by or aggravated by the use of one amino acid in isolation (which may have been contaminated in the factory).

The problem with megavitaminitis is that it distorts your view of vitamins, minerals, and nutrients that occur naturally in foods. If pills are contaminated or removed from the market, users of the product begin to fear the naturally occurring variety, staying away

▲ Food Skills   ● Behavior Skills   ◆ Exercise Skills

from food. Hardly a day goes by without some vitamin or mineral being singled out for abuse. This is *not* caused by the use of food as a vitamin/mineral source, but by abuse in pill form, then sadly transferred to food.

Dieters are the population most susceptible to megavitamin hype. Weight is an emotional issue, and the desire is always there for a magic formula or pill to take it all away. It is also part of a problem created by poor diets that promote one enzyme, one vitamin, or one mineral as the cure-all for weight problems. Some of these programs even have doctors' names on them, but you should notice that, regardless of the gimmicks, the enzyme, vitamin, or mineral usually occurs in the presence of a calorie-balanced diet. You are being sold a miracle pill idea, when the miracle is really in your food.

This magic cure idea is perpetuated by dieters themselves. The problem is *these gimmicks sell.* If they didn't sell, companies wouldn't keep producing them. It's up to you, as a dieter, to stop supporting these gimmicks and fads. You owe it to yourself to turn your attention back to real food. That's where the success rates are greater. That's where the only side effects are losing your fat, not inviting other, greater health risks.

The final problem with isolated vitamin or enzyme plans is doubly sad for people with weight problems. They fail, and you continue to gain weight.

METABOLIC RATE

Your rate of heat production, measured in specific units, or calories—usually calories per hour, or kilocalories per day (a kilocalorie equals 1,000 calories). All of your body processes produce heat as a byproduct of chemical reactions that are occurring at all times. Eating, digestion, motion, body maintenance, and metabolism itself release heat. For your heart to beat, a chemical reaction takes place that releases heat. To breathe, a chemical reaction releases heat. This heat can be measured as it escapes your body, and that measurement is your metabolic rate.

There are two ways to measure your metabolic rate, but don't go running to your doctor, because these methods are expensive and reserved for research.

1. There is a machine called a metabolic calorimeter that measures the amount of heat escaping from solid bodies. You

---

⟫ How-to Skills ❤ Good for Heart

could be put inside that machine, and your heat production could be measured. This is a very costly and complicated process.

2. Since the first process is costly and complicated, a more practical method was devised. Heat and oxygen have a unique relationship. When heat is released from your body, oxygen is consumed. A liter of oxygen is consumed for every 4.8 kilocalories of heat produced. Therefore, you can measure metabolic rate by measuring the rate of oxygen that is consumed and by calculating the heat from that. It's a back door approach that allowed scientists to calculate thousands of metabolic rates. In this test, if you were a laboratory subject, you would be required to breathe into a mouthpiece or face mask that is hooked up to a device that measures oxygen. Your metabolic rate would be added to the pool of metabolic rates that give dieters all the values for calories, heat expenditure in exercise, and all those measurements in books that are taken so lightly.

Factors that influence your metabolic rate are:

1. Your age. Your metabolic rate decreases with age, regardless of your sex.
2. Your sex. Men have a slightly higher metabolic rate than women, because of their higher body muscle content. Women's metabolic rate is slightly lower because of their higher body fat content, needed to insulate a potential baby.
3. Temperature. In colder climates, your metabolic rate is higher. In warmer climates, it's lower.
4. Activity level. The more you move, the higher your metabolic rate.
5. Time of day. Your metabolic rate slows down toward the end of the day. It goes into a very slow state while you are sleeping, called a fasting state. This means you should not eat your heaviest meals at night, when you can't burn calories as well.
6. Your state of health or dis-ease. Your metabolic rate can be affected by certain conditions. Stress will give you a higher metabolic rate, but it will also burn you out faster. Weight will give you a lower metabolic rate. Heavier people have lower metabolic rates per unit of body weight than lighter people. This is caused by the higher body-fat content and lower muscle content, since the muscle tissue is the site for fat burning.

7. Food intake. The food you eat can increase your metabolic rate. This is called specific dynamic action, and you can use that to your advantage. After you eat, your metabolic rate rises for several hours, even if nothing else occurs. The effect is greater after eating low-fat protein and carbohydrates, and last comes fat. This is caused by the biochemical reactions (heat producing) that go on in your cells to process the nutrients derived from food and to use those nutrients to build up your body.

To discover all these facts about basal metabolic rate, scientists had to find a way to measure it without the variables or interferences, such as individual activity levels, eating styles, and climate. To do this, they measured metabolic rates in resting states and came up with a standard for basal metabolism, or the heat production required for your body to maintain itself on the most basic level—to keep your lungs functioning, heart beating, eyes opening and closing, ad infinitum.

Basal measurements were taken with the following requirements:

1. The people had to be at rest but not sleeping.
2. The temperature couldn't be too hot or too cold.
3. No food could be eaten twenty-four hours prior to the test.

In this way, the figures were derived for your body's basic need to maintain itself or keep itself alive, without added activity, temperature differences, or internal food processing occurring. This is how the figures for basal metabolic rate were determined. After that, activity levels could be calculated, exercise levels tallied, and calorie levels determined by the way they affect basal metabolic rate.

Your daily metabolic rate can be increased by adding on the factors that increase it—more activity, better eating, more exercise. That's how you drive up your metabolic rate to produce more heat and burn more calories daily. That's how you retrain your body not to hold on to its fat.

METABOLISM

The biochemistry of life. At all times during the day, thousands of chemical reactions are occurring in your cells. The nutrient molecules from digestion are circulating in your blood, ready to be taken up for metabolic work—repair and maintenance of your entire body system, from your heart to a nerve impulse. Different cells take different nutrients, depending on the jobs they have to do.

For instance, your muscles are made of two different proteins. Cells have to make these muscle proteins, and each one has to be different from each other and different from the amino acids floating in your bloodstream after digestion. A cell can make some of the amino acids for its new protein by itself, by breaking the bonds of a sugar molecule and converting it to an amino acid. But the cell cannot make eight of the possible amino acids needed for its new protein. It has to get them from you, through your food. The cell takes the amino acid provided from your food and breaks its bonds, freeing up the amino acids it needs to complete its chain. This metabolic process is called *catabolism*—the breaking down of available compounds.

When the cell makes its new protein and you have some new muscle molecules, this metabolic process is called *anabolism*—the building of new compounds from others. These two processes, anabolism and catabolism, are going on simultaneously all over your body. All of the materials of your body are being created in cells that are breaking down the nutrients from food.

If the amino acid isn't available to the cell, no muscle will be made today. One-half of your body protein is rebuilt every three months by your cells. A blood cell lives for four months, then has to be destroyed and replaced with a new one.

Your body is what you give it on a daily basis.

When the bonds of any molecule are broken, heat is produced. You can't use the heat as energy, and it leaves your body. The collective heat from these processes of breaking nutrient bonds to build new materials for your body is your *metabolic rate, basal.* The better you eat, the more you accelerate this process, because the nutrients are there for the cells to take. It takes approximately 60 percent of your calories to operate these processes, calories you don't store as fat. If you don't provide the nutrients, the reactions don't take place as often or as well, and you burn fewer calories.

When the bonds of a nutrient are broken, some energy escapes and isn't used by the cell. It's picked up by the chemical ADP (adenosine diphosphate) and stored in the bonds of its big sister ATP (adenosine triphosphate). This chemical circulates around

---

▲ Food Skills ● Behavior Skills ◆ Exercise Skills

your body bringing energy where it's needed. Every movement and motion requires that the bonds of ATP be broken, to get the energy out. This releases heat. The heat from these reactions are the heat of your metabolic rate over the basal rate. If you are active and exercise, you are stimulating many more chemical reactions that release heat. These are calories that don't store.

If you don't do much moving around and don't do much exercise, the excess sugars and amino acids are converted to fat for storage in your adipose tissue. The major sites of adipose tissue are directly beneath your skin, in your abdomen, and in your buttocks. The major storage sites for glycogen (from carbohydrates) are in your liver and in your muscles, to be used for energy, but the carbohydrate stores are small compared to fat.

As time goes by, your adipose mass gets larger from these stores, and your muscle mass has to perform all of the chemical reactions it takes to support that fat mass and the added pressure on your system. Cells are waiting for nutrients to build their proteins and other body materials, but sugars and fatty acids seem to predominate. And there aren't enough vitamins and minerals to get the process activated. The cells sit waiting. No muscle protein is made today, or tomorrow. Your metabolic rate slow down. Your cells don't have the nutrients they need to make new materials. (And that is just the protein materials. Your body needs many more).

▥➡ *Dieting and Your Metabolism*

When you diet to correct this problem, the first priority is to provide these nutrients in the form your body needs. That may not be the form provided in some of the diets you can find in your neighborhood, but you can find it in the food groups and in the Problem Solver Diet (pages 69–85). That's the beauty of science. It's based on the energy of metabolism.

MINERALS

Organic or inorganic nutrients found in your body and food. Less than 5 percent of your total body weight is minerals, but their role is crucial. They are part of your body fluids and tissues, protecting your muscle tissue and nervous system. They aid digestion, metabolism, and hormone production; they also help create antibodies, and many are responsible in catalyzing enzymes to facilitate metabolic processes. There are seventeen essential minerals, and all of them need to be supplied by your food daily. Some are called macro-minerals, because they are present in high amounts (for a mineral) in your body. These are calcium, chlorine, phosphorous, magnesium, sodium, and sulfur. They're measured in milligrams (1/1000 gram). Others are called trace minerals, because they are present in your body in very small amounts, but some are very essential. They're measured in micrograms (1/1,000,000 gram).

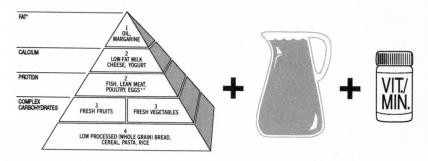

All of your minerals work together, and excesses of one mineral can throw off the balance of the others. Distilled water removes minerals. Excess fiber can bind with minerals, and you excrete them.

When you are on a low-calorie diet, it's essential to take a vitamin/mineral supplement. Otherwise, you get all your minerals from the food group eating plan.

Dictonary of Minerals

Aluminum   trace/toxic in excess
Beryllium   trace/toxic
Cadmium   trace/toxic
  Antidote—Zinc
Calcium   essential/macro
Chlorine   essential/macro
Chromium   essential
Cobalt   essential
Copper   essential/trace
Fluorine   essential/trace
  Sodium fluoride in water
  can be harmful
  Antidote—Calcium

▲   Food Skills   ●   Behavior Skills   ◆   Exercise Skills

Iodine	essential/trace
Iron	essential
Lead	trace/toxic
Antidote—Zinc	
Magnesium	essential/macro
Mercury	trace/toxic
Molybdenum	trace/essential
Nickel	trace/essential
Phosphorous	essential/macro
Potassium	essential
Selenium	trace/essential
Sodium	essential/macro
Sulfur	essential/macro
Vanadium	trace/essential
Zinc	trace/essential
Others: boron, lithium, silicon, strontium, tin, tritium	trace/essential. Their role in nutrition isn't known.

● MIRROR EXERCISES

Techniques for evaluating and changing your negative inner perceptions; body image issues in a glance. Mirrors are two-dimensional; they do not give you a realistic view of yourself. When you look in the mirror, how you see yourself is a reflection of your inner views about yourself, your weight, and your attitude. How you respond to what you see is a body image issue.

➠   _How to Do a Mirror Image Appraisal_

Stand in front of the mirror in underwear or nude.
What do you look at first?
Your face or your body?
When you look at your body, do you look at your whole body or at parts of your body that are fatter than other parts? Which parts do you look at? The thin parts or fatter parts?
Most people with weight problems tend to look at themselves from the neck up first and not at their whole image in the mirror.
Most people with weight problems also tend to look at _parts_ rather than the whole image. They will single out their heavier parts and forget to look at their slimmer parts. Or they will avoid

_____

➠   How-to Skills   ❤   Good for Heart

their heavier parts and concentrate on their thin parts. Either way, this is fragmented thinking, because it singles out specific problems, whether you look at the problems or avoid them. To have this fragmented image, you don't necessarily have to be overweight. Many thin people look at themselves as parts that need to be fixed, rather than as a person in the mirror who is unique in life.

◗ _Creating a Positive Mirror Image_

Your view in the mirror is subjective and often fragmented. To make your weight goals more objective, get a notebook and pen. Stand in front of the mirror again.

First, look at your whole self, taking in your height, length of your trunk and legs, and even your feet. Turn a shoulder to the mirror, so you can get a more three-dimensional effect.

Next, objectively evaluate what areas you would like to change with weight loss. List them in your notebook. Hips, buttocks, belly. Make the list as short or as long as you need.

Now look in the mirror again and study each of the parts you listed. If you listed your hips, look at your hips. Write down the first thought that comes to your mind about your hips, using these guidelines:

My hips look like _____.
This makes me feel _____.

Use this format for each of the body parts you listed. Be honest. This record is for you. You may continue to write the things you start feeling, and you can write as much as you like. But try to answer the two questions for each body part you listed.

After you are finished, stand in front of the mirror again.

Read your response to the mirror for each part.

Then change each negative response to a positive one.

For instance:

My hips look like tankers.

Change: My hips look like the hips of a strong woman (man).

My hips allow me to turn quickly. They support my upper body. I used to hold my baby on my right hip when I was shopping.

Say anything you want to switch your response to a positive response.

Follow this procedure with all the parts you listed.

▲ Food Skills   ● Behavior Skills   ♦ Exercise Skills

How does it make you feel to say something nice about yourself?

If it makes you uncomfortable, ignore the discomfort. Practice this exercise again tomorrow, and try to feel good and light when you say something nice about a body part you think you don't like.

If it makes you feel light and surprised with the feeling, you've accomplished this exercise. But that doesn't mean negative thoughts won't creep back in. Every time you think something negative about a body part, use the positive substitution process, until the negative feeling lets go.

If you don't believe what you're saying, it doesn't make any difference. Your brain is a recorder of your responses and feelings. It will repeat back to you what you feel and see. It may take time to get your brain used to the idea that you are not insulting yourself regularly. But it will learn it. And you will lift a great weight off your self-image. This will give you support to achieve your goals.

Whole-Self Appreciation

Stand in front of the mirror in underwear or nude and look at yourself.

Absolutely and unequivocally love who you see. Say *I love you* to the person in the mirror. Tap the mirror to assert it. Repeat it until you believe it. If you don't believe it the first time you do it, keep doing it. Eventually, you will feel what it feels like to love yourself in the mirror. It does not matter how much fat you have or where you have it, how long you've had it, who likes it or doesn't, or if you ever intend to let go of it. This has nothing to do with external weight. This has to do with you as a person in the world. You are uniquely and distinctly you, and that is uniquely and distinctly beautiful. Do this exercise at least two times a day, once in the morning and before bed at night.

Every time your mind wanders to a body part, stop it.

Breathe deeply and look at your whole self again and love yourself.

You may get a number of negative-sounding thoughts to try to take you away from your purpose, which is learning to love yourself exactly as you are. You can explore those thoughts at your leisure, because they will reveal interesting reasons you think you don't like yourself. Always assume power over the thought. For instance, you might look in the mirror and say *I love you* to yourself, and in the back of your mind you'll hear: *No you don't*. Or *You shouldn't wear your hair that way*. Or *You're getting crow's-feet*. Or even, *You never do what I tell you to do.* Or even *You don't deserve something.*

You can listen to these thoughts, but realize that they don't own you anymore. They are trained thoughts. You do not have to go through years of psychoanalysis to stop them. You can change them every time they come up. You can change them in the mirror every time you look at yourself. When you do this, it begins to change you. Gradually, you stop dealing from negative places and negative viewpoints and you begin to look at things differently. You begin to look at things almost as if you were a child amused with life again. This is the person you really want to own, that amused child grown up. That child was born to love herself/himself. When you deal with yourself from a place that is loving and positive, you can accomplish anything you set your mind to.

● MODERATION

The midpoint between extremes; a behavior key for extreme thinkers. Dieters tend to think in extremes, especially ones who have been trained to do it by deprivation diets. A diet is seen as a short-term affair that is unpleasant. Therefore the sooner it's over the better. Unfortunately, this kind of thinking leads to failure and weight regain. The reasoning is that if a diet can take off ten pounds in a month, then stricter dieting will take off twenty.

Food

Extreme thinkers see foods in two categories:

Good foods/bad foods, their foods/my foods. Diet foods are good, all other foods are bad. The only trouble is each diet has foods they say are good and others say are bad. This leads to food confusion and generates anxiety about food. Every time a new food arrives in the supermarket, it's seen as a curse or a cure. This also leads to abnormal eating habits, which remove whole categories of food from the daily plan. Often carbohydrates are removed from diets, when the natural complex carbohydrates are the best fat burners and fiber sources for dieting.

Moderation means developing a whole new philosophy about food. Food is your energy and primary source of nutrients. It's not the food that gives you trouble, it's how you use it. Using food wisely gives you more variety and flexibility in your diet; it opens up a world of pleasures, instead of a limited menu of food monotony. A new relationship with food is like a new lease on life.

▲ Food Skills   ● Behavior Skills   ◆ Exercise Skills

Programs

Extreme thinkers tend to choose extreme programs, the stricter the better. The more miserable you are on a diet, the more it reinforces the idea that you should be punished for having weight. That leads you to want sweet treats and fats for reward. This also separates the diet from real life, as if they have nothing to do with each other. You bring this separation into your daily routine and habits, and before you know it, your perspective on other things begins to change too.

Moderation lifts you out of this pattern. You begin to see extremes for what they are: stress-promoting habits. Your daily life should be less stressed on your diet, and there should not be such a gap between the diet phase and maintenance. When you practice moderate habits during your diet, you wind up at ideal weight with the skills you need to stay there. That leads to a healthier outlook on everything in life.

Exercise

Extreme thinkers go all out on exercise, or they don't do it at all. Everything on the weekend and nothing during the week. Jump in fast, and get out fast. This can cause injury, and it can use the wrong kind of energy for your exercise. You can be doing most of your activity on an anaerobic level—not getting oxygen uptake.

Moderation means that you gradually increase your activity and aerobic exercise, learning to experiment with options, to find choices that give you pleasure, not strain, pulled muscles, and fatigue. This is the original intent of exercise, physical and cardiovascular conditioning, and it makes everything run more smoothly in your life.

MONOUNSATURATED

A type of unsaturated fat, or OK fat. *See* Cholesterol.

MUSCLE

Body protein or muscle tissue; also called lean body mass. *See* Weight.

N

● **NEGATIVE THINKING**
A mindset that subverts your success. The solution to this is found in positive self-statements. Every time you express a negative or think in the negative, you change it to its positive counterpart. You don't even have to believe it. It works anyway. For examples, *See* Mirror Exercises.

● **NETWORKING**
A support skill for dieting and weight maintenance. Networking means finding booster systems to help you through the rough spots while you are dieting and trying to stay fit. Going it alone can be difficult, but it is not impossible. Networks of friends, organizations, or even positive-thinking tapes can help you get the incentive you need to keep going. *See* Buddy System.

◆ **NORDIC TRACK**
Stationary aerobic machine; simulated cross-country skiing.

Benefits:
• Best cardiovascular training
• Best calorie-burning exercise
• No orthopedic injury; no shock to joints and muscles
• Works upper and lower body (especially buttocks); can adjust tension for greater strength building and higher intensity.
• Builds coordination and rhythm

Guidelines:
• Slip feet into stirrups on skis, which glide along track.
• Lean slightly forward, balancing pelvis against pelvic cushion.
• Grasp handles on arm pulley.
• Position arms and legs in opposite positions (i.e., left leg forward, right leg back—toe bends up—right arm pulled up, left arm pulled back).

▲ Food Skills   ● Behavior Skills   ◆ Exercise Skills

- Then switch positions, gliding opposite leg forward and simultaneously pulling arm pulley, switching arm positions.
- If you struggle with either leg or arm movement, decrease tension on either or both gauges.
- The goal is to develop a comfortable, gliding stride. The opposition of arm and leg movement keeps your balance while you lean forward against the pelvic cushion.
- Handlebars are also attached so you can start out just learning leg coordination, yet in the long run it's easier to balance when the machine is used as designed with arms and legs in opposition. It's a natural stride, like walking. Don't outthink your stride, just glide! *See* Exercise.

NORMAL WEIGHT

Your ideal weight, based on height/weight tables. This gives you a weight *range*, not simply one set weight or one number for ideal pounds. Some people are comfortable with a higher weight, and as long as it doesn't involve weight-related risks, a higher weight in your weight range would still be safe and normal. *See* Ideal Weight.

▲ NUTRIENT DENSITY

The ratio of nutrition-to-food-unit; the energy it provides. Eating for nutrient density means getting the most nutrient power for the least calories. For instance:

½ CUP FRESH STRAWBERRIES	½ CUP FROZEN STRAWBERRIES (SYRUP)
30 calories in addition to standard nutrients	125 calories standard nutrients plus empty calories (sugar)
NUTRIENT DENSITY	CALORIE DENSITY
1 BAKED POTATO MEDIUM 125 calories standard nutrients and low fat	6 FRENCH FRIES 125 calories standard nutrients, excess fat, perhaps saturated fat
NUTRIENT DENSITY	CALORIE DENSITY

⇒ How-to Skills ♥ Good for Heart

Choosing your foods for nutrient density is the easiest way to stay satisfied on a diet while you lose fat.

▲ NUTRIENT NEEDS

The carbohydrates, protein, fat, vitamins, minerals, and water required to maintain your body and burn fat better; RDAs, required daily allowances. The best sources for complete nutrient satisfaction on a daily basis are the food groups, which give you fifty essential nutrients, along with your daily vitamins and minerals in an easy-to-use system. They include complex carbohydrates for energy and fiber; low-fat proteins for energy, muscle protection, and balanced amino acids; and calcium for strong bones. Anything less is not the best. _See_ The Problem Solver Diet for a balanced foot group plan.

▲ NUTRIENTS

Nourishment that produces energy or aids in the production of energy. The essential nutrients for your body energy and calorie burn are:

Carbohydrates	Body nutrients are derived from food nutrients.
Protein	
Fat	Food nutrients become nutrient supplements, such as vitamins and minerals.
Vitamins	
Minerals	It all starts with food.
Water	That's the source to return to.

This is ideal nutrition and ideal nutrition for fat burn. There's no better way to diet. _See_ The Problem Solver food pyramid.

▲ Food Skills   ● Behavior Skills   ◆ Exercise Skills

▲ NUTRITION

Achieving daily nutritional status at optimum. That means meeting your recommended daily allowances for protein, carbohydrates, fats, vitamins, minerals, and water. *See* The Problem Solver food pyramid for your nutrition guide.

O

OBESITY
Excess weight to the degree of 20 to 30 percent over ideal body weight. Obesity is generally regarded as a disease, since excess body weight over 30 percent of ideal weight usually involves other complications such as diabetes and hypertension. However, people can be obese without any overt signs or symptoms of disease.

Obesity is a disease of malnutrition, not necessarily overeating. Studies have shown that obese people can eat the same amount of calories as a normal-weight person but still gain weight. Part of this problem is due to the oversized fat mass that steals nutrients and keeps the body malnourished or imbalanced nutritionally. Part of the problem is activity, which is decreased with obesity. The heavier you get, the more you tend to slow down and avoid exercise. As a result, you burn fewer calories. And one of the biggest factors is the content of your daily diet: it is often imbalanced in the direction of sugar and fat.

On page 274 you'll see the problems in context, and how to resolve them. While obesity is a higher degree of weight gain than *overweight*, the problems with food and activity are similar, and the solution is the best one for any weight problem.

▲ OILS
Vegetable oils or unsaturated fats. These are considered good sources of fat because they help remove cholesterol, rather than add to it. *See* Cholesterol.

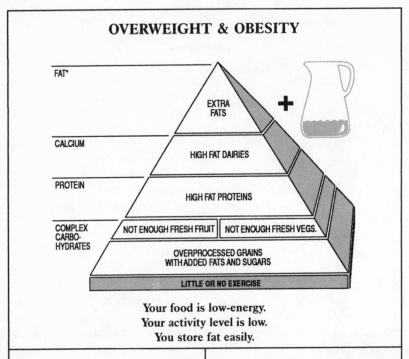

OVERWEIGHT & OBESITY

FAT*

EXTRA FATS

CALCIUM

HIGH FAT DAIRIES

PROTEIN

HIGH FAT PROTEINS

COMPLEX CARBO-HYDRATES

NOT ENOUGH FRESH FRUIT | NOT ENOUGH FRESH VEGS.

OVERPROCESSED GRAINS WITH ADDED FATS AND SUGARS

LITTLE OR NO EXERCISE

**Your food is low-energy.
Your activity level is low.
You store fat easily.**

Your food intake is not balanced. Even if you get your baseline nutrition, it is depleted or overshadowed by poorer energy sources, like sugar, fat, and sodium. Stress depletes your nutrients even more. Your fiber intake is low, and fat doesn't mobilize. Your metabolism is slow, so you gain weight even if you eat less. It's a cycle that continues to escalate until you balance your food intake.

Your activity level is not sufficient to burn the calories you eat. Because you carry fat, you tire easily and exercise seems like a chore, so you put it off. The more you sit, the more you eat, the more you eat, the more your gain. Even when you limit your calories, you still gain, because your body composition is tilted in the direction of fat. If you lost muscle on a poor diet, this compounds your problem, because it helps you to store fat instead of burn it.

YOUR GOAL: Fix your food intake first, because that will give you more nutrient energy for more activity. Begin with a low-impact aerobic program and work your way up to greater exercise levels as you lose your excess fat.

IDEAL DIET WEEK

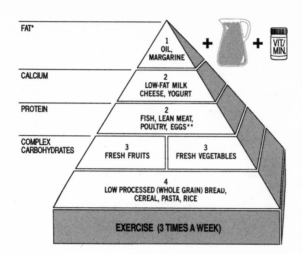

FAT*
1
OIL,
MARGARINE

CALCIUM
2
LOW-FAT MILK
CHEESE, YOGURT

PROTEIN
2
FISH, LEAN MEAT,
POULTRY, EGGS**

COMPLEX
CARBOHYDRATES
3
FRESH FRUITS
3
FRESH VEGETABLES

4
LOW PROCESSED (WHOLE GRAIN) BREAD,
CEREAL, PASTA, RICE

EXERCISE (3 TIMES A WEEK)

**Your food drives up your energy.
Your activity drives up your calorie burn.
You burn more than you eat.**

Your food burns calories too from thermogenesis—the heat of eating. The pyramid provides the fifty essential nutrients you need to feed your metabolism, to activate its chemical action to repair, rebuild, and maintain all of your body processes, from the largest organ to the smallest cell. When you take the pyramid to its low-fat format, the result is fat burns and burns.

Your thirty-minute aerobic routine, three times per week drives up your metabolism to burn more calories (15% +). It also builds muscle, the vital body protein you lose from poor dieting and need to rebuild, in order to be a better fat burner for life. These factors combine to revive your sluggish metabolism, align your body composition, and set you up with the status you need to stay lean after your diet.

Overall result: While fat is burning, muscle is restored. You get superior weight loss and a body composition to match. In maintenance, you will be able to raise your calorie level without regaining.

YOUR GOAL: TO GET BACK IN BALANCE

▲ Food Skills   ● Behavior Skills   ◆ Exercise Skills

OSTEOPOROSIS

Reduction in bone mass and density; brittle bones. The more weight you have, the greater your tendency for osteoporosis, from the pressure of weight, dietary deficiencies, and sedentary tendencies that go along with weight.

The major causes of osteoporosis are:

1. Calcium-deficient diet, usually over a long period of time. When you eat too little calcium, your body takes the calcium it needs from your bones. These losses can't be restored to your bones, except by meeting your daily calcium needs in your food.
2. Lack of weight-bearing exercise. Calcium absorption is increased with exercise, and lack of it means less calcium absorption. Weight-bearing exercises are ones where your body bears the weight, such as walking (instead of swimming). This increases your bone strength along with your calcium absorption.
3. Calcium-phosphorus imbalance. You need equal amounts of calcium and phosphorous for calcium to absorb properly. How do you get it without worrying? Balanced meals from the food groups.
4. Intestinal absorption problems. This may be the result of dietary deficiencies of phosphorous, vitamin D, and protein along with lack of exercise, or it can be caused by underlying medical conditions and hormonal issues.
5. Cigarette smoking inhibits calcium absorption, along with many other nutrients, which is a good reason to stop. (If you don't intend to stop, you need more calcium, exercise, and vitamins/minerals than a nonsmoker.)

The primary nutrients needed for calcium absorption are: vitamins B12, C, D, E, copper, flouride, magnesium, phosphorous, and protein. *See* Calcium.

Caution! Dieters are notorious for casually eliminating milk and other diary products from their diets, thinking that they're major sources of fat. Don't diet if you're going to do that! Use 1 percent or 2 percent low-fat milk and other low-fat dairy products and eat plenty of vegetables daily to get your calcium requirements. What's a good body without good bones!

OUTPUT

Calories burned, specifically on a daily basis. Output is one-half of the energy scale that determines your weight, or weight regulation. The balanced state is:

Input Equals Output
Calories Eaten Equal Calories Burned

Output is a combination of heat-producing processes that include body maintenance and repair (cellular), activities you do in your everyday life, and exercise you add on for greater heat production and calorie burn. *See* Exercise and Metabolic Rate, for the total picture.

OXYGEN UPTAKE

The ability of your blood to pick up and carry oxygen. Since oxygen is vital to all body processes and increases fat burn, increasing your oxygen uptake is important. This can be accomplished with exercise and deep-breathing exercises. Relaxation and meditation can also improve oxygen uptake, since they relax your body and that naturally causes you to breathe more deeply. *See* Breathing; Exercise; Meditation; Relaxation.

P

▲ **PECTIN**

A soluble fiber. It prevents blood sugar swings and lowers blood cholesterol. *See* Fiber.

● **PERFECTIONIST THINKING**

Needing everything to be ideal, or your perception of ideal. This is a trap. It's like driving to your vacation with the map in your mind, instead of the view. You think you're in control, but if you had to stop and spend the afternoon in a strange town, you'd completely lose your grounding. Needing perfection can prevent you from trying something because you think you already know how it goes. And it can prevent you from succeeding, because life has a way of putting obstacles in your path. Flexibility is the only way to bypass obstacles and get on with your priorities with both feet on the ground. Dieters who set goals that have to be met by a certain date, regardless of the stress, are often perfectionist thinkers. You want to do it once—perfectly—and never again. The trouble is, it backfires. You do it once and perfectly, and you have to do it again because you regain. You don't have the habits you need to deal with all the changing situations of daily life. All you learned were the habits to lose weight in isolation.

The best route to ideal weight is to set standards that are realistic to live with, instead of ones that make your daily life so rigid that a minor crisis can throw off your diet. It takes the pressure off you and makes the process more interesting. Then, if you're caught in a strange town on the way to your vacation, you will know how to eat in a restaurant there as well as anywhere, and you will know how to find the high school track there as well as anywhere. You've learned how to be flexible, to adapt.

♦ **PHYSICAL ACTIVITY**

A means to burn calories. *See* Exercise.

● PLATEAU

A weight you reach during dieting that you can't seem to get below. Often this weight is the last ten pounds, but a plateau can occur at any time in the weight-loss phase.

It's a sign to review your food and exercise patterns.

➡   *How to Overcome a Plateau*

There are two basic steps to overcoming a plateau:

1. Review your food. Keep a food diary for a week to see if fat and sugar are creeping into your diet, while fiber is falling out. Check your carbohydrate, fat, and protein levels to see if they are up to par for the best fat burning. Make sure you're not skipping water. Make sure you're taking your vitamin/mineral supplement. If you find out that your food intake is perfect, you *can* make an effort to reduce the fat content to a lower level. This will increase the fat that is taken from storage. But don't reduce any other servings in your diet. Less is not best when it comes to nutrition and fat burn. Less means less weight loss, from a reduced metabolism.

2. Review your exercise. If you are loyally exercising three times per week for thirty minutes per session, then you will have to add an extra session or two of a low-impact aerobic exercise to your program too. You can take a one-hour walk each night to drive up your calorie output. The combination of these two factors will take you over the plateau.

Plateaus on Low-Calorie Diets

If you are on a very low-calorie diet, you've got a problem, and it won't be easy to resolve, but you can do it. You have to go off the very low-calorie diet and on to a full-food program of at least 1,200 calories, and you have to put up with the water weight that will occur in the first week or so. If you stay on the low-calorie diet, you may stop losing weight all together. The only way to drive up your metabolism is to reintroduce food, while continuing to exercise and trust in the fat-burning effects of real food. This also means that you can't go back to rapid weight-loss diets for quick results. You've gotten your metabolism down to such a low ebb that another rapid weight-loss diet may cause you to regain beyond your expectations. Don't cheat your body of its natural potential to use food for fat burn. Follow a balanced diet formula and keep your fat intake as low as you can. Fat loss will happen. Be prepared

▲ Food Skills   ● Behavior Skills   ◆ Exercise Skills

to wait for it. Celebrate the fact that you've finally broken the habit of weight regain while you're waiting. It's the plateau for a new life.

POLYUNSATURATED

A type of unsaturated fat, or OK fat. *See* Cholesterol.

● POSITIVE SELF-TALK

A self-strengthening technique. The simple key is to change every negative thing you say to yourself and about yourself to its positive counterpart. *See* Mirror Exercises and Rationalizations for examples.

● POSITIVE THINKING

A success-oriented outlook. This means more than a good attitude going into a diet. It means developing skills that enhance your overall perspective on life. A diet is a part of life, not a separate time away from life. The more lifelike your diet is, the better you will be able to adapt to ideal weight maintenance, which means eating well for life. The skill of positive self-talk is a vital one, along with imagery and relaxation. *See* Imagery; Mirror Exercises; Rationalizations; Relaxation for examples of how to do it.

▲ POTASSIUM

An essential mineral. Potassium is 5 percent of the total mineral content of your body, and its role is crucial. In partnership with sodium, potassium regulates the fluid balance on both sides of your cell walls.

Water is the medium for all of your body's reactions. Your cells are surrounded by water, and they contain water. They're the sites for metabolism and building body compounds. Keeping the sodium/potassium balance is vital to a healthy life.

The recommended daily doses of sodium and potassium are:

SODIUM	POTASSIUM
1,100 = 3,300 mg/daily	1,800 = 5,600 mg/daily

⇒ How-to Skills   ♥ Good for Heart

Sodium & Chloride   **Potassium & Phosphate**

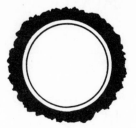   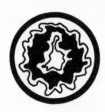

EXTRACELLULAR FLUID   **INTRACELLULAR FLUID**

Sodium excess is one of the major problems in diets. These excesses cause potassium losses through urine. Excessive use of sugar, alcohol, and caffeine can also add to potassium losses. This upsets the balance of sodium and potassium and inhibits the benefits of potassium. These benefits include:

- healthy nerve impulses and muscle contractions
- conversion of glucose to glycogen for storage
- efficient metabolism
- efficient enzyme reactions
- synthesis of muscle protein from amino acids
- normalized heartbeat
- healthy oxygen supply to brain
- healthy skin
- acid/alkaline balance
- stimulation of kidneys to secrete toxins

Potassium is usually lost through perspiration or excessive sweating. Refined sugars make your urine alkaline, and this means mineral instability. Other causes of potassium deficiency are:

- existing on starvation diets
- use of diuretics
- excessive vomiting
- malnutrition
- diarrhea
- injuries, burns, or surgery

Potassium supplements are not recommended as a solution, except in serious cases. The best source is daily replacement of potassium in your food. Potassium supplements contain potassium

SODIUM/POTASSIUM BALANCE

SODIUM	POTASSIUM
Daily Dose 1,110–3,300 mg	1,800–5,600 mg

AVOID	HIGH POTASSIUM FOODS	
Salt	1 Potato (especially skin)	556 mg
	1 cup	
Substitutes	Grapefruit juice	420
w/Potassium	Orange juice	503
Chloride	Tomato juice	549
Excess Salt	Prune juice	602
	Skim milk	355
	½ cup	
Excess Caffeine	Banana	221
Excess Alcohol	Broccoli	207
	Brussels sprouts	212
	Lentils	249
Potassium	Squash	473
Chloride	2 ounces	
Supplements	Tuna in water	158
Excess Sugar	Chicken (skinless)	246
Not Rx Prescribed	Lean beef	292

chloride, which can cause bowel lesions and corrode your intestinal lining. The FDA set the following regulations on potassium chloride:

- Tablets with more than 100 mg of potassium chloride must be given under a doctor's supervision
- Liquids with more than 20 mg of potassium chloride must be given under a doctor's supervision.

There are rare cases where misuse of potassium supplements, along with liquid protein diets, led to death. While this isn't the average situation, it's vital to keep in mind, especially for dieters.

Potassium chloride can be found in salt substitutes, which is why they should not be used without your doctor's approval. Often potassium chloride is used as a flavoring agent, flavor enhancer, stabilizer, thickening agent, or for acid control. Read the labels in order to limit your intake of potassium chloride. Turn to real food, the richest source of potassium, and the natural way to keep your sodium/potassium ratio in line. If you are on a very low-calorie diet that is high in sodium, this can deplete your potassium and create weakness, headaches, poor reflexes, saggy muscles, nervousness, and irregular heartbeats.

POUNDS
Weight. *See* Weight.

POWDERED PROTEIN
A protein supplement used as a meal replacement in a diet plan. *See* Meal Replacements; Supplements.

POWDERED PROTEIN DIETS
Programs that use protein supplements in powder form as meal replacements. *See* Meal Replacements; Supplements.

PRESERVATIVES
Chemicals used to prevent spoilage in processed foods. *See* Additives.

▲ PROCESSED FOODS
Factory versions of real food. Also called refined foods. The most common features of processed foods are high sugar, high salt, high fat, low fiber, high additives, little texture, and low nutrition. Even when they're fortified, these foods can't match the fat-burning effects of fresh food. The typical combination of ingredients in processed foods is the formula for storing fat. *See* Sugar.

▲ PROTEIN
The word *protein* comes from a Greek word that means "of first importance." It is a constituent of every cell and the functional element in glandular secretions, enzymes, and hormones. Protein is essential for tissue growth and repair, regulation of your fluid balance, and stimulation of antibody formation to combat infections.

▲ Food Skills   ● Behavior Skills   ◆ Exercise Skills

It is particularly critical for dieters who are cutting back on calories to consider the quality and quantity of protein they need to meet daily requirements.

Proteins are complex substances made up of a series of amino acids or structural building blocks that are chemically bound together. There are twenty or more different amino acids that occur naturally, with the amino acid combinations creating the nature of different proteins. This is the same as forming different words from different combinations of letters. If you were in the middle of the ocean in a sinking boat with a plane flying overhead, and you had only six flag letters to signal the plane, you might spell R-E-S-C-U-E or S-E-C-U-R-E. The arrangement of the letters is of first importance. It's the same with amino acid combinations that form proteins.

Some combinations of amino acids are essential; some are not. Essential amino acids are the ones that cannot be made by your body and therefore must be obtained from your food. The foods that contain all of the essential amino acids in the proper proportions are good-quality proteins, or complete proteins. Animal sources of protein—meat, fish, fowl, eggs, and dairy products— are complete, with the exception of gelatin. Plant proteins, such as grains, beans, fruits, and vegetables, are incomplete, because they lack one or more of the essential amino acids or have insufficient amounts.

You can combine the incomplete plant proteins, such as beans, dried peas, lentils, nuts, and seeds, with complementary proteins, such as grains, potatoes, and corn, to form a complete source of protein. This is mandatory for vegetarians to ensure adequate protein intake. Many people think there is no such thing as a fat vegetarian, but in fact vegetarians often eat too much fat, since vegetable protein sources include seeds and nuts, which are high-fat foods. Eating too much food fat adds up to body fat, no matter whose calculator you use. If you are a non-red-meat vegetarian, you might consider eating only low-fat fish and fowl, instead of cheese for protein, to avoid excess fat. If you are a no-meat vegetarian, you might rely on soy, bean, and grain casseroles, and soups. It is essential for you to get your protein daily and cut out the high-fat cheeses and nuts.

Red-meat eaters must also be cautious of fat. The most common sources of protein are meats and cheeses, but the best sources for fat loss are the lowest-fat meats and cheeses. In fact, meat is the major source of fat in the average American diet. If you are a red-meat eater, you would be wise to switch to the lower-fat fowl and fish and use red meat as a protein source less frequently.

⭢   How-to Skills   ❤   Good for Heart

Protein Truths and Falsehoods

It is a common misconception that you can eat a lot of protein without gaining weight. This way of thinking stems largely from the high-protein diets, which were supposedly good fat burners. When high-protein diets first came out, they were well received because people dropped weight fast. Actually, they were losing weight simply because they were eating fewer overall calories, but eating a lot of protein felt like more eating, mostly because of the fat and bulky quality of meat. Even after the death scares from high-protein liquid diets, many people forgot that the false notions about protein came out of a decade that supported fast weight loss with high protein.

It's time to erase all the faulty information and start fresh. Not only does excess protein store as fat, but when you fill your diet primarily with protein, you are stripping away something else, and usually that's carbohydrates, your main brain food. When you eat a high-protein diet without protecting your daily dairy need, you are inviting calcium leeching from your bones, and you could wind up with bone deformities or osteoporosis. To stay safe, remember that anything eaten to excess is a dangerous practice.

On the flip side of the coin, protein deficiences are the last thing a dieter wants. When you do not have enough protein in your diet, your body will break down your muscle tissue to meet its protein needs and perform its basic functions. These muscle losses can be life threatening if prolonged. Muscle is what you should gain on your diet.

Another false belief about protein exists among athletes. Strenuous exercise does not require—and is not enhanced by—increased intake of protein. Rather, you need an increase in the total amount of calories you eat in the form of carbohydrates to meet the energy demands of higher levels of output through exercise.

Your ideal body weight is measured by the amount of lean body mass or muscle you have, and it can never be ideal unless you have enough muscle. During weight loss, you need adequate protein to protect your muscle and ensure that you lose only fat.

PSMF

Protein Sparing Modified Fast; a diet designed for morbid obesity. The term *sparing* doesn't mean that it uses food protein sparingly, rather that it relies on protein as a primary energy source, since protein is necessary to *spare* or save your body's lean muscle tissue, which is too often lost on a diet. The PSMF is a low-calorie diet that was developed specifically for use in medical settings for people who were very severely obese, facing medical risks that endangered their lives. For this reason, the rapid weight loss was justified, because the weight itself was life threatening. However, commercial imitations of this *type* of diet began to appear in the consumer marketplace, and have been used for minor weight loss and mild obesity. In these cases, the diet is not used safely and isn't justified. The PSMF should only be administered under a doctor's supervision, and it is generally agreed that the diet should be restricted to extreme cases of obesity.

● **PSYCHOLOGICAL HUNGER**
Desire for food, as opposed to a *need* for food. *See* Hunger.

Q

● **QUICK-FIX MENTALITY**

Wanting instant solutions, immediate results; a Band-Aid approach to weight loss. The desire for instant slimness leads dieters to try fads and gimmicks that promise fast results with little or no effort. Ads appeal to this desire for magic, miracles, and instant cures with claims about secret formulas and miracle vitamins or enzymes. Patches go on wrists, pins go in ears, and fat continues to go into storehouses. The lure of the quick fix is understandable, because overweight or obesity causes tension and anxiety, and as pressures mount, you need an outlet. The best outlet is exercise, an excellent stress reducer and fat burner. In one aerobic session, you can burn 500 calories. Seven sessions will burn a pound. That's the quickest fix you can find.

One of the difficulties about a quick-fix mentality is how you limit your options and deplete your health. When you want to lose weight *fast*, you choose diets that promise seven to ten pounds of weight loss per week. They are the same diets that caused weight regain that is rounder all over. But because you believe that *fast* weight loss is acceptable, you never get to the safer programs, because the safe programs don't make false claims, so they don't sound exciting to you.

Do yourself a favor. The next time the urge comes over you to try a gimmick or program that promises fast results, remind yourself that they *mean both fast weight loss* and *fast weight regain*. Then go for a walk, or do fifteen minutes of a relaxation exercise. Afterwards, congratulate yourself for breaking an unhealthy habit!

▲ Food Skills   ● Behavior Skills   ◆ Exercise Skills

R

◆ **RACQUETBALL**
Skill-sport aerobic exercise. *See* Exercise.

RAPID WEIGHT LOSS

Weight loss that exceeds 2 to 3 percent of your body weight per week. If you go on a diet and lose five to seven pounds in a week, that's rapid weight loss. Most of your losses are water in the first week, but after a few weeks, more of your losses will be muscle. On the average rapid weight-loss diet, you don't lose a significant amount of fat, compared to your total weight loss. Most rapid weight-loss diets show wide fluctuations in weight loss, if you stay on them for a long time. The first few weeks you lose five to seven pounds and it may keep up for a few more weeks, then suddenly the weight loss drops to a lower level. That's because your body has adjusted to living on fewer calories, and it will try to hoard the limited energy it's getting. The most common problems with rapid weight loss are muscle losses that cause you to regain weight, bouts of binge eating after the diet, and hunger that doesn't seem to turn off. The weight you regain is rounder or plumper-looking than before using the rapid weight-loss plan, because you are regaining fat fast, and you have less muscle, which is needed for tone.

Habit patterns are a special concern after rapid weight-loss diets. In order to develop a diet that takes weight off fast, the food plan must be very restricted, and this leads to good food/bad food attitudes in dieters. A reentry phase is necessary after a very restricted diet to teach you how to cope with more food options, but it's often too late, since the habits learned during dieting were not supportive of food variety and learning how to choose foods wisely. The most common habit that emerges after severe food restriction is to eat and eat, similar to the behavior after famine.

The faster you lose your weight, the harder it will be to maintain your weight loss. If you are very obese and in your doctor's care, the difficulties with rapid weight loss can be managed and monitored, but that doesn't mean that they won't be there. If you

---

are not in your doctor's care, you shouldn't be on a rapid weight-loss diet. *See* Yo-Yo Syndrome.

● **RATIONALIZATIONS**

Reasons or excuses to postpone self-care, such as weight loss and stress management. Rationalizations and excuses usually take the form of "I don't . . ." or "I can't. . . ." A simple change of perspective from negative to positive can turn your rationalizations into positive action. To do this, you use *affirmations,* or positive self-statements. This process removes your own defenses and helps you learn how to solve problems creatively.

Problem: I need to lose weight. Therefore I need to diet and exercise.

RATIONALIZATIONS	AFFIRMATIONS
I don't have time.	I don't need extra time. I just have to use my time differently: five minutes a day for food review, fifteen minutes a day for self-strengthening, thirty minutes every other day for exercise. Where will I get the time? I'll take it from negative time. The time I take to think I can't is easily thirty minutes a day, so I'll start now.
I don't have the energy.	Getting better daily nutrition will give me more energy. Exercise will give me more energy. So I'll just start, in order to get more energy.
I don't have support.	Eating better and exercising will be very supportive. In addition, I can add further support with imagery and relaxation. These things will make me stronger. I'll start so I can feel like I'm supporting myself.

▲ Food Skills   ● Behavior Skills   ◆ Exercise Skills

I don't have the money.	I don't need extra money. I buy food anyway. I'll just make leaner choices. Leaner choices are cheaper. I'll actually save money without all the expensive processed foods with added sugar and fat.
I don't like dieting.	I don't have to feel like I'm dieting and being deprived. I can still have pleasure and enjoy wide varieites of food. In fact, I'll be eating better than I have in a long time. I'm going to enjoy this experience, I'm going to develop a new relationship with food.
I'm lazy, I admit it.	Nutrition and exercise are going to give me energy and a sense of well-being I haven't felt in a long time. I'll just start. I need a pick-me-up.
I was born to be fat.	I was born to be lean. This issue about fat might be less personal if I say *I have fat*, or *I temporarily have fat*, instead of *I am fat*. Fat isn't part of my identity. It's just something I have, and I can let it go.
I don't know how to do it.	I'll just start eating better and exercising more, and by a week or two I'll be losing fat and I'll know how to do it.
I don't like exercise.	I love to feel the air on my skin during a walk outdoors. I like to feel my muscles getting strong while rowing. I love the feeling of exercise because it makes me feel young.

To develop affirmation or positive feedback to yourself, you also need a positive outlook on life. It's hard to have that if you are always criticizing yourself. Stop all criticism and begin to tell yourself only positive things. You can build up the strength you need to stay positive by beginning to practice behavior techniques like relaxation and deep breathing for stress control. You'd be surprised how strong they can make you feel in a very short time. Start your exercise program with walks or one aerobic selection that pleases you. When it begins to bore you, switch to another. Increase your activity and exercise gradually as you get stronger and more nutritionally fit.

The simplest way to get the drop on your rationalizations is to start tomorrow by fixing your food day. That alone will give you unexpected energy, and you'll feel better about everything. *See* the Problem Solver Calendar for guidelines to an ideal program.

▲ RDAs

Recommended daily allowances for nutrients, vitamins, and minerals based on your body's need for growth, repair, and maintenance (metabolism). Rather than worry, the best way to get them is to meet the serving requirements in the food group system on a daily basis. Only after that should you consider eating other foods.

● REGAIN

A relapse following a diet, entering the yo-yo syndrome and gaining weight back. *See* Rapid Weight Loss; Relapse; Yo-Yo Syndrome.

● RELAPSE

Weight regain immediately following a diet. This occurs more frequently after diets that are too low in calories, too restrictive, and used for rapid weight loss. It is particularly true of diets that remove carbohydrates or use any form of imbalanced food plan. The major reason for regain after these types of diets isn't your eating habits; it's your metabolism and body composition. You're at ideal weight with a very low-burning metabolism caused by the dramatic calorie restriction. And you've lost muscle, which doesn't give you the body composition you need to keep fat away.

▲ Food Skills   ● Behavior Skills   ◆ Exercise Skills

If you're coming off a plan that was very restrictive, and you're starting to regain, you have to stop the regain in the first stages. It will take a little work, but you can do it. The last thing you should do is go back on a low-calorie plan that is very restrictive. It will create the same problems, and you may not see weight loss at all. You have to retrain your body to burn more calories, and that means eating from all food groups, keeping your calories in a range that is more like the diet you should have tried in the first place. You need to exercise while you diet. Food energy is the source to rebuild muscle protein you lost on the rapid diet, and the exercise keeps the process stabilized. Food kicks up your metabolism, especially in the proportions identified in the Problem Solver food pyramid, when you eat the leaner versions of those foods.

At first, you'll see some water weight, and you have to get through that stage; but after a week or two, your body will start to stabilize if you diligently replace your water, and eat a balanced diet. Use the plan to get yourself back to ideal weight, which needs to be slow, not rapid, to keep your metabolism at a higher burning level. When you get back to your ideal, remain on the diet for a week or two, until you are sure you've stabilized, then you can move on to maintenance.

This acts as a reentry phase to help you repair the damage caused by losing weight too rapidly. Don't use this as permission to go on a rapid weight-loss diet again, thinking you can pull yourself out again the next time. Each time you use rapid weight loss, your regain potential gets greater, and it's not healthy to keep throwing your metabolism out of balance. If you find yourself regaining again, go back to a full food diet at no less than 1,000–1,200 calories for women, no less than 1400–1600 calories for men, to bring yourself back into line.

● **RELAXATION**
A self-enriching skill. It's the backbone of success, used to renew yourself, beat stress, and drive you forward to success.

There are two basic approaches to relaxation.

Body to mind: Using physical techniques to relax your body, which in turn relaxes your mind. Examples are deep muscle relaxation, stretches, callanetics, yoga, Akido, Tai Chee, massage, diaphragm breathing.

Mind to body: Using mental techniques to relax your mind, which in turn relaxes your body. Examples are deep muscle relaxation (mental), meditation, relaxation, response, biofeedback.

Both seek the same result: harmony of body and mind through release of tension. Since your body and mind are a team, it is difficult to separate one from the other in either process of relaxation, and the best programs include both aspects. For instance, in the body to mind video program *Callanetics*, while you are using stretches to release your tension, the music creates a soothing mood, the voice is caring and comforting, and the lighting and visuals are not distracting. The result is a combined mind and body relaxation, or deep muscle meditation. This is an example of relaxation as an art.

However, it is possible to do one without achieving the other. You can use stretches for relaxation and fail to quiet your stressed mind (mental resistance). Or you can use meditation and fail to relax your stressed muscles (physical resistance). Your goal is to learn how to do *both* simultaneously. The art of relaxation is achieving it, feeling it. One moment of release can compensate for hours, if not days, of stress.

The benefits of relaxation are also interrelated:

- Your pulse, heart rate, and respiratory rate decrease (relieving stress).
- Your breathing becomes more even and deeper (oxygen uptake is more effective).
- Your brain emits soothing alpha waves (well-being waves).
- Your blood lactate decreases (an ester of lactic acid, which is associated with neurosis).
- Your body is refreshed.
- You are more receptive to learning in this state.
- You are more capable of doing imagery or visualization in this state (claiming or owning a more positive future).
- Everything works better because you do.

How to Do Relaxation

The Relaxation Initiator

The first part of relaxation is the technique that sets the stage for fuller relaxation and use of other skills. In a sense, it's like an enzyme—it catalyzes other responses.

You can use this technique by itself or use it to initiate other, deeper suggestions.

Find a quiet spot were you won't be disturbed, in a soft, comfortable chair. Dim the lights. Sit straight, but not tensed. Close

▲ Food Skills   ● Behavior Skills   ◆ Exercise Skills

your eyes and clear your mind. If your mind wanders, allow the thoughts to pass through; float them on a cloud.

Breathe in to the count of three: one, two, three. Hold it lightly for the count of three: four, five, six. Exhale to the count of three: seven, eight, nine. As you exhale, let all of your muscles relax; repeat. As you continue to breathe deeply, let yourself go deeper and deeper into relaxation . . .

The Relaxation Adjuncts
Choose one skill at each session to add on to the relaxation initiator.

DEEP MUSCLE RELAXATION
Starting with your toes, progressively relax each muscle group from your feet to your scalp. Feel relaxation spreading through your body. Use the feeling of heat or warmth to enhance the release. "My toes are warm and limp . . . My feet are warm and limp. . . ." Feel your muscles loosen up and expand. Continue to the top of your scalp.

FULL BODY RELEASE
Imagine your body as a sack of sand. Picture pin holes in the bottom of the bag. Sand is seeping out the holes. As the sand seeps out, you feel more and more relaxed. Picture a situation during the day that caused you tension. Let it flow out of the bag with the sand.

FINDING YOUR PERFECT PLACE: Visualizing Your Place
Find a scene from nature that gives you joy and pleasure. An ocean vista. A wheat field in the wind. A garden of flowers. Hills in Vermont. Put yourself in the picture. You are lean and light in this picture. Your weight doesn't go with you. Become part of the scene. Feel the air, the sun. Be there. . . . If people or animals come into the place, wave to them and let them pass through. You own this place. . . . It's your space to be completely protected and safe. . . . Nothing can hurt you in this place. . . . Smile at anything that arrives and wave goodbye to it. . . . Feel the air as you do it. . . . Inhale and exhale evenly. Relax and enjoy this place as long as you want to.

Later: When something or someone stresses you, bring up the picture of this place. . . . Feel the air and comfort. . . . Breathe deeply. . . . None of the stresses go with you into this place. . . .

They can't get in because the place won't let anything stress you. . . . It's your perfect place.

VISUALIZATION FOR PROBLEM-SOLVING
Eating. Picture a situation where you are ready to eat something very fattening or very sweet. Then picture yourself not eating it, and laughing.

Stress. Picture yourself covered in a mountain of paper, stressed. Picture a wind coming in and blowing the paper away like day moths.

Stressors. Picture your boss stressed at you. Picture the stress falling off him/her like feathers. Picture him/her smiling and congratulating you.

Mental Rehearsal. Invent your own problem scene and resolve it. For instance, create a scene where you might feel angry, helpless, afraid, or upset by something and picture the same scene with a positive resolution.

Exercise. Picture yourself lying on the couch too tired to move. Picture air coming in and lifting you up. Picture yourself walking, running, rowing, or cycling, and loving it.

Mental Rehearsal. Invent your own sedentary scene and resolve it with a picture of yourself being active.

IMAGERY ON PAPER
See Fear of Failure to learn how to draw positive imagery pictures to resolve negative emotions.

RISKS

Conditions associated with excess weight. The more weight you gain, the greater the strain on your body system. Weight-related risks range from mild disorders to major diseases. This does not mean that an overweight person can't be free of disease or disorders. It means there is a greater tendency for these conditions to occur. If specific conditions are already present, excess weight can aggravate conditions. If family history shows a tendency toward a specific disease, excess weight can increase the likelihood of acquiring this disease.

▲ Food Skills　　　● Behavior Skills　　　◆ Exercise Skills

WEIGHT-RELATED RISKS

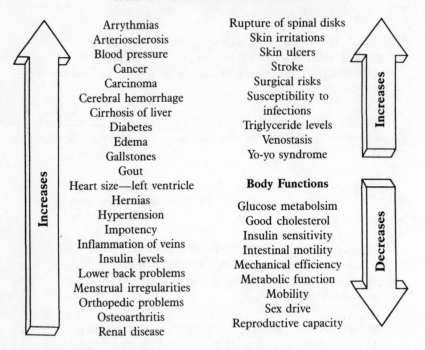

Increases

Arrythmias
Arteriosclerosis
Blood pressure
Cancer
Carcinoma
Cerebral hemorrhage
Cirrhosis of liver
Diabetes
Edema
Gallstones
Gout
Heart size—left ventricle
Hernias
Hypertension
Impotency
Inflammation of veins
Insulin levels
Lower back problems
Menstrual irregularities
Orthopedic problems
Osteoarthritis
Renal disease

Rupture of spinal disks
Skin irritations
Skin ulcers
Stroke
Surgical risks
Susceptibility to
infections
Triglyceride levels
Venostasis
Yo-yo syndrome

Increases

Body Functions

Glucose metabolsim
Good cholesterol
Insulin sensitivity
Intestinal motility
Mechanical efficiency
Metabolic function
Mobility
Sex drive
Reproductive capacity

Decreases

Based on 40–90 pounds of excess weight

▲ ROUGHAGE

Fiber. *See* Fiber.

◆ ROWING

Stationary aerobic exercise machine or outdoor aerobic sport.

Benefits:

- Excellent cardiovascular training
- Great calorie-burning exercise
- Works upper and lower body, improving strength and mobility
- No orthopedic injury
- Pace and tension easily adjusted
- Very portable; stores in small space
- Can be used for additional strength-building exercises

➠ How-to Skills   ❤ Good for Heart

Guidelines:

- Adjust the tension of the arm pulls to the lowest level.
- Sit on the seat cushion and strap feet into stirrups.
- Make sure handles of the rowing arms are parallel to your foot pads.
- Position the seat up to your feet so that you're in a crouched position. Keep your back straight and grasp the handles of the rowing arms.
- Glide the seat backward, straightening your legs, and pull the rowing arms until your legs are fully extended and your hands are parallel to your body. (For a full arm extension, bend your arms past your body and fully extend.)
- Return to starting position by gliding the seat forward, bending your knees and simultaneously pushing the rowing arms back to the start.
- The pace at which you row and the rowing arm tension determine the intensity of your workout. Start slowly.
- Wear gloves to prevent or minimize blisters. *See* Exercise.

S

● **SABOTEURS**

Cues (people, situations, things) that cause you to feel less secure about success. A saboteur can be a person who tries to tempt you to break your diet, situations that lure you to eat excess food, or unexpected events that cause extra stress, with the effect that you think you might fail.

When you are on a diet, it can seem as though everything and everyone is trying to subvert your success. A family member might say, "I liked you better when you weren't dieting." A friend might comment, "Go ahead and have dessert. I won't tell." Even though these people might not intend to subvert you, inadvertently they do. Events can compound your stress during a diet. For instance, the week you start dieting, you find out that your best friend is getting married and wants you in the wedding party. That means parties and food. Or work pressures increase, family crises develop, and that means added stress. It might seem that Murphy's Law is running your life when you start a diet: If things can go wrong, they will.

It's important to remember that any change in your life—such as a diet—will create its own set of problems in the first phases. After all, it's notice to people that *you intend to change,* and that upsets their old familiar routines with you. This can be particularly threatening to people who have centered their relationship with you around food, with you as the food preparer or you as the companion for all-you-can-eat lunches. The key to solving these upsets is found in your attitude. You can face these issues as challenges to your *skill power,* not threats to your *will power.* When it comes to successful dieting, skill counts, not will. Skills are positive sets of solutions you can use to strengthen your resolve and make you self-sufficient. Learning to be assertive about your decisions is an important skill. That means you can say no thanks to dessert without getting angry at the person who is offering it. It means you can ask your best friend to include low-fat alternatives to the standard wedding buffet without feeling embarrassed about speaking up for yourself. Remember whom you are

---

trying to change—you, not everyone else—and keep a sense of humor about their responses to your diet.

Use crisis situations as opportunities to learn how to gain control over your eating patterns and emotional habits, rather than triggers to let go. Review your goals each day, and reaffirm your commitment to succeed. Reinforce yourself daily with relaxation exercises for stress reduction, and behavior techniques for positive self-support—skill power! Keep a journal of problem situations that occur and the strategies you used to combat them. Review your journal regularly, adding new possibilities for creative solutions as you progress. Most of the behavior skills developed for successful dieting are strength giving and will enrich your whole life. Each time you triumph over a difficult situation, congratulate yourself with a reward that isn't food, such as tickets to a play you've wanted to see or a walk with a close friend. Your goal on a diet is to become a successful problem solver. Eventually, you won't have to keep a journal about problems and solutions; the solutions will snap into play when problems emerge, because they will be ingrained and natural. *See* Food Cues.

SACCHARIN

A crystalline compound used as a sugar substitute, more than 300 times sweeter than sugar. Studies differ about whether it causes cancer. It has no energy value. No evidence suggests it aids in weight loss. *See* Artificial Sweeteners.

SAFE WEIGHT LOSS

Removing fat from its stores, while providing the nutrition that's needed for muscle protection and health. Safe weight loss is generally regarded as losing 1.5 percent of your body weight per week. It means fat loss, not muscle losses. To accomplish this, the diet you choose must provide your essential daily nutrients. Without these nutrients, nothing works right. The preferred calorie level for women is 1,000–1,500 calories per day, but not below 1,000. The preferred calorie level for men is 1,400–1,800, but not below 1,400. The best choice is real food, not the processed variety with added sugars and salts (and fats). The program should fit into your lifestyle so you'll keep doing it. You should go for the maximum, not the minimum, in variety, personal pleasure, and a positive diet

---

▲ Food Skills   ● Behavior Skills   ◆ Exercise Skills

experience. You should exercise simultaneously, which is why you need more energy from carbohydrates, your body's preferred source of energy. Your weight loss should be slow and steady to ensure that you are only losing fat. You can see water fluctuations, but if you learn to gauge your weight loss *range*, instead of your weight loss each day, you won't be fooled by water changes. You must drink plenty of water while you are on a diet to facilitate all of the metabolic processes and mobilize your fat. And you should always take a vitamin/mineral supplement any time you diet as a secondary support for nutrition.

The decade of the eighties was the age of the rapid weight-loss diets. The lessons that were learned were based on failure. These lessons were: rigid calorie restriction, strict rules and deprivation, no- and low-carbohydrate menus, abnormal eating patterns, your foods and my foods. All of these techniques create rapid weight regain. *See* the Problem Solver food pyramid for guidelines to evaluate or create a balanced food plan.

▲ SALT
See Sodium.

SATIETY
Nutrient satisfaction, or the *off* signal that follows hunger when it is abated. *See* Appetite.

SATURATED FAT
The fat in food that is considered poor fat, because it raises the level of LDL or bad cholesterol in your body. *See* Cholesterol.

◆ SAUNA SUITS
Rubberized outfits promoted as "slimming" gear. The only thing they slim is your potential for healthy weight loss. These suits provide an artificial weight loss from water displacement. If you wear a sauna suit and exercise for twenty minutes, you'll feel perspiration dripping from your body, and you'll weigh less when you get on the scale. You're seeing temporary water losses, not fat losses, and you could be courting danger.

These suits should never be used in hot, humid weather because they prevent your body from cooling naturally by trapping perspiration next to your skin. For proper evaporation to occur, your skin needs to come into contact with a steady circulating stream of air, which rubberized suits prevent. In hot weather, these suits can cause heat stroke, heat exhaustion, chronic dehydration, and even death. A better bet is to skip the suit and do the twenty minutes of exercise. That way, you get the benefits without the risks.

● SCALE, BODY WEIGHT

A combination of your fat, muscle, and water in pounds. Your scale tells you more about the flow of water in and out of your body than it does about fat. Water is approximately 60 percent of your body weight. When you are looking down at that number in the metal box, you could be reading water retention from too much salt. Or you could be reading water losses from an active exercise session on a hot day. The numbers can trick you into actions that might not be appropriate. For instance, if your scale reads that you lost three pounds of water, you might think you lost fat, so it's OK to have a dinner at your local restaurant (where you know they cook with fat). Or you might feel frustrated when your scale reads the same after a week of dieting, and you might stop. A day later, you lose the water that you were retaining and you see a sudden drop in weight (last night you quit your diet and ate everything in the refrigerator because you were sure your diet wasn't working). Relying on your scale to measure your weight-loss success is like asking a mirror in a fun house to tell you how you look tonight. The scale is responsible for more diet headaches than appetite suppressants on an empty stomach.

Rely on getting looser in your clothing and tightening your belt a notch, instead of standing on the scale every day.

If the scale were perfect, this is what it would tell you:

Body Fat				
	Men		Women	
Thin	8	percent	15	percent
Lean	11	percent	18	percent
Average	15	percent	22	percent
Plus	18	percent	25	percent
Excess	22	percent	28	percent
Obese	25 +	percent	30 +	percent

Based on underwater weighing of athletes

▲ Food Skills   ● Behavior Skills.   ◆ Exercise Skills

It would tell how much body fat is standing on the box. Then you could subtract that from 100 percent, and the rest would be your lean muscle.

Because the scale isn't an accurate indicator of your body composition, you have to outsmart it.

How to Weigh Yourself

1. Weigh yourself before breakfast, after your bladder is emptied.
2. Weigh yourself at the same time every day, in the same way.
3. Wear light clothing (or underwear) and no shoes.
4. Add up your daily weights for one week and divide by seven to determine your average weekly weight. For your average weight range, compare that average to the lowest and highest weight of the week. Your average weight range will tell you how much weight variation you can expect on a weekly basis (usually from water fluctuations).
5. The pounds lost below your average weekly weight are as close as you can come to reading your actual fat loss, using your scale.

If you are on a healthy diet that uses lean protein for muscle protection, low-fat for fat removal, and carbohydrates for energy, the actual weight loss will be fat loss.

If you are on a rapid weight-loss diet that is very low calorie, you can see dramatic water losses and muscle losses, so there is no way for you to tell what's going on when you stand on the scale.

If you are a woman, you have to take your monthly ovulation cycle into account, when you can see greater fluctuations in water weight.

If you are retaining too much water, diuretics are not the best choice. Reduce your salt intake and drink more water to bring yourself back into balance.

If you find that your clothing is looser, but the scale doesn't register any difference, don't despair. You could be increasing your muscle content and muscle is heavier than fat.

If you are starving yourself to lose weight, the losses you see on the scale are primarily muscle and water. You are going to make it easier to gain back your fat.

If you are watching the numbers go down slowly (say two pounds per week) and you are sticking to your diet, congratula-

---

tions! You know how to play the numbers and win. You're losing your fat. The interesting thing about fat loss is how it appears on your body. Five pounds of fat loss *looks like* ten pounds of weight loss (which can be water, muscle, and fat). That's the real benefit of aiming for fat loss with a healthy diet. You lose fat slower, but you look better faster. And you set yourself up for lean body maintenance for life.

● SCALE, FOOD

A kitchen device to weigh your food to conform to serving sizes recommended by a diet.

You do not have to use a measuring scale for your food if you are not on a diet that limits your food to the maximum. You can use average serving sizes indicated in the food groups. If you want to be sure you're not overdoing your protein, weigh your proteins for a week, and teach yourself how to calibrate portion sizes with your eye. Then retest yourself every few weeks to see how good your eye is. If you eat more than your share of vegetables and fruits, it isn't going to pack on fat. In fact, it will help to keep you lean. Studies indicate that complex carbohydrate foods take so long to digest that extras don't store as fat. This is how athletes stay slim, when they seem to eat so much more than the average person. Their *extras* are complex carbohydrates. The foods to watch closely are the fats and oils and sweets. They're the ones that take you over your fat maximum and sugar maximum. They combine to store fat. Keep your fiber content high, and limit the amount of processed foods you eat. Make sure you get your daily calcium from low-fat milk and dairy products. Your measuring scale should be the proportions of food you eat: 60 percent complex carbs, 20 percent lean proteins, 20 percent fat. When you get it down to a routine, you get lean.

SCREENING

Tests to determine if you are able to go on a particular diet program. Most of the diets that need medical screening are very strict diets with low-calorie formats. You should never embark on a diet like that without proper screening. Under 800 calories should always be monitored by a doctor, especially if the diet doesn't include enough carbohydrates. Balanced food diets (1,000–1,500 cals/day for women; 1,400–1,800 cals/day for men) don't require screening, because these are the same standards your doctor would ask you to adhere to for safe weight loss.

▲ SEASONINGS

Taste enhancers for dieters. *See* Herbs and Spices for the list.

● SELF-ESTEEM

A feeling of self-worth. Lack of self-esteem is usually associated with the overweight state, especially in obesity. This may not have been a problem before weight gain; but nevertheless, after weight is gained and held for long periods of time, your sense of self-worth begins to be more closely linked to food issues and fat problems. This is a form of projecting emotions and feelings into food. Regardless of your self-esteem issues, it's vital to learn how to like yourself as you are, as you begin dieting. The success of your diet and fitness efforts are strengthened by a sense of self-worth at the outset. If you start with too many negative feelings about yourself, then weight loss is viewed as the miracle solution, and all you've done is transfer all of those emotions and feelings to being thin. This is a form of extreme thinking that will not serve you well during or after your diet.

It's important to realize that no one is immune to negative self-criticism, or low self-opinions, even thin people. In fact, many thin people spend excessive energy finding fault with themselves. Their small pads of fat are as large to them as your weight is to you. The weight problem has to be put in perspective. It's a situation you can deal with, but it doesn't have to be your identity. You *have* fat; fat isn't your identity. Even if you think that fat is part of your identity, you can use mirror exercises and relaxation exercises to let go of this misconception. Many people make the mistake of identifying with their fat. If you have a headache, you don't say, "I am a headache." And yet, the language of weight suggests that you're supposed to take fat on as an identity and say, "I am fat."

Perhaps our society won't change, and thin will always be perceived as a sign of greater self-esteem. But thin isn't identity either. A thin person can have just as many identity issues as a fatter person. In the meantime, practice relaxation and mirror exercises, and social pictures of self-worth will have less of a hold. In the end, what really counts is what you think of yourself. *See* Imagery; Mirror Exercises; Relaxation.

● SELF-IMAGE

How you see yourself from inside, regardless of the view from the mirror. *See* Mirror Exercises.

SERVINGS

Standard measurements for food portions based on nutrient value and healthy eating (to stay lean). The food group system sets the requirements for standard servings, based on the needs of your metabolism to maintain your body, repair its cells, and facilitate all processes. These serving recommendations are the ones that are used for most eating plans and healthy diet programs across the country. However, it is important to note that the meat group serving size has gotten a bit out of line, even in diet books and calorie counters. Most people think that a standard serving of meat is four to six ounces, when it really should be two ounces. This mistake can add a great deal of excess fat. The food industry isn't consistent with servings, and a TV dinner might have four to six ounces of meat. The labels usually have the correct serving size per total weight of the product, but it's best to check to be safe.

Your carbohydrate servings (complex carbohydrates) do not have to be as carefully watched as your protein and fat servings, because protein and fat add the most fat to your body, and the carbohydrates tend to burn off. Carbohydrates also have fiber, which helps to prevent fat storage. This only refers to the natural carbohydrates such as fruits, vegetables, and whole grains, since the processed varieties contain fats, sugars, salt, and very little fiber.

It's a good idea to learn the standard servings, even memorize them. That way, you can be sure you're getting accurate information. A serving size mistake can cost you a lot of fat. For instance, you might read a calorie counter that gives the fat content of a candy bar, but it's a one-ounce serving, while the standard candy bar is two ounces. In addition, most diet programs adapt the serving sizes to their overall calorie level, so that their serving size may be different from the required one. Because of all the variations in sources, few people know what the accurate requirements are. *See* The Problem Solver Diet for standard serving sizes.

SETPOINT

A theory about metabolism that was popular in the 1980s; an idea rather than a scientific fact. The setpoint idea claimed that your

---

▲ Food Skills ● Behavior Skills ◆ Exercise Skills

body has an inner thermostat determined to keep you fat or at a weight you will return to despite a diet. This theory sprang out of research on the failure rates of diets, specifically rapid weight-loss diets, which are notorious for causing rapid weight regain. It's a result of *poor* dieting that was taken out of context and sold as a fact of life.

If you think about a thermostat, you'll see the flaw in reasoning for setpoint. A thermostat only reads what is happening, it can't read what can happen. The thermostat in your car reads the existing heat level. If you stop the car and restart it later the thermostat will read that your car engine is cooler. The same thing applies to your metabolism. Your metabolic rate (thermostat) only reflects what you give it to work with. When you lose weight rapidly, your metabolic rate is reduced from calorie restriction and muscle losses. It reads cool. When you eat less fat, more fiber, and adequate protein, you generate more metabolic heat from eating, even on a diet. The thermostat reads warm. When you exercise, you raise the heat production in your body by 15 percent, and the output continues after the exercise is over. Your metabolism is never set, or static. The combination of exercise and a heat-producing diet can drive up your metabolism to burn fat and build muscle, and that prevents weight regain. The thermostat reads *hot*.

▲ SIMPLE SUGARS

Naturally occurring sugars in carbohydrate foods. *See* Carbohydrates; Sugar.

♦ SKIING

Skill-sport aerobic exercise. *See* Exercise.

♦ SKILL SPORTS

Aerobic exercises including tennis, racquetball, squash, handball, skiing, basketball, volleyball, and so forth.

_____

⇒ How-to Skills   ♥ Good for Heart

Benefits:
- Easily combined with a more regular aerobic routine
- Add variety and excitement, challenging a partner or joining forces with a team
- Considered play rather than workout

Guidelines:
- Play as frequently as possible to improve skill, since skill level determines intensity.
- Couple these games with other aerobic activities to equal half an hour at least three times per week.
- Try to stay in continuous motion and minimize nonactive time.

SKIN-FOLD CALIPERS

The metal instrument that resembles a giant tweezer used in anthropometric tests for body fat and muscle composition. *See* Anthropometric Measurements.

▲ SNACKS

Energy boosters between meals. *See* Snacks in the Problem Solver Diet section (pages 69–85).

▲ SODAS (DIET)

Drinks with artificial sweeteners are usually considered dieters' sodas, but they shouldn't be. They have no nutritional value and are simply sugar drinks with additives, even when they are low calorie. When you're on a diet, you want to get the most nutrition for your calories, and artificial sweeteners have no value. The long-term effects of artificial sweeteners have led to warnings about saccharin and have banned cyclamates, and the newest one, aspartame, is still being tested. Many dieters drink sodas by the six-pack, thinking they're an acceptable way to ward off hunger. But they're not. Studies indicate that sweet drinks lead to an increased tolerance for sugar. If you're drinking sodas with artificial sweeteners, all you are getting is sweetness in a condensed form. This can make you want and need more sweets to be satisfied. Evidence shows that artificial sweeteners have no benefit for weight control.

▲ Food Skills   ● Behavior Skills   ◆ Exercise Skills

What's the real diet soda? Club soda spritzers (lime, lemon, cranberry). Water, plain or fruited. Fresh fruit juices for super-nutrition. Cold herbal teas provide an interesting change of pace. Low-fat milk is excellent and essential. Start limiting your use of diet sodas and turn to the drinks that give you greater nutrient density. That way, you get better fat burn and health.

▲ SODIUM

A naturally occurring mineral; also called salt. In your body, sodium is found in body fluids and bones—50 percent in your extracellular fluid, arteries, veins, capillaries, intestinal fluids, around your cells; and 50 percent in your bones.

In your diet, you get sodium in five ways:
- occurring naturally in foods (best source)
- added during processing (worst source)
- added during cooking (habit to limit)

SODIUM IN BALANCE 1100–3300 mg per day	SODIUM TO EXCESS 3300–6000+ per day
It works with potassium to balance blood acid/alkali content.	Causes losses of potassium which create fluid retention, swelling, and dizziness.
It helps to regulate fluid balance on both sides of cell walls.	Causes high blood pressure, which leads to heart attacks and strokes.
It's vital to muscle contraction/ expansion	Leads to kidney disease.
It's vital for nerve stimulation.	
It keeps minerals soluble so they don't form deposits in your blood-stream.	
With chlorine, it purifies your body of carbon dioxide and aids digestion.	
It maintains blood volume and pressure by attracting and holding water in blood vessels.	

• added at the table (habit to eliminate)
• from medications (source to control, where possible)

Don't forget that sodium and potassium need to be balanced. *See* Potassium.

Sodium excesses are extensive in our modern-age microwave and TV dinner diets. It's second to sugar in additives used in processed foods as a preservative and flavor enhancer. Most of us are getting double the recommended daily dose, primarily from table salt misuse, cooking abuse, and reliance on processed foods as a diet staple.

If you diet with fresh food sources as your primary foods and use a pinch of sodium, instead of a pour from the salt shaker, in cooking and at the table, you won't find sodium excesses in your diet. It's the easiest way to take control over sodium without doing endless calculations. And you gain another benefit from fresh foods—better fat burn and health.

If you are on a low- or no-sodium plan for your heart, use an herb salter to replace your regular salt for eating and cooking needs and eliminate sodium-rich processed foods from your diet. Check our sodium-at-a-glance guide to find the foods highest in sodium, and beware that they don't sneak into your menus. Rely on natural foods, avoiding processed cheese foods and cured meats.

Shaking Off the Salt Habit

Sodium is a learned habit. Over time, as you increase the level of sodium in your food, you increase your taste for it. This process can easily be reversed by gradually reducing your sodium intake,

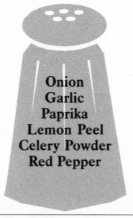

Onion
Garlic
Paprika
Lemon Peel
Celery Powder
Red Pepper

▲ Food Skills ● Behavior Skills ◆ Exercise Skills

SODIUM AT A GLANCE
SOURCES OF EXCESS

Average Intake
2300–6900 mg/day

ELIMINATE OR MODERATE SOURCES OF EXCESS SODIUM

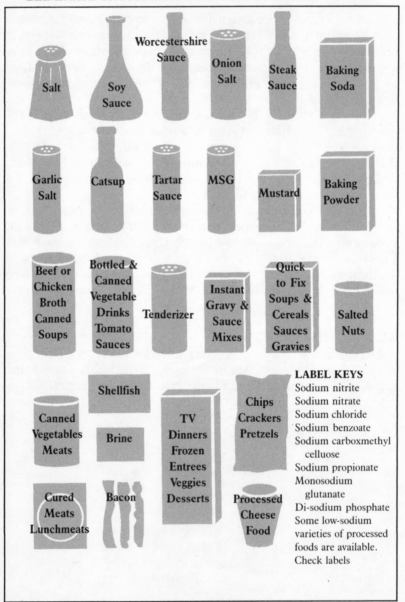

Salt

Soy Sauce

Worcestershire Sauce

Onion Salt

Steak Sauce

Baking Soda

Garlic Salt

Catsup

Tartar Sauce

MSG

Mustard

Baking Powder

Beef or Chicken Broth Canned Soups

Bottled & Canned Vegetable Drinks Tomato Sauces

Tenderizer

Instant Gravy & Sauce Mixes

Quick to Fix Soups & Cereals Sauces Gravies

Salted Nuts

Shellfish

Canned Vegetables Meats

Brine

TV Dinners Frozen Entrees Veggies Desserts

Chips Crackers Pretzels

Cured Meats Lunchmeats

Bacon

Processed Cheese Food

LABEL KEYS
Sodium nitrite
Sodium nitrate
Sodium chloride
Sodium benzoate
Sodium carboxmethyl
  celluose
Sodium propionate
Monosodium
  glutanate
Di-sodium phosphate
Some low-sodium
varieties of processed
foods are available.
Check labels

1 teaspoon table salt = 2000 / mg sodium, ⅔ of daily maximum

⟶ How-to Skills   ♥ Good for Heart

❤BEST REPLACEMENTS

Recommended Dose
1100–3300 mg/day

RELY ON SODIUM THAT OCCURS NATURALLY IN FOOD

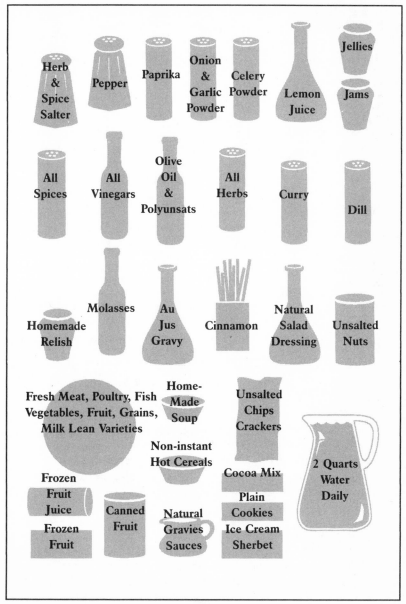

Herb & Spice Salter · Pepper · Paprika · Onion & Garlic Powder · Celery Powder · Lemon Juice · Jellies · Jams

All Spices · All Vinegars · Olive Oil & Polyunsats · All Herbs · Curry · Dill

Homemade Relish · Molasses · Au Jus Gravy · Cinnamon · Natural Salad Dressing · Unsalted Nuts

Fresh Meat, Poultry, Fish Vegetables, Fruit, Grains, Milk Lean Varieties · Home-Made Soup · Unsalted Chips Crackers · 2 Quarts Water Daily

Non-instant Hot Cereals · Cocoa Mix

Frozen Fruit Juice · Frozen Fruit · Canned Fruit · Natural Gravies Sauces · Plain Cookies · Ice Cream Sherbet

2 teaspoons herb & spice salter = 0 mg sodium = more sodium options

▲ Food Skills ● Behavior Skills ◆ Exercise Skills

thereby reducing your taste and desire for it. Many people find that it's better to go all out against sodium, enduring a saltless week or two, because it purifies your system and palate for salt, and you will immediately find salty foods undesirable, with your own taste buds acting as a regulator. Every so often, compute an average day's use of sodium to see if you're keeping within your limits. Sodium, like fat, has a tendency to sneak in when you let down your guard.

Shopping Low Sodium
- Read labels for sodium content. Look for the exact content in milligrams. The label can say lower sodium and mean lower than the former version of that food.
- If sodium is not listed in milligrams, remember that label ingredients are listed first to last by weight. Sodium should be very low on the list, for safety.
- Learn to recognize high-sodium ingredients that can be listed on labels without saying sodium, such as baking soda or baking powder.
- Don't buy foods that don't have the sodium content listed. They aren't worth your trust.
- Don't forget to check labels on medications for sodium.

Diet/Sodium Sense
- Eat fresh foods whenever possible.
- Cut salt in your recipes to one-half or less.
- Replace high-sodium condiments with low-sodium versions.
- Replace your salt with an herbal shaker for seasoning★ in cooking and salting at the table.
- Taste your food before salting.
- In restaurants, ask for your food to be prepared salt-free.
- Ask for sauces and salad dressings on the side, so you can control the amount you use.

★Herb and Spice Salter
You can make your own salt replacer that has no sodium. Mix your favorite herbs and spices to taste. Suggestions: onion powder, garlic powder, paprika, lemon peels, celery powder, red pepper, and other spices of your choice. Experiment with blends until you achieve the perfect mix. Use it for cooking and table salting. No salt doesn't have to mean no taste.

▲ SOY

Vegetable protein; nature's protein. Soy is a major source of protein for weight-conscious dieters who are looking for a replacement for red meats or animal sources. Even though soy is listed as a grain, it is best to view it as a protein food since it is the only natural grain that has about ten grams of fat in a cup. When compared to an equivalent *protein*, soy is very low-fat. When you use it as a grain source, be aware that it's fatter than other grains, but it's still a remarkable food. Consider these important ingredients in soy:

High protein
Unsaturated fat
Low sodium
High fiber
Rich source of B complex, calcium, phosphorus, potassium, magnesium, iron, lecithin

❤ Lecithin in soy helps reduce cholesterol buildup by keeping cholesterol/calcium deposits in suspension. This prevents the deposits from adhering to artery walls.

Soy milk is a low-fat substitute for people who have allergies to regular milk. Soy oil is a good source of linoleic acid. Soy flour has a nutty taste for breads, gravies, and sauces. Soybeans take a little time to soak overnight and cook. But they're worth it. *See* Grains.

SPARE TIRE

Midriff weight, common to men. Men are primarily upper-body fat distributors, depositing their fat in the midriff, chest, and neck. This weight is easier to lose than lower-body fat; but it's medically more risky, since it has been linked to heart disease. Weight lifting doesn't remove this fat, unless your diet is adjusted to remove fat in your food. Men get more of their fat from high-fat proteins, particularly steaks and red meats. The best plan is to switch to the leaner proteins such as chicken, turkey, and fish, using the red meats less frequently and choosing the lean ones. Fiber increases are important too, since fiber aids in fat loss and reduces the levels of bad cholesterol in your system—a heart saver. Men lose weight faster because of their greater percentage of muscle tissue, so a low-fat, high-carbohydrate, lean-protein diet will flatten that tire. Women can be upper-body fat distributors too,

---

▲ Food Skills ● Behavior Skills ◆ Exercise Skills

but they tend to get more of their fat from gravies, sauces, and sweets. Removing these excesses and improving your overall diet, along with exercise, will trim that tire and give you back your hourglass curves.

▲ SPICES

Seasonings and taste enhancers for dieters. *See* Herbs and Spices for the list.

SPORTS

Aerobic or nonaerobic exercises, depending on the level of intensity. *See* Exercise, Skill Sports.

♦ STAIRMASTER

Stationary aerobic exercise machine that simulates stair-climbing, a weight-bearing exercise. For total fitness, be sure to add an upper body routine to your workout with this machine. *See* Exercise.

STARCH BLOCKERS

A fad of the 1980s which consisted of a protein extracted from kidney beans. Chemical tests indicated that this form of protein blocked starch digestion by inhibiting the enzyme amylase (the enzyme in saliva that begins to break down carbohydrates). Supposedly, this caused starch (from carbohydrate foods) to pass into your intestines undigested like fiber, instead of being converted to glucose for absorption by your blood. However, human studies didn't show the same results as chemical studies. In humans, starch blockage was only about 10 percent of the total starch in the diet. It seems that the blockers couldn't hold their own when they met gastric juices and the acid composition of the stomach. Even if they worked, starch blockers would hardly be useful to a dieter, since starch in complex carbohydrates is one of the least fattening sources of energy. Remember, the starches are lean, calorie-burning foods, but the fats you put in them aren't. Your body requires starch for metabolism, and blocking can cause nutrient imbalance and digestive disorders. When starch breakdown is inhibited, your body uses protein and fat, and your metabolism can be distorted. The FDA put a halt to the sale of starch blockers for safety reasons, but a number of people paid the price in fat gain. Because they thought starch was not digesting, they ate more of everything and gained weight.

It's never wise to interfere with the natural processes of metabolism, which require the nutrients in carbohydrates, protein, and fat to function properly. You also need vitamins, minerals, and water on a daily basis. This not only protects your health, but it also gives you the best fat burn.

STARVATION (TOTAL FASTING)

Chronic nutrient deficiency that causes severe metabolic stress. When you go without food for one day, your body's glycogen storage is used up. (Glycogen is the name for stored glucose, derived from carbohydrates in digestion.) But your brain *needs* glucose for its energy and maintenance. With no glucose or glycogen stores, your body has to steal protein from its own cells, in order to make glucose (glucogenesis). At this point, starvation causes a gradual depletion of body parts, called muscle wasting. After a few weeks of starvation, your brain adapts and can then use fat as a fuel (ketones from fatty acid breakdown). This temporarily stops the breakdown of body protein for fuel. After your fat stores are depleted, there's nowhere else to turn for energy, and your body uses its remaining protein for all of its fuel needs. If food is not introduced, drastic muscle losses occur and death follows.

If food is introduced, it takes months of nutrient therapy to rebuild body protein, and it's seldom rebuilt fully unless exercise is included along with a low-fat diet. Often, metabolic and psychological changes can occur that were not present before starvation.

How does this relate to a diet? Many diets use a mild form of starvation to achieve weight loss. While the results are not as extreme, the process is similar. Many dieters stop eating for a few days at a time, thinking they can take off weight fast. It's the worst thing you can do for your health. It only takes a day of starvation for your body to begin to steal its own protein. And that means less muscle, which in turn leads to poorer calorie burn.

▲ Food Skills ● Behavior Skills ◆ Exercise Skills

STEP AEROBICS

Aerobic exercises using a step device on the floor and combining that with calisthenics or dance aerobics. This is a good workout for strength and endurance, but be sure your program involves the upper body too, for a full routine. *See* Cross Training.

STIMULANTS

Chemicals or substances that speed up your nervous system. *See* Appetite Suppressants; Caffeine.

STOMACH

One of the primary organs of digestion. Your stomach breaks down food into smaller units to prepare them for the small intestines where digestion continues and absorption of the nutrients takes place. Your stomach is J-shaped and muscular, with three areas that perform specific functions. The upper part acts as a storage center for food, while digestion takes place in the middle and lower parts. The upper part continues the breakdown of carbohydrates that began in the mouth with an enzyme from your salivary glands. The midpart is where primary breakdown of proteins take place, and the lower part has a pumplike muscle action to move food into your small intestines. It takes from four to seven hours for food to pass through your stomach. *See* Digestion.

STOMACH STAPLING

Surgery for serious obesity problems. Part of the stomach is sealed off to make the stomach capacity smaller. This prevents intake of excess food, because fullness occurs sooner.

♦ STRENGTH TRAINING

Building muscle strength and endurance by using resistance exercises, such as weights.

If you tend to believe that weight training is only for the ultra fit or devout body builder, you're in for a delightful surprise. Not only is weight training the key to the fit appearance you desire at the end of a diet, it is also a fat reducer. Since muscle needs more

---

energy to sustain itself than fat, building your muscle mass means you burn more calories to maintain that muscle on a daily basis. This has a double benefit for a dieter: you get to the end of your diet sooner by burning more calories overall, and you have the higher-muscle body you need for maintenance. This means you can eat more calories without regaining your weight.

There also is a bonus for your bones. Bones get stronger and thicker when they are used, and strength training has been shown to help restore *density* to them. This is a crucial factor to help prevent arthritis and osteoporosis, particularly in women.

If your muscles are not used, they can shrink, atrophy, and even disintegrate. Since muscle losses lead to fat gain, this is a situation you want to avoid in order to keep yourself leaner through life. It's also particularly important news for dieters who have lost muscle on unhealthy diets, since strength training gives you the means to rebuild your lost muscle and rebalance your body composition.

There are other important benefits as well:

- Strength training protects you from injury or strain, since stronger muscles help you perform your daily tasks easier, such as lifting, pulling, pushing, and carrying. Since daily activity can count for 15 percent of the calories you burn daily, this also helps to increase your overall calorie burn.
- Strength training protects you from back injury and pain, since stronger muscles provide better support for your spine. This improves your mobility and makes activity easier and more pleasurable. It's also an important consideration for people who carry a great deal of extra weight, since weight and back problems have been known to go together.
- Strength training improves your posture and overall body balance, and that gives you a greater sense of self-esteem, self-confidence, and well-being.
- Strength training maintains your bone mass and even helps restore calcium to your bones. This keeps you fitter and younger as you age. When you keep your muscles stronger, particularly in your upper body, you avoid the weaker, shortened appearance you can get from upper-body muscle losses with aging.
- Strength training improves your blood flow and circulation. This not only makes you feel healthier, but makes you look healthier as well.

▲ Food Skills ● Behavior Skills ◆ Exercise Skills

➡ *How to Do Strength Training*

The key to strength training is found in two factors:
1. Resistance—weight or opposing force;
2. Repetitions—number of times you repeat the exercise.

The American College of Sports Medicine recommends using eight to ten exercises for strength training that use your body's major muscle groups, and aiming for one set of ten to fifteen repetitions (reps) for each exercise. The best plan for muscle maintenance is strength training two times each week, and for muscle development three times each week. Your goal is gradually to increase the resistance weight while you gradually increase the repetitions, using the recommended limits.

Form is more important than the amount of weight you use. It's better to lift less weight with more "form" than to lift more weight with less form, since injury or strain can defeat the purpose of your training, which is to build stronger muscles. You should never lift more weight than is comfortable or do one more repetition for the road, since that, too, can cause strained or pulled muscles.

You can do a very effective strength training program at home with one-pound to five-pound weights. There is a rule of thumb to remember: Lifting ten pounds one hundred feet is the same effort as lifting one hundred pounds ten feet. This means that you can use ten-pound weights and by using more repetitions, you can achieve the same strength training benefits as a body builder who lifts one hundred pounds once.

Your concentration should be focused on exercising one muscle or muscle group at a time with "form," gradually working up to exercising all of your body's muscle groups in a workout session.

You can use any machine that uses resistance, such as weights, cams levers, or pulleys to work specific muscle groups. Nautilus machines use cam or pulley resistance; Universal machines use lever resistance; and hydraulic machines use rubber bands or elastic tubing for resistance.

At home, portable weights are also effective, such as hand or leg weights, bar bells, and smaller devices such as Thighmaster. Remember, the key is in resistance and repetition (reps).

This is how you would approach your strength training session.

If you are using bar bells, for instance, you start with a lower weight and gradually work up to lifting that weight ten to fifteen times slowly, concentrating on the muscle group you are exercising. When the repetitions become easy to do at fifteen reps, then you increase the weight again.

_____

➡ How-to Skills ❤ Good for Heart

You can stop at a weight that provides a good workout, or you can go on to a gym for more advanced weight lifting. However, even with higher weights, the same rules apply.

An at-home beginner might start with one-pound weights and work up to ten to fifteen reps with each muscle group of the body, then increase the weight to two pounds and work up to fifteen reps, and ultimately to five pounds.

It is believed that the best way to work your muscle groups is from the *ground* up. Since most of your weight rests on your lower body, that gives you the grounding you need for a strong foundation.

A basic program to work the major muscle groups would be these, from the ground up: calves first, then thighs, abdomen, lower back and stomach, upper back, arms, and shoulders. This can be followed by a good full body stretch to relax your muscles and reward yourself for a job well done.

An excellent resource for strength training is *The Strength Connection*, by the Aerobics Institute, Dallas. There are many books at the library that can guide you through a basic program.

The following exercises may serve as a guide to a basic at-home program.

Begin by lightly stretching the muscle or group of muscles you will be using. Then do your strength exercises with low weights to begin, working up to ten to fifteen repetitions for each exercise.

Calves: Sit firmly on the edge of a straight-back chair. With leg weight on ankle and leg out straight, lift leg slowly in the air. Don't tense knees or try to lift your leg too high. Work up to ten to fifteen reps. Repeat with other leg. (Grasp chair base for support as necessary.)

Thighs: Lying face down on the floor with weight on ankle, lift heel of leg toward buttocks. Work up to ten to fifteen reps. Keep knees relaxed. As you get stronger, you can try this exercise with your leg straight as you lift it from the floor (with relaxed knees). Repeat with other leg.

Abdomen: Lie on the floor on your side. Rest your head on your arm or on your hand. With weight on ankle, lift top leg to strengthen outer thigh, now lift lower leg to meet it and strengthen entire thigh area. Work up to ten to fifteen reps. Repeat on opposite side.

Lower Back and Stomach: Lie on floor face up, with your knees bent to take pressure off back. Curl head and shoulders up into your trunk (no weights for this). Work up to ten to fifteen reps.

▲ Food Skills ● Behavior Skills ◆ Exercise Skills

Upper Back: Raise arms to shoulder level, holding weight. Bend your elbows up. The exercise is to lower weight slowly to straight arm position (don't tense elbows). When you get stronger, you can start with the arms out at shoulder level, holding weights, and gradually press your arms backward (keeping elbows relaxed, not locked). Work up to ten to fifteen reps.

Arms and Shoulders: Standing straight th weight in hand, flex elbow. The exercise is to slowly extend your arm straight down to your side again, to strengthen upper arms. Work up to ten to fifteen reps. Repeat with other arm.

People with arthritis have special needs and should always talk to their doctor before beginning any exercise program. A wise course would be to have an exercise physiologist outline a safe program for you. If you are very overweight, build yourself up with this type of program without the use of weights.

● STRESS

A high-tension system, speeded up; also called the fight or flight response because that's the way you feel when you're under stress, as though you want to run or fight, and most of the time you can't do either one. Stress is a series of physiological changes that can be brought on by shock, change, or threat in your environment, or the perception of it in your mind. When stress occurs, you pump more adrenaline, your heart beats faster, your breath is short and shallow, your blood pressure is elevated, and blood rushes to your muscles (to run). Your blood vessels constrict to keep your system pressure up (to fight).

In emergency situations, stress can save your life. You can respond quicker, move faster, lift more weight, do things you thought you were afraid of. Some stress is necessary for growth and change to motivate you to seek new challenges, set new goals, start new businesses, feel excited by life, or reach optimal levels of performance in sports. Athletes face stress regularly, but it's considered good stress because it has a physical outlet.

In nonemergency situations in daily life, stress often has no outlet. A traffic jam every morning, money constraints, time deadlines, job pressures, a sudden family crisis, any major change, threats to your security—all of these conditions bring on stress. Any situation that requires you to alter your behavior is stress producing. Your thoughts and feelings can exacerbate stress. Nutrient depletion puts you in a defenseless position against stress.

Dieters have to face two levels of stress: the normal, everyday stress that everyone else is facing and stress peculiar to dieting.

Calories and Stress

Calorie reduction is stress. Your system adapts to using a certain calorie level for metabolism, and a sudden calorie decrease upsets the status quo. Your body has to work harder for its energy. If your diet doesn't provide the nutrients you need to meet that stress biochemically, your metabolism has to work at a deficit. Metabolic stress is one reason deprived diets are so dangerous for a dieter.

Nutrition and Stress

Daily stress also depletes your nutrients. When your heart beats faster and your blood pressure rises, so does your metabolism. It burns nutrients faster. You have to replace the nutrients in your daily diet, or your body will take them from your muscles and bones. Daily nutrient insurance is a must for anyone facing stress, but particularly for a dieter.

Behavior and Stress

Dieting means changing your standard eating *patterns* into different ones. Change causes stress, even when the change is for the better. That's why it's important to choose a diet that uses natural eating patterns in a low-calorie format, instead of an unnatural diet that causes a great disruption in your lifestyle. The more unnatural the diet, the greater the stress to adhere to it.

Food and Stress

Stress leads to eating, particularly for a person who uses food for rewards or consolation. The more stressful your diet program, the greater the likelihood that you will eat to compensate for the feeling of deprivation and isolation from the world of food. That's why real food programs are better for you than low- or no-food programs with food substitutes. They create less food stress. Some programs say that removing people from food helps them resist food cues, and this allows greater weight loss. It also allows greater weight regain. The shock of reentry into the world of food after months of deprivation is too stressful. You can't learn about eating and dealing with food by removing yourself from it, and you can't find good food habits in a prepackaged mix or drink. You have to use food to practice. You learn by doing, then repeating it until it becomes a habit.

▲ Food Skills ● Behavior Skills ◆ Exercise Skills

Body Image and Stress
An image change occurs during dieting, and even when it's desired, it can be stressful. When you lose weight too fast, your image changes rapidly. In a sense, it runs ahead of you, and you're left with a thinner body that looks as though it belongs to someone else. Rapid weight loss can disrupt your sense of self and create image disturbances that leave you insecure about the results. This creates a great deal of emotional stress.

Your goal at the end of a diet is too important to be taken lightly. You shouldn't be scared out of your fat. You should move toward your thinner image gradually, using all the self-strengthening you can get to make the experience *feel* valid. Slow, steady change is far more genuine and more supportive for long-term personal security. Often dieters set weight loss as their only goal, forgetting that there's a person on the diet and that person needs to let go of his or her inner sense of weight, along with the outer one. When you get to ideal weight on strength instead of stress, that creates image balance, not disturbance.

Your World vs. the World
The diet you choose should help you cope with the world of food opportunities, not remove you from them. When you choose deprived diets with special foods, you won't be able to find those foods in your supermarket. You can't adapt those foods to your ethnic background. If you have a family, you have to cook one thing for them and have another food for you. Your food won't be found in restaurants, in vacation spots, and at family gatherings. You've got to carry a lunch box through life. This creates stress every time you face a vacation, party, or restaurant. You might stop going out for the duration of your diet, because these situations are too threatening. Diet isolation is an extreme form of stress. The solution isn't found by compounding your sense of separation. The solution is to form a new relationship with food.

Sudden Maintenance Stress
The more natural your diet, the easier it will be to shift into weight maintenance. The more abnormal your diet, the greater the gap between weight loss and maintenance. You can fall into that gap between your diet pattern and a lifestyle pattern and stay there for a long time when you diet too differently from everyday life. If you spend a few months eating oddly on a diet, you've ingrained odd eating habits, and they are hard to shake. How do you go home and suddenly eat and live creatively with your thinner body? You

---

         ⇒   How-to Skills   ❤   Good for Heart

don't. You go home and eat to compensate for eating oddly for several months.

When your diet eating plan is too different from normal eating plans, it cannot be fixed by a six-week maintenance program that tries to jam in all the things that make a positive lean life. It's too late by then. You have to start all over again or face months of reentry. This creates stress at ideal weight, when the stress should be abating. A balanced food diet is the best for a maintenance program, because it's a dress rehearsal for the way you will live for life at higher calories. The food skills you learn during dieting carry over to maintenance, and you can eat more calories with an

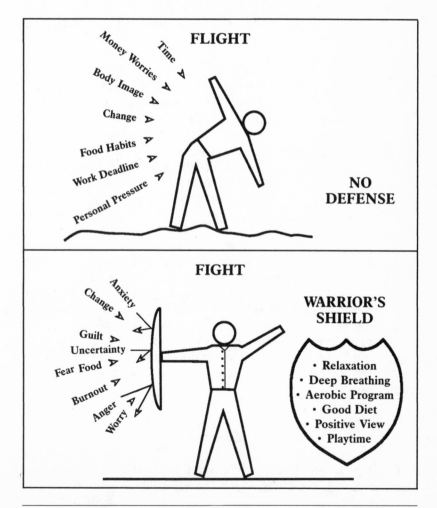

▲ Food Skills   ● Behavior Skills   ◆ Exercise Skills

awareness of food content, sources of better food energy, and how to use food as your friend, not your enemy.

Minimizing diet stress is essential, since stress has been linked to most of the major lifestyle diseases including hypertension, heart disease, and cancer. Stress reduction techniques, such as relaxation, meditation, and deep breathing exercises, are as important as nutritious food. They recharge your mind, attitude, perceptions, and belief systems. Not only do they make your diet experience less stressful, they're tools to use in other areas of your life.

If you think about stress and the fight or flight feeling it gives you, you have two choices to make. You can run from it or fight. If you stand there and take it, stress will get the best of you. The best way to fight stress is to build a defense or shield. The material that follows shows you how.

Creating Your Lifestyle Shield

If you face stress without defenses like nutrition, exercise, relaxation, and personal pleasures for yourself, you'll have to take flight, because your system isn't built to handle stress.

But when you create a lifestyle shield for yourself, using a regular routine for self-enhancement, you can face stress like a warrior. When you learn these skills for dieting, you've got them on your side for life. It's a life defense for stress.

◆ STRETCHING

Exercises to lengthen or elongate muscles and spine, loosen joints, and increase overall coordination. Stretches are usually combined with breathing exercises for the best oxygen uptake. The effect of stretching is excellent for total body energy and grace. Excellent start-up exercises for obesity.

The following workout will provide a basic stretching program for building overall body flexibility. Avoid bouncing or jerking when stretching. Concentrate on making smooth, graceful movements, letting go of the tension in every specific area being stretched.

➠ *How to Do Stretching Exercises*

The key to an ideal stretch is found in the combination of stretching and breathing. Don't hold your breath while you

---

➠ How-to Skills   ♥ Good for Heart

stretch. This creates strain and tension instead of relaxation and a good physical release.

Here's how to breath properly:

1. Before each stretch, *inhale.*
2. *Exhale slowly* as you stretch, exhaling a bit more as you hold the stretch for a count of three;
3. *Inhale and exhale* once more as you return to the starting position.

If you find yourself needing to breathe in and out while you are holding the stretch, just breathe naturally. Eventually you will become more proficient in combining stretching and breathing in one smooth movement.

Spine Stretch

Stand straight with your feet about one foot apart on the floor, hands on hips. Inhale.

Exhale as you raise your arms straight up toward the ceiling, grasping your thumbs lightly as your arms meet. Add one inch to your upward stretch, and hold for count of three. Return your hands to your hips. Repeat five times.

Neck Stretch (1)

Stand straight with your feet about one foot apart on the floor, hands loosely at your sides, your whole body relaxed. Inhale.

Exhale and slowly bring your chin to your chest, concentrating on allowing your neck muscles to let go of tension. Don't strain or try to stretch too far. Hold for count of three, and return to the starting position. Repeat five times.

Neck Stretch (2)

Stand straight, with your feet about one foot apart on the floor, hands loosely at your sides, your whole body relaxed. Inhale.

Exhale and slowly turn your head to the right while exhaling, holding for a count of three and returning to center. Then repeat to the left side. Imagine that you are trying to look at something behind you, but slowly and gently, never overstretching. Repeat five times.

Shoulders and Arms Stretch

Stand straight with your feet about one foot apart on the floor, arms out to the sides at shoulder level with your palms *up.* Inhale.

Exhale as you stretch out an extra inch; slowly circle your arms clockwise three times and return to your starting position. Repeat

▲ Food Skills   ● Behavior Skills   ♦ Exercise Skills

the exercise counterclockwise. Repeat five times. If you need to relax your arms during the exercise, let them hang loosely at your sides for a minute, then continue.

Shoulders and Upper Back Stretch

Stand straight with your feet about one foot apart on the floor, arms out to the sides at shoulder level with your palms up. Inhale.

Exhale and slowly press your arms backward. Hold for count of three, and return to starting position. Repeat five times.

Trunk Stretch

Stand straight with your feet about one foot apart on the floor. Raise your right arm toward the ceiling, and rest your left hand on hip for support. Inhale.

Exhale as you reach your right arm up an extra inch and slowly bend to the left, being sure to let your muscles relax as you bend your trunk. Return to starting position. Repeat five times. Repeat the exercise with your left arm raised and right hand on hip, and bending right as you exhale.

Lunge Stretch

Stand straight with your feet together, hands on hips for support. Inhale.

Exhale as you slowly lunge forward, then slowly straighten back leg, being careful not to lock your knees when your back leg is straight. Return to starting position. Repeat five times. Repeat with other leg.

Hip Stretch

Stand straight with your feet about one foot apart on the floor, arms out to the sides at shoulder level. Keep both feet flat on floor, but don't lock your knees. Inhale.

Exhale and twist slowly to the left as far as possible. Don't stretch beyond your comfort zone. Hold for a count of three, and return to the starting position. Repeat five times. Repeat by twisting to the other side.

Thigh Stretch

Lie on your back on the floor, knees bent toward your chest and arms bent at the elbow, palms up, lying flat on the floor. Inhale.

Exhale as you slowly bring your knees to the left side, as far as comfortable. Hold for count of three, and slowly return to the starting position. Repeat five times. Repeat by bending knees to the right side.

⟫ How-to Skills   ♥ Good for Heart

Abdomen Stretch

Lie on your back on the floor, arms straight and pointed over your head, without locking your elbows. Inhale.

Exhale as you slowly bring your knees up toward your chest and press your legs to the left, while stretching your arms in the opposite direction. Hold for count of three, and return to the starting position. Repeat five times. Repeat exercise to the other side, knees going right and arms going left.

Leg Stretch

Stand facing the back of a chair, holding chair for support. Inhale.

Exhale and bend left leg, bringing your knee to your chest, then swinging leg out in back (slowly). As you reach the back, add an extra inch of stretch to your leg, and return to the starting position. Repeat five times. Repeat exercise using opposite leg.

Heel Stretch

Stand on a stair, holding the bannister for support, and position the balls of your feet on the stair, with heels hanging slightly over edge. Inhale.

Exhale as you slowly lower your heels below the edge of the stair. Don't stretch too far, only to the comfort zone. Hold for a count of three, and return to the starting position. Repeat five times.

All-Over Stretch★

Stand straight with your feet about one foot apart on the floor.

Exhale and *slowly* bend over at the waist, letting your head and arms sink to the floor. Lightly grasp the insides of your lower legs. Let everything go. Imagine you are a rag doll with everything sinking to the floor. When you return to the starting position, do it slowly, feeling each vertebra in your spine slowly straightening up, from your lower back to your upper back. Repeat five times.

★Note: You can use this stretch for an instant relief technique when you are stressed.

Reminder: Even though stretching exercises seem easy and your tendency therefore would be to forget about doing them, don't fall into this pattern. The benefits of these simple stretches are tremendous. They free up trapped energy, elongate your muscles, improve your circulation, and make you feel great. So stretch those muscles toward success and fitness.

▲ Food Skills   ● Behavior Skills   ◆ Exercise Skills

● SUBLIMINALS

Audio or visual tapes that contain underlying messages for unconscious teaching or training; self-help tapes. Subliminal tapes usually contain affirmation messages under pictures, music, or talk, but it is a good idea to be sure the messages are positive. The best choice is one that allows you to turn up the volume and hear the message or turn up your TV screen to see the message. Written scripts aren't suitable, since a script is a separate entity. Subliminals have been used for relaxation training, stop-smoking programs, and motivational training in many areas. Subliminals are based on studies of the unconscious, where perception and learning are different from the normal waking state. Sleep learning is a part of this category, but most subliminals available on the market are not sleep training tapes. Those that can put you to sleep usually indicate that they are not to be used while driving or doing other active work.

Subliminal tapes can be helpful as an adjunct to diet and exercise, but it's not a good idea to rely on them as a solution. There is evidence that this form of training is easily forgotten and therefore must be repeated regularly. Anything positive is a good support aid, but it might be better to train yourself in positive thinking and affirmations on a more conscious level. That way, you're making a conscious choice to make positive changes, and you can enjoy the process of self-awareness that is associated with conscious choice. For instance, when you change negative statements you make about yourself to positive ones, in a conscious way you can feel the effect on your system, and you can notice some interesting things about yourself. What you think, how you react, how you talk back to yourself—all of these responses lead to self-awareness. If you leave that process to a subliminal tape, it's not your voice and your process, and the effect is less permanent. The best plan would be to combine both.

● SUBSTITUTION BEHAVIORS

Habits replaced for other habits, such as substituting exercise or relaxation exercises for eating binges. Substitution behaviors are the basis of behavior modification for weight loss and positive lifestyle change. *See* Lifestyle, for an easy way to use this powerful technique.

⥤   How-to Skills   ❤   Good for Heart

● SUCCESS

Goal achievement. Successful dieting is viewed differently by the scientific community and dieters themselves. In science success means maintaining your weight loss for at least two years after dieting. This is called medically significant weight loss. To the average dieter, success means losing weight (preferably as soon as possible). This is a very important issue because it influences the diet you choose. If you expect success to be weight loss only, you can probably achieve your goal on a number of diets, even poor ones that allow you to lose body muscle. But you can't expect to maintain your weight loss unless you choose a balanced diet that includes exercise, habit change, nutrition education, food cue control, and self-strengthening components. These fall into the category of lifestyle diets.

The least promising diets for weight loss and maintenance are rapid weight-loss diets, since regain is highest in this diet group. Despite this fact, dieters buy into them again and again, repeating patterns of failure that are physically harmful and emotionally draining. Dieters are left feeling there is something wrong with them, when there is something wrong with the diet. One of science's goals is to make people realize that slower weight loss is ideal weight loss. But this is hard to do in a fast-paced society where everything is expected A.S.A.P.

The best course for you is to redefine your expectations, to want more out of a diet than short-term slimness, because it's painful to get there after a lot of hard work only to find you're losing the one thing you really wanted—stay there and enjoy the fruits of your efforts. In addition, you don't want to repeat failure too often, as you can with rapid weight-loss diets, because failure can become ingrained like a habit on automatic pilot, and fear of failure can inhibit other decisions you make in your life. Keep in mind that dieting is something you are doing *for* yourself, not *to* yourself. The more skills you gain during your diet phase, the better equipped you will be to sail through maintenance and celebrate your life.

Success Keys

When you are planning to lose weight, you are standing in front of three doors. One door is Diet, one is Exercise, and one is Behavior of you in the diet. Many programs are like the old TV show "Let's Make a Deal." You only get to choose one door. When

---

▲ Food Skills   ● Behavior Skills   ◆ Exercise Skills

you do that, you can lose the big prize. That's a gamble you shouldn't take with your body. You need the keys to open all three doors, and success is yours.

▲ SUGAR

A sweet tasting, water-soluble carbohydrate. There are three ways you get sugar in your food, but only one way to ensure that you're not getting the *empty calorie* version of sugar.

All-natural Sugar

This is sugar that is an indigenous part of a food, such as sugar in an orange or apple. In this form, sugar is a naturally occurring carbohydrate in low-fat format that provides vitamins, minerals, essential nutrients, and fiber, a perfect diet food. The calories are packed with nutrition and metabolic clout.

Refined Sugar

This is sugar removed from its source food, increased in potency, and used as a garnish or ingredient in processing. Table sugar is double-barreled sucrose—one-half fructose and one-half dextrose. Corn syrups are also refined and combine high-fructose and dextrose. Refined sugars can be the entire calorie content of a food or beverage, such as jelly beans or cola, which are 100 percent sugar. These varieties of sugars are the ones that give sugar its empty calorie reputation, not the naturally occurring ones. Stripped from its source food, sugar has no vitamins, minerals, or nutrient benefits, even though it is still energy.

Processed Foods with Refined Sugars Added

These are the foods that spell trouble for dieters. The sugar isn't the biggest problem, even though processed foods typically have sugar to excess. The problem is *all* of the ingredients taken together—they add up to fat.

Take a look at the following comparison between a fresh-food carbohydrate (pasta salad with vegetables) and a processed imitator (boxed pasta salad with vegetables). The fresh-food version is a natural complex carbohydrate made with fresh-cut vegetables and any plain pasta, garnished with a no-fat, spicy salad dressing (genuine carbohydrate). The imitator is a premixed pasta salad in a box.

⇒ How-to Skills ❤ Good for Heart

WHAT DEFINES A CARBOHYDRATE FOOD?	
GENUINE CARBOHYDRATE	**CARBOHYDRATE IMITATOR (PROCESSED)**
Fiber content is high	Fiber is stripped out
Fat content is low	Fat is added in (sauce)
Simple sugar occurs	Double-barreled sugar added
High vitamin/mineral content	Nutrition stripped out
Protein (when it occurs is intact)	Protein damaged in processing
Chewability (activates digestion)	Smooth and easy to swallow
Low calorie overall	High calorie

You decide. Do processed carbohydrate foods look like the real thing to you? A decade of confusion and misinformation has centered around carbohydrates. Dieters learned to fear them and the sugar in them, when the foods that caused this confusion weren't even legitimate carbohydrates. They were fats in carbohydrate costumes.

You do not get fat from eating natural carbohydrates, even with sugar in them. You get fat from eating processed imitators with refined sugar added. Before we had processing—freezing, drying, canning, pickling, sweetening, preserving, coloring, texturizing—sugar wasn't a problem in our diets. Today, 70 percent of our foods are processed, and these foods have created a sugar excess in our diets. They've also dramatically increased our fat problems, because the combination of ingredients in refined foods is the formula that makes fat store easily.

This doesn't mean that all processed foods are bad for you. There are many new versions arriving in the supermarket every day. But don't be fooled by the names or claims. For instance, a cereal called "Natural Grain" might make you think it's made from whole grains and isn't fattening, but you can get six teaspoons of sugar in every cup and no real fiber. You can see a food

---

▲ Food Skills   ● Behavior Skills   ◆ Exercise Skills

HOW SWEET IT IS

Current Average Use
1 cup per day
or 48 teaspoons

PRIMARY SOURCES OF REFINED SUGARS

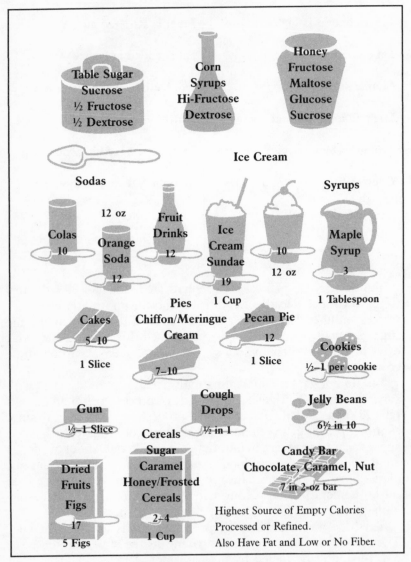

Table Sugar
Sucrose
½ Fructose
½ Dextrose

Corn
Syrups
Hi-Fructose
Dextrose

Honey
Fructose
Maltose
Glucose
Sucrose

Ice Cream

Sodas

Syrups

12 oz

Colas
10

Orange
Soda
12

Fruit
Drinks
12

Ice
Cream
Sundae
19
1 Cup

10

12 oz

Maple
Syrup
3
1 Tablespoon

Cakes
5–10
1 Slice

Pies
Chiffon/Meringue
Cream
7–10

Pecan Pie
12
1 Slice

Cookies
½–1 per cookie

Gum
½–1 Slice

Cough
Drops
½ in 1

Jelly Beans
6½ in 10

Cereals

Dried
Fruits
Figs
17
5 Figs

Sugar
Caramel
Honey/Frosted
Cereals
2–4
1 Cup

Candy Bar
Chocolate, Caramel, Nut
7 in 2-oz bar

Highest Source of Empty Calories
Processed or Refined.
Also Have Fat and Low or No Fiber.

Empty Calories = 100% Sugar

Recommended diet dosage: Cut intake of refined sugar.
Rely on fresh food sources from food groups.
Select others sparingly.

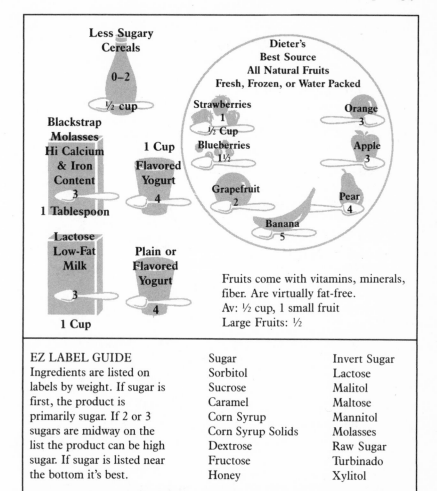

Less Sugary Cereals
0–2
½ cup

Dieter's Best Source
All Natural Fruits
Fresh, Frozen, or Water Packed

Strawberries
1
½ Cup

Orange
3

Blueberries
1½

Apple
3

Blackstrap Molasses
Hi Calcium & Iron Content
3
1 Tablespoon

1 Cup Flavored Yogurt
4

Grapefruit
2

Pear
4

Banana
5

Lactose Low-Fat Milk
3
1 Cup

Plain or Flavored Yogurt
4

Fruits come with vitamins, minerals, fiber. Are virtually fat-free.
Av: ½ cup, 1 small fruit
Large Fruits: ½

EZ LABEL GUIDE
Ingredients are listed on labels by weight. If sugar is first, the product is primarily sugar. If 2 or 3 sugars are midway on the list the product can be high sugar. If sugar is listed near the bottom it's best.

Sugar	Invert Sugar
Sorbitol	Lactose
Sucrose	Malitol
Caramel	Maltose
Corn Syrup	Mannitol
Corn Syrup Solids	Molasses
Dextrose	Raw Sugar
Fructose	Turbinado
Honey	Xylitol

ARTIFICAL SWEETENERS*
ASPARTAME. 200 times sweeter than sugar. Synthetic. Combines 2 amino acids—aspartic acid and phenylalanine. Unstable in high heat such as baking. Not for people with phenylketonia (metabolic disorder). Still being tested. Avoid or limit use to 1–2 servings daily.
SACCHARIN 350 times sweeter than sugar. Synthetic. Studies vary as to its possible connection to cancer.

*No indications that artificial sweeteners are beneficial to weight control.
»Not Safe

▲ Food Skills ● Behavior Skills ◆ Exercise Skills

that claims "lower sugar" on the box or can, but you have to ask, lower than what? Lower than it was when it jumped off the scale for sugar content, meaning it can still be too sugary and too fatty. And the term *natural* can be misleading when it refers to sugar, because double barreled table sugar (sucrose) is allowed to be called natural, since it once occurred in beets and sugar cane. Even the processed diet foods can be high in sugar, giving you empty calories.

It's up to you to do some serious investigating of processed and refined foods with a magnifying glass in the supermarket, if you have to. It will save you pounds of fat and sugar each year.

Your best plan for dieting is to avoid them as much as possible since they can't give you the kind of fat burn that you get from fresh food. You can save fast-lane foods for emergency situations if you must, but only use fat-free, low-sugar, and low-sodium varieties. And even then, you're losing fiber.

Diet/Sugar Smarts
- Sugar in processed foods provides empty calories, meaning you get calories but no nutritional benefits. When you're on a limited calorie plan (say 1,200 calories) and you eat 400 calories per day as sugar, you're sacrificing 400 calories you could eat in fat-burning, filling foods such as vegetables, pastas, or grains. In vegetables or grains, 400 calories is high nutrition. You get more for your calories and feel more satisfied too.
- Sugar-rich foods are usually fat-rich foods and nonfibrous foods. That combination adds up to weight gain, not weight loss.
- Sugar-rich foods usually include additives too. When you're on a diet, additives can cause symptoms that might not occur when you're eating more calories. It's best to avoid as many additives as you can.
- Because high-sugar foods have low or no fiber, they can be eaten in a flash, with no chewing and minimal salivation, and no time for hunger to abate naturally from eating (it takes twenty minutes). You might get a quick sugar boost that causes your blood glucose to rise, then drop again quickly. This doesn't give you steady, dependable energy, and it doesn't keep hunger at bay for long.
- Food tolerance tests suggest that eating high-sugar diets dulls your sensitivity to fats. In other words, you can eat more fat

without being aware of it. Part of this is related to taste and part habit, since fat and sugar often get double billing in low-nutrition foods. To stay on the lean side, make sugar one of the first habits you break.
• Don't cut sugar by *increasing* your use of artificial sweeteners.

Don't forget that eating too much sugar can give you the epinephrine effect. *See* Epinephrine.

SUPPLEMENT, DIETS

Powdered or liquid food plans. Many diets are built around food supplements that act as meal replacements. These supplements can be liquid drinks in cans that are premixed, powdered formulas in cans or packets that must be added to another liquid.

Advocates of food supplements claim they're a good way to get the benefits of a full meal (nutritionally) while avoiding the calories. A standard lunch might be 400 calories or more, while a standard supplement lunch is 50–100 calories. For fast-lane people who don't eat regularly and *won't* eat regularly, supplements can provide needed nutrition, but the quality of a supplement is a critical issue. If you are getting a lot of sugar along with reduced calories, the supplement isn't a good diet bet. Most of the supplements are used to provide low-fat sources of protein, but check the labels. If you're getting 5 grams of fat in one shake, along with sugar, this doesn't add up to dietary sense. Check the labels for additives or imbalanced amino acids.

Drawbacks to Supplement Diets
The problem with supplements for dieters is varied. They haven't got the metabolic clout of real food. Fiber content, if any, is minimal, and too many rely on sweeteners to make the supplement palatable. The right combination of amino acids is tricky and not sufficiently researched, and imbalances can occur. This can prevent the absorption of your protein, defeating the purpose of the supplement. In addition, you can start to rely on these supplements as food substitutes, which doesn't help you handle your real food issues. People develop emotional dependencies on supplements, seeing them as a form of medication, thinking they're responsible for the weight loss, which isn't true. It's the calorie restriction that is creating the weight loss, not the formula in the

▲ Food Skills   ● Behavior Skills   ♦ Exercise Skills

supplement. Most of the diets that use supplements are very low-calorie ones, and that can promote rapid weight loss and rapid weight regain.

● **SWEET TOOTH**

Desire for sweets, as opposed to a *need* for sweets; a part of emotional hunger. The more sweets you eat, the easier it is to tolerate higher levels of sugar. And the surprising fact is that a sweet tooth may be caused by a fat tooth in the background. Since sweet foods provide no real nutrition, you're wasting calories that you could get from fat-burning foods such as complex carbohydrates. If you feel you must have sweets, make sure you're not using them in place of nutritious foods. First, insure that you're getting your daily food requirements met, then see if you have the room or desire for the sugary foods. You'll find that your desire for sugar will be decreased when you eat more fruits, vegetables, grains, and water. Balanced nutrition keeps that sweet tooth satisfied, not sweets. *See* Fat Tooth; Sugar.

SWEETENERS

Sugars, natural and synthetic. *See* Sugar.

▲ **SWEETS**

Sugar-rich foods such as candy, cola, ice cream, baked goods, processed foods. They provide empty calories and little nutrition and are usually the foods you use to appease emotional hunger. Real hunger isn't abated by high-sugar foods. You get a quick rise in blood sugar, then a quick drop, and hunger returns quickly. Ten extra pounds per year can be attributed to high-sugar foods. The first step to slimness is to find substitutes for sugary foods that satisfy your desire for something sweet while providing needed nutrition. Best substitute: fruit—something sweet and fat free with fiber, essential vitamins, and minerals.

➡ How-to Skills ❤ Good for Heart

◆ SWIMMING

Aerobic exercise, nonweight bearing.

Benefits:
- Excellent cardiovascular training
- Good calorie-burning exercise
- No injury to joints
- Works upper and lower body
- Improves range of arm motion
- Pools available at most community centers
- Good exercise to combine with other activities

T

♦ **TARGET HEART RATE**

The recommended heartbeats per minute that give you maximum oxygen uptake during aerobic exercise. This is considered cardiovascular conditioning because it lowers your daily resting heart rate, which helps to avoid heart disease. The benefits are also muscular, since greater oxygen to your muscles increases their efficiency and increases your fat burn. Also called training rate.

The target heart-rate zone is the range that is recommended for aerobic conditioning. It is 70 to 80 percent of your maximum heart rate. Figures for maximum heart rate were derived from stress tests on thousands of individuals, with the formula for target heart rate derived from those studies. Your maximum rate is not a *desired* rate, and if you find yourself nearing maximum, it's best to slow your heartbeat by walking around the room, allowing it to decrease gradually. Sitting down or falling into an exhausted heap on the floor immediately after an aerobic exercise is not a safe way to bring your heart rate back to normal. A program of cool downs is usually the best routine to ensure gradual heart-rate recovery.

⠿➡ *How to Measure Your Heart Rate*

Find your pulse on your wrist or neck, just below your jaw. Place your four fingers (not thumb) lightly over your pulse and count the number of beats for ten seconds. Multiply that number by six (for sixty-second rate).

Use your sixty-second rate to compare with the table for target heart rate.

AGE	TARGET ZONE 70%	85% of Max	MAXIMUM HEART RATE Heart beats/min
20 (or under)	140	170	200
25	137	166	195
30	133	162	190
35	130	157	185
40	126	153	180

| AGE | TARGET ZONE | | MAXIMUM HEART RATE |
	70%	85% of Max	Heart beats/min
45	123	149	175
50	119	145	170
55	116	140	165
60	112	136	160
65 (or older)	90	132	155

Heartbeat too fast? You started too fast and are pushing too hard. Walk around the room to slow your heartbeat. Don't sit to do it. You want to bring your heartbeat down gradually. When you return to your exercise, keep it more fluid and steady. Don't strain or push yourself. *See* Interval Training.

♦ TENNIS

Skill sport aerobic exercise (if you stay active). *See* Exercise.

▲ THERMOGENESIS

The thermic effect of food or heat from eating. Eating, digesting, and absorbing food takes metabolic energy. You burn calories by eating too. Some foods cause a great rise in your metabolism, needing more energy to be broken down into the form for absorption by your blood. By choosing more thermic foods, you can burn 10 to 15 percent more calories each day.

Complex carbohydrates are very thermic foods. They use approximately 23 calories out of every 100 calories to be digested and absorbed. If you eat 700 calories of complex carbohydrates daily, you burn 161 calories because you ate them. To a dieter trying to lose fat, that's a significant amount of calories. Fat is barely thermic. It only uses 3 calories out of every 100 to digest and absorb. If you eat 400 calories of fat daily, that's only 12 calories burned from eating fat. The remaining 388 fat calories are easily stored. Protein is also a very thermic food, but it has a higher fat content than carbohydrates, and the fat can be stored. The leaner proteins are the best thermic bet.

● THIN FROM WITHIN

Using your inner resources to help you achieve your weight-loss goals. *See* Imagery.

▲ Food Skills   ● Behavior Skills   ♦ Exercise Skills

TRACE MINERALS

Organic or inorganic materials found in small amounts in your body, and also found in food. Some are essential. *See* Minerals.

♦ TRAMPOLINE

Aerobic exercise device for rebounding. You can use a regular trampoline or a minitrampoline for at-home rebounding.

Benefits:
- Excellent cardiovascular fitness
- Great calorie-burning potential
- Easily accommodates all levels of fitness
- Develops coordination and balance
- No injury to muscles and joints

♦ TREADMILL

Stationary aerobic exercise machine.

Benefits:
- Superb cardiovascular training
- Excellent calorie-burning exercise
- Great for all levels of fitness, accommodating beginners to seasoned exercisers
- Available in motorized and manual (motorized is usually better for the beginner because there's less tension and the speed and grade are easy to adjust; manual machines are more appealing to the advanced treadmiller because of the greater challenge of motorizing it yourself).

TRIGLYCERIDE

Another name for lipid, or fat in your cells or blood.

TRYPTOPHAN

An essential amino acid that occurs naturally in food proteins, such as meat, poultry, fish, peanuts, and dairy products. The naturally occurring form of tryptophan is not only safe but essential. It is one of the eight amino acids that cannot be produced by your body and must be derived from your food.

➠ How-to Skills ❤ Good for Heart

▲ TV DINNERS

Preportioned meals in heat-and-serve packages. These aren't the best foods to eat in front of the TV or anywhere else. They're usually low in fiber and high in sugar and fat. The TV is one of the major cues to eat, and an entire industry of microwave and oven entrées capitalized on that. Food commercials appear on TV every fifteen minutes on most stations, and the models eating fats and sugars are always thin and toned. Most dieters are told to stop eating in front of the TV, and in a clinical world that would be ideal. But home isn't a clinical world, and TV is a part of many people's lives. If you don't feel you can stop eating in front of the TV, adjust your couch eating to a healthy habit. Instead of eating a processed dinner, make your own variety of TV entrées and freeze them in one-meal servings for reheating. You can make casseroles, pasta salads, stews, and soups with complex carbohydrate vegetables and grains. That way you won't have the extra fat, sugar, and salt. This kind of TV dinner can make a couch potato lean.

U

● **UNDEREATING**

Eating less than the required nutrition for healthy body maintenance. This can be a mild form of undereating for a few days or a
week of starvation. Either way, your body is malnourished and,
over time, this leads to serious illnesses and metabolic disturbances. Undereating or starving for a few days is often perceived
by dieters as a way to make up for days of eating poorly or overeating. Dieters think that *not eating* will lead to faster weight loss. In
fact, the reverse is true. Not eating, or nutrient starvation, will
throw your body into a calorie-conserving state, and your metabolism will reduce to hold on to the few calories you eat. This causes
you to burn fewer calories overall, and it forces your body to go
after its own muscle protein for energy. Calcium is taken from your
bones, muscle is broken down for protein, and you wind up with
an undermined metabolism and risk osteoporosis. You are less
resistant to stress, which further depletes nutrient stores, and illness often results.

When undereating is prolonged, you will see weight loss, but it's
water and muscle being wasted, and the appearance of this form of
weight loss is dragged out, both externally and internally. In a
literal sense, your body drags out every nutrient it can find before
it goes after fat. You can remain fat and be depleted, which will
lead to more fat gain. If more dieters understood this simple
Catch-22 about *not* eating, it would save them serious conse-
quences in weight regain. In the end, undereating will lead to
more fat gain.

UNDERWATER WEIGHING

A method for determining body fat content, usually in major athletic centers. The method uses a tub of water that is attached to a
scale. You get in the tub, and water is displaced. The more fat you
have, the more water displacement since fat is lighter than water.
This makes the scale lighter, and it lifts. Slimmer bodies sink
lower because muscle is heavier than water. Your "water" weight is

then compared to your dry weight to calculate your body-fat content.

UNDERWEIGHT

Ten percent below ideal body weight. Any weight loss beyond that degree is usually accompanied by physiological problems, particularly in women. Being underweight without lack of daily nutrients is generally considered safe, if not good prevention, since weight tends to increase with age. However, underweight with malnutrition is a serious condition that makes the person more susceptible to infections and disease. Underweight people who are malnourished lose muscle tissue, and a main priority should be replacing these losses. The recommended therapy is a well-balanced diet with extra protein to rebuild muscle tissue, frequent small meals, and exercise to gain muscle, not fat. The diet should not seek to increase the fat level, promoting fat gain as weight gain since the low-muscle body will gain fat easily. An increase up to 500 calories per day is recommended in lean proteins, complex carbohydrates, and low-fat dairy products. The goal is to gain weight slowly, up to one pound per week. This is achieved by eating 500 more calories per day.

❤ UNSATURATED FAT

The fat in food that is considered OK fat, since it helps reduce the level of LDL or bad cholesterol in your body. _See_ Cholesterol.

V

▲ VARIETY

Diversity in food energy, specifically from the four major food groups. When dietary guidelines suggest that you "eat a variety of foods," it has a very literal meaning. Not just any variety, but the *science of variety* furnished in the food group system, where foods are grouped according to their highest-yield nutrients. No two foods yield the same nutrients and many nutrients need to be in the presence of, or in combination with, other nutrients to work properly. The science of variety insures that you receive the fifty essential nutrients you need on a daily basis when you eat the required servings in each group: two servings meat, two servings milk, four servings fruits and vegetables, four servings grain. This applies even if you are on a diet for weight loss. If you omit one or two groups during a diet, you could lose one-fourth to one-half of the nutrition your body needs on a daily basis to supply healthy, nonsaggy fat loss.

Many dieters have the misimpression that eating balanced meals is a tired idea, and they look instead to some magic food or magic combination of foods as the solution to their weight problems. The fact is that may be a good reason why their weight problems continue. Eating for variety means eating for power and health.

The Benefits of Variety

- You get the protein you need for lean muscle protection—and that means better fat burn.
- You get the fiber you need for fullness and better intestinal transit time—and that means less calorie absorption.
- You get the fifty essential nutrients automatically—and that means health and disease prevention.
- You get the calcium you need to prevent bone deterioration as you age.
- You get the textures you need for chewing—and that means better appetite control.

- You get pleasure from variety—it's more palatable and less likely to make you break your diet from boredom.
- You get an automatic maintenance plan—all you have to do is increase your calories across the board.
- You're set for a healthy, slimmer life.

The science of variety is the real magic combination. *See* the Problem Solver Diet for a program that meets these requirements.

▲ VEGETABLES

Carbohydrate sources of fiber, vitamins, and minerals; one of the food groups for healthy eating; diet foods. *See* Food Groups.

● VISUALIZATION

The ability to picture success before it occurs in order to increase the likelihood that it will occur. *See* Imagery; Relaxation.

VITAMINS

Organic nutrients from food that have no calories or energy. Vitamins are the building blocks of your enzymes, the chemicals needed to break down your foods for energy. Your body can't make most vitamins on its own, and they must be provided daily in your food. One of the reasons you eat for variety and need all food groups to do it, is that no one food or group provides all of the essential vitamins in the ratios your body needs.

Your vitamin needs are based on many factors: your age, sex, health status, weight, genetics, stress level, activity level, and even the climate. For this reason, it's best to take the easy route and get them from your daily food, as recommended in the food groups. Trying to study vitamins and figure out isolated needs could take a lifetime, and it often leads to confusion, if not vitamin excess.

There are two forms of vitamins: water soluble (can be excreted) and fat-soluble (can be stored). It's fairly easy to tell the difference. Fat-soluble vitamins like A, D, E, and K are measured in IUs (international units) and that's listed on the label. Water soluble vitamins are measured in milligrams (mg) on labels.

More than fifty vitamins and nutrients are needed in the presence of water for healthy body balance. To make it easier to get them, ten leader nutrients were identified as essential in your diet. When you get these leader nutrients, you automatically get the rest of your vitamins.

The ten leader nutrients were used to design the food groups. They are: calcium, carbohydrates, protein, fat, vitamins A, C, B1 (thiamin) and B2 (riboflavin), niacin, and iron.

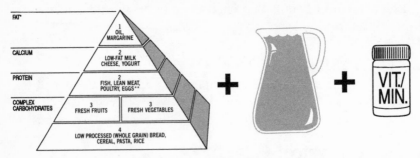

Best sources for vitamins

The Vitamins

Vitamin A
Vitamin B complex
  B1 thiamine
  B2 riboflavin
  B6 pyridoxine
  B12
  B13 orotic acid
  Biotin
  Choline
  Folic acid
  Inositol
  B17 laetrile
  Niacin
  Para-aminobenzoic (PABA)
  B15 pangamic acid
  Pantothenic acid

Vitamin C
Vitamin D (food and sunlight)
Vitamin E tocopherol
Vitamin F unsaturated fatty acids
  Linoleic acid
  Arachidonic acid
Vitamin K
  K1
  K2
Vitamin P
Bioflavonoids

VLCD

Very low calorie diet; 600 to 800 calories (or less) per day; also called hypocaloric diets. The most common variety of these diets are fasts, modified fasts, meal replacement diets, ketone diets, and often one- or two-food diets that dramatically limit your calories.

⇒ How-to Skills   ♥ Good for Heart

The only way to make an 800 calorie (or less) diet meet the requirements for essential daily nutrients is to provide part or most of the diet in the form of a food substitute or meal replacement, which concentrates protein in a low-fat liquid or powder. These are rapid weight-loss diets and produce the effects associated with rapid weight loss—refeeding problems and rapid weight regain. Some studies indicate that they also produce greater hunger afterward and can lead to bouts of binge eating that may not have been a problem in the prediet state. The one- or two-food diets that achieve a very low-calorie format are imbalanced diet plans, often without adequate protein, which cause extreme muscle losses and nutritional deficiencies. All very low-calorie diets allow muscle losses to occur, and the weight regain that follows appears rounder, as a result.

♦ **VOLLEYBALL**
Skill sport aerobic exercise (if you keep moving). *See* Exercise.

W

♦ **WALKING**

Low-impact aerobic exercise. Walking develops muscle tone, strength, endurance, flexibility, and agility. Joggers say that running puts them in touch with their bodies, but walking goes one step further: it gives you time and space to reflect on yourself and your environment. The visual stimulation of walking is less stressful than jogging with fast-forward films running across your eyes. You can enjoy nature or your city, noticing things that might otherwise have passed you by.

➡ *How to Do Aerobic Walking*

- In the beginning, duration is more important than distance.
- Begin with modest distances and gradually increase your speed as walking becomes more comfortable.
- Swing your arms rhythmically and try to breathe deeply.
- Strike the longest stride that is comfortable for you.
- Keep your momentum steady and think about being light, putting less weight on your feet.
- Wear light, comfortable clothes and shoes that don't slip or rub.

To turn your walking routine into an exercise that also builds strength, you can do *power walking*, with hand weights. This extra *resistance*, created by the weight, gives an upper-body workout to the exercise.

In addition, to build lower body strength, along with the exercise, try *varied terrain* walking. Climb hills, walk on sand, gravel, grass, over obstacles—all without decreasing your stride.

Avoid putting weights on your ankles to walk, since that will defeat the purpose of a low-impact exercise, putting too much stress on your ankle joints.

♦ WARM-UPS

A mild exercise or stretching routine for eight to ten minutes to precede strenuous exercise. If you've ever reached to one side too quickly and pulled a muscle, you know the effect that sudden movement can have on tight muscles—strain. This can happen when you jump into a vigorous workout routine or aerobic exercise without warming up. Tight muscles feel cold, and your goal is to elongate them, which raises your body temperature, stimulates your circulation, giving you a warm feeling. This increases the efficiency of muscle contractions and makes you more supple, protecting you from injury or strain. The increase in blood circulation is especially important to older or sedentary exercisers because it prevents myocardial ischemia (insufficient blood supply to the heart). In a pinch, walking is an ideal warm-up, or you can use an overall body stretch, flexing and relaxing one muscle group at a time, from your head to toe, while breathing deeply. Or you can follow the example of many athletes who prefer yoga for a great overall stretch. *See* Cool Downs; Stretching.

▲ WATER

Essential body fluids; also any liquid excreted from your body such as urine, sweat, tears. Your body is about 60 percent water. Men tend to have 10 percent more body water than women: slender men, 65 percent water; slender women, 55 percent water. Obese people tend to have less body water than normal: obese men, 55 percent; obese women, 45 percent. Two-thirds of your body water is located inside your cells, and the other one-third is outside your cells.

Your body-water content is regulated by three mechanisms:

1. thirst, which causes you to drink when your water level is low;
2. pituitary gland, which releases or withholds an antidiuretic hormone (ADH) that acts as a water monitor and stabilizer;
3. kidneys, which expel water and waste products.

You lose about one-half gallon of water each day, through sweating, body excretion, and breathing. You can lose more than one-half gallon if you exercise, if outside temperature rises, or if you experience fever, vomiting, or diarrhea.

Your goal is to replace the water you lose daily.

▲ Food Skills ● Behavior Skills ♦ Exercise Skills

The easiest way to ensure that you get your daily water requirement is to fill two one-quart pitchers with water and make sure you drink them each day. It is preferred that you drink at least two glasses with each meal and two in between meals.

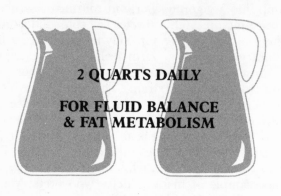

2 QUARTS DAILY

FOR FLUID BALANCE & FAT METABOLISM

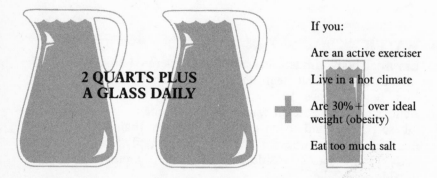

2 QUARTS PLUS A GLASS DAILY

If you:

Are an active exerciser

Live in a hot climate

Are 30% + over ideal weight (obesity)

Eat too much salt

The magic formula: water and why you need it for weight loss

- It improves your fat metabolism. More water leads to less fat stored.
- It suppresses your appetite. You can use it as a no-calorie snack.
- It's necessary for proper digestion.
- It binds with fiber to create a feeling of fullness.
- It acts as a natural diuretic to prevent water retention.
- It supplies oxygen to your muscles, which are the home of your fat burn. More oxygen means better metabolic fire. More water to your muscles means better muscle function, since muscles are 72 percent water.

➠ How-to Skills　　　❤ Good for Heart

- It maintains normal bowel function. This allows food to move through your intestines with ease and prevents excess calories from being absorbed. The longer food stays in your intestines, the more calories you can store as fat.
- It removes wastes, which are increased during weight loss.

♥ Water is vital to your heart, since it maintains blood volume and blood pressure. Note: If you only drink water when you are thirsty, you are already in 2 percent dehydration. In a 130-pound person, that means you are down one and one-half pounds of essential water. Don't wait until you are thirsty.

Drinking less water will not prevent water retention. In fact, the opposite is true. If you don't have enough body water, the hormone ADH will be released to act as water conservator.

WATER RETENTION

Holding water. This is usually caused by excessive sodium intake or inadequate intake of drinking water, or both simultaneously (presuming absence of disease). Diuretics are not advised for mild or periodic water retention in healthy people, since cutting back on salt and drinking more water is the best medicine. Do not confuse mild water retention with edema, which usually indicates an underlying disorder which needs specific medical attention. *See* Sodium; Water.

WEIGHT

A combination of water, fat, and muscle (lean body mass). Your basic body composition breaks down this way:

- Water is typically 55 to 60 percent of your total body weight.
- Fat ranges from 10 to 30-plus percent of total body weight in women. Fat content can be lower than 10%, but it is rare and dangerous. Fat ranges from 8 to 25-plus percent of total body weight in men (they have less fat to begin with).
- Muscle (muscle tissue and bone is the rest).

Muscle weight is also called lean body mass and is usually measured along with water, muscle, and bone, because they are difficult to separate. Muscles are approximately 72 percent water, while fat has very little water content—approximately 3 percent.

▲ Food Skills ● Behavior Skills ◆ Exercise Skills

Measurement of muscle, therefore, take in everything that is *not* fat, and is called your fat-free mass.

The ideal weight combination is low fat, high muscle, and balanced water.

◆ WEIGHT LIFTING

Exercises for muscle building or body building. The only caution, besides possible strain or injury, is to watch protein and fat levels. Excess fat in your diet can be a detriment to your results. Muscles can be built up under a layer of fat and the look appears too bulky. It also can inhibit your flexibility. It's best to combine muscle building with stretching exercises and a low-fat diet, so the look is lean, toned, muscular, and flexible. *See* Strength Training for guidelines.

WEIGHT LOSS

Water, muscle, or fat reduction. This is an important definition to keep in mind. Weight loss can be any of the three losses, but the only one you need is fat loss. Water facilitates fat removal, so losing water won't help you get slim. And water losses aren't *real* indicators of successful weight loss, since water displacement in early phases of a diet will eventually stabilize.

You want to avoid wasting muscle on a diet, because muscle is the home of your fat burn. The more muscle you lose, the greater your tendency to store and gain fat. This becomes very apparent in maintenance after a muscle-wasting diet, because you'll see your weight come back *fast*, and you'll be gaining only fat. Muscle-wasting diets cause rapid weight regain that's hard to stop. One of the reasons men are good calorie burners is because of their higher content of body muscle. Women start out with a higher body-fat content, and when muscle losses occur with dieting, they exacerbate fat problems.

The most common diets that can cause muscle losses are:

- imbalanced diets that rely on one or two foods as primary fuel, or diets with entire food groups missing;
- starvation diets;
- very low-calorie diets;
- diets with inadequate protein;
- any combination of the above, without exercise.

The two known ways to protect muscle during a diet are: (1) eating adequate food protein (along with a balanced diet). This prevents your body from going after its own muscle to burn for energy. (2) Exercise. This protects existing muscle and builds new muscle for ideal weight maintenance. That's why the best diets advocate exercise at the start of calorie reduction.

WEIGHT MAINTENANCE
Energy balance. Your output equals your input. You burn what you eat. *See* Maintenance, for guidelines.

WEIGHT-RELATED
Created by or associated with excess weight. This covers a wide spectrum of science, including diseases or disorders that are advanced by fat gain, personality issues that emerge from fat gain, habits and behavior that center around weight, in addition to any discipline that advances treatment. Specifically, this means factors that have been validated by research or clinical study to have a direct relationship with weight gain and weight loss. *See* Risks.

● WELLNESS
Absence of disease. This means more than not having an illness. It means being in a health state that minimizes the risks of future illnesses that are lifestyle diseases—hypertension, diabetes, heart disease, and cancer. The concept of wellness didn't quite catch on as a movement in health and has been primarily used in the corporate sphere. It involves two phases: the evaluation phase and resolution phase.

The primary issues involved in a wellness evaluation are:

1. Weight problems. Are you 10 percent away from your ideal body weight?
2. Energy level. Are you tired, and do you lack stamina? Do you exercise regularly?
3. Habit problems. Do you use medications or alcohol too frequently?
4. Stress problems. Do you have difficulty concentrating, feel anxious, or have a quick temper? Are your sleep patterns regular?
5. Food problems. Do you have digestion problems? Do you use diet aids or digestive aids frequently?

▲ Food Skills   ● Behavior Skills   ◆ Exercise Skills

● WILL POWER

Mind over matter; the ability to use strength of mind to support your desires, wishes, and goals. Too often in dieters, this strength of mind is seen as the power to say no. But that's not the whole story with willpower. It's also the ability to say yes. And it implies the ability to make self-enriching choices. The concept of willpower has been so abused with deprivation diets that it isn't its old self. To get back to a state of self-initiation—the ability to drive yourself forward—use skill power. This will help you regain your perspective on will, and simultaneously it will drive you to your goal. For skill power, *See* all behavior keys ●.

X, Y, Z

X-FACTOR DIETS

Programs that promote one vitamin, mineral, enzyme, amino acid, or an odd combination of them, as the cause for weight loss; alphabet diets that use any letter to symbolize the unknown x. In mathematics, the x factor is a variable, a solution you can derive in a number of different ways, if you assign different numbers to the x. That holds true for x-factor diets. These diets often use the words "secret formula" and "our laboratory," and they often rely on testimonials for promotion. These diets are no secret. The poorest ones only use certain vitamins or nutrients in isolation, and the better ones are simply disguises for normal low-fat diets. The danger is believing the claims about certain components taken in isolation and used as a supposed cure-all. They foster a fad mentality, which doesn't help you deal with weight problems from a realistic perspective. The worst ones cause serious problems from nutrient imbalance; the best ones make you think that something other than dieting is responsible for weight loss. *See* Food Groups.

◆ YOGA

A specialized exercise which concentrates on slow stretching movements performed in harmony with breathing. The discipline can range from beginner stretching to advanced techniques, all designed to relieve stress from the spine, elongate muscles, toning your entire body system. Yoga also increases the oxygen supply to your body and achieves the effects of relaxation. *See* Exercise.

● YO-YO SYNDROME

Rapid weight loss followed by rapid weight regain, often to weights higher than the original weight. This syndrome is common to, if not created by, very restrictive diets that last for several months. Why?

▲ Food Skills   ● Behavior Skills   ◆ Exercise Skills

Drastic Calorie Reduction

When you go on a very low-calorie diet for months or more, you are retraining your body to exist on fewer calories. Your body holds its energy in store because it "reads" that it will not be receiving more. The pattern of your everyday eating gives your body its information for a "reading." When you suddenly increase your calories back to average levels (it doesn't have to be excessive levels), you see weight regain because average levels are dramatic increases when compared to the calorie level your body has adjusted to eating and burning. Very low-calorie diets can reduce your metabolic output by as much as 30 percent. That means you are teaching your body to get by on 600 to 800 calories per day. When you go off the diet and eat 500 calories more per day (an average level of eating or dieting), you don't have any metabolic power to burn the new calories, and they head for storage. You also have another problem that compounds the issue.

Lean Muscle Losses

Your body protein mass (lean body muscle) is reduced on very low-calorie diets. You lose vital body muscle along with your fat. This creates imbalanced body composition, with a fat mass that is too high and muscle mass that is too low, even though you may be slimmer. With a low muscle body, you gain fat more rapidly. When you gain, you gain fat, not muscle, and you could wind up with a very high-fat body that has been trained to get by on 600 to 800 calories per day. Your weight gain gives you the appearance of being soft and round all over, because you have too much body fat and not enough body muscle. Your weight gain after a rapid weight loss diet *appears* plumper than average weight gain. Physiologically speaking, it is plumper. And there's another problem that compounds the issue.

Repeat Dieting

The second time around, your rate of weight loss is slower, because of your reduced metabolic rate. If you choose another very low-calorie diet, you can escalate your problems and might not lose weight at all, even though you are only eating 600 to 800 calories. Your body reads less calories coming in, and it holds back its energy again.

⟱ How-to Skills　　　❤ Good for Heart

How to Get Out of the Yo-Yo Cycle

If you are a person who has suffered with yo-yo cycling, your best course is absolutely to avoid drastic solutions and bring your body back into shape in steps. This is called step goals, and it means losing five pounds, then stabilizing, losing five more pounds, and stabilizing, until you get down to your ideal weight. The diet you choose should be one with a higher calorie level, such as 1,000 to 1,200 calories, and it should be based on the following ratio of food energy:

Carbohydrates: 60 percent of total calories
Protein: 20 percent of total calories
Fat: 20 percent of total calories

Be patient and persistent in your body retraining. You don't want to see rapid weight loss, because that led to your yo-yo problems. You want to see slow, steady weight loss, which is fat loss, and you want to see a firmer appearance from your weight loss. The point to remember is that your body is very forgiving when you give it the right energy and give it a way to output that energy: with exercise, it will reward you by functioning more normally. Top off your diet plan with strong behavior skills that will hold you in good stead for ideal weight maintenance. This will prevent you from falling back into the old habits of eating that helped to create your weight in the first place. *See* Yo-Yo Syndrome in the first section of this book.

ZERO FAT

No fat calories; a dieter's dream food. Is a zero-fat food the perfect food? Not necessarily. Consider these zero fat foods: sugar, alcohol, coffee, tea. Foods can have no fat and be poor food choices, because they provide no nutrients. Diet sodas have no fat, lots of artificial sugar, and additives. They deplete your diet rather than enhance it. Perfect foods are the ones that provide the most nutrient density for the least calories. It's the quality of the total composition that counts. A food can have fat and still be an ideal source of nutrition, such as the proteins in meats. Fruits have sugar, but they're packed with vitamins and minerals and are ideal sources of fiber, which helps to remove fat. Excess fat is a major problem in our diets, but it doesn't stand alone as the cause for

---

▲ Food Skills ● Behavior Skills ◆ Exercise Skills

body fat. Not eating complex carbohydrates and not getting sufficient fiber are equally the causes of body fat. The point to remember is that no food, or source of energy, stands alone as the
cause or cure of fat and fat-related disease. It's the balance of foods
that solves fat problems, food working in harmony to provide
essential nutrients along with variety and pleasure, varied taste
and texture. This provides the right ingredients to make a perfect
diet for weight loss and a perfect diet for life.

CALORIE COUNTER

These are estimated values of standard foods. Your average daily intake of protein and fat are important on a diet. Protein protects your muscle and fat needs to be limited, so you lose your stored fat. *Legend:* PRO = protein; CARB = carbohydrates; CALS = calories; T = trace (a very small amount).

Average Protein Daily
60–65 grams

Average Fat Maximum
Women: 30–45 grams
Men: 45–60 grams

You should meet the protein *maximum* daily for muscle protection and *not* exceed the fat maximum to get lean and healthy on a diet.

	AMT	PRO	FAT	CARB	CAL
Ale	8 Ozs	T	0	8	100
Alexander	Cktl Glass	1	1	1	225
Alexander, Brandy	Cktl Glass	1	1	1	240
Allspice	⅛ Tsp	0	0	0	0
Almond Cake	1 Sm Serv	2	4	27	160
Almond Choc. Bar	1	1	10	17	150
Almond Coffee Cake	1 Serv	4	7	35	200
Almond Cookies	2 Med	T	2	9	50
Almond Extract	2 Tsps	0	0	0	6
Almond Fudge	1" Sq	1	4	22	130
Almonds, Salted	12 Med	3	9	3	100
Anchovies	6	5	3	T	50
Anchovies, Canned	2 Ozs	11	6	T	100
Anchovy Paste	1 Tbsp	5	3	1	50
Angel Food Cake	1 Serv	3	T	22	110
Animal Crackers	6	1	1	12	50
Anise	⅛ Tsp	0	0	0	0
Anise Cookies	3 Sm	T	2	9	50
Anisette Cordial	1	0	0	7	80
Apple	1 Sm Serv	T	T	11	75
Apple, Baked	1	T	T	47	200
Apple Betty	4 Ozs	2	4	34	175
Apple Butter	1 Tbsp	T	T	9	35
Apple Cake, Dutch	1 Serv	T	1	65	270
Apple Cobbler	1 Sm Serv	1	2	44	200
Apple Crumb Cake	1 Serv	T	1	49	200

	AMT	PRO	FAT	CARB	CAL
Apple Dumplings	1 Med	1	2	63	275
Apple Fritter	1	1	16	12	205
Apple Jelly	1 Tbsp	T	T	13	50
Apple Juice	4 Ozs	T	T	14	55
Apple on Stick	1	T	T	55	230
Apple Pie	1 Serv	3	11	42	275
Apple Pie à la Mode	1 Serv	4	19	58	425
Apple Pie, Deep Dish	1 Serv	5	8	44	270
Apple & Raisin Salad	½ Cup	1	T	25	200
Apple Salad, Diced	1 Serv	T	T	18	80
Applesauce Bread	1 Sl	3	1	21	110
Applesauce Cake	1 Serv	4	12	63	400
Applesauce, Canned	4 Ozs	T	T	13	55
Applesauce, Fresh	4 Ozs	T	T	11	50
Apple, Stewed	1	T	T	29	120
Apple Strudel	1 Serv	3	9	34	225
Apple-Carrot Salad	4 Ozs	T	T	11	50
Applejack	1 Shot	T	T	0	100
Apricot	1	T	T	4	20
Apricot Brandy	Cord.	T	T	7	75
Apricot Cordial	1 Gl	0	0	7	75
Apricot Jam	1 Tbsp	T	T	14	50
Apricot Nectar	4 Ozs	T	T	17	65
Apricot Pie	1 Serv	3	11	31	250
Apricots, Candied	4 Ozs	T	T	96	380
Apricots, Canned w/Syrup	4 Ozs	T	T	19	75
Apricots, Canned, Water	4 Ozs	T	T	10	40
Apricots, Dried	5 Hlvs.	1	T	13	60
Apricots, Frozen, Sweetened	4 Ozs	T	T	26	110
Arrowroot	1 Tbsp	T	T	8	30
Arrowroot Cookies	1	T	1	4	25
Arrowroot Flour	2 Ozs	8	1	40	200
Artichoke	1 Med	2	T	10	50
Asparagus	4 Ozs	3	T	3	20
Asparagus, Canned	4 Ozs	3	T	3	20
Asparagus, Cream Soup	4 Ozs	3	1	9	60
Asparagus, Frozen	4 Ozs	3	T	3	25
Aspic, Seafood	1 Serv.	34	2	2	170
Aspic, Tomato	1 Serv	T	T	9	35
Aspic, Tomato Salad	4 Ozs	4	T	4	40
Avocado	4 Ozs	2	18	7	190
Bacon, Canadian, Broiled	2 Ozs	16	10	T	155
Bacon, Crisp	3 Strips	5	8	T	100
Bacon Fat	1 Tsp	2	4	1	50
Bacon, Lettuce & Tomato	1 Av	10	10	29	245
Bagel	1	2	1	23	110
Baked Alaska	1 Serv	8	14	26	350
Baked Beans	4 Ozs	8	T	24	135
Baking Powder	1 Tap	T	T	2	10
Bamboo Shoots	4 Ozs	3	T	5	30

	AMT	PRO	FAT	CARB	CAL
Banana	1 Med	1	T	23	95
Banana Bread	1 Sl	4	2	22	120
Banana Cake	1 Serv	2	5	36	200
Banana Cream Pie	1 Serv	5	8	56	300
Banana, Fried	1 Med	1	6	35	200
Banana Split	1 Av	8	25	75	560
Barbecue Sauce	1 Tbsp	2	5	T	50
Barley	4 Ozs	10	1	80	390
Basil	⅛ Tsp	0	0	0	0
Bay Leaf	¼ Tsp	0	0	0	0
Bean Sprouts (Mung)	4 Ozs	4	T	7	40
Bean Sprouts (Soy)	4 Ozs	8	5	8	115
Beans (Look up by name)					
Beef, Boiled	2 Ozs	17	4	0	110
Beef, Chuck (Pot Roast)	2 Ozs	16	8	0	145
Beef, Corned	2 Ozs	20	5	0	125
Beef, Dried	2 Ozs	19	4	0	115
Beef, Filet Mignon	2 Ozs	18	4	0	125
Beef, Flank, Cooked	2 Ozs	17	4	0	110
Beef, Hamburger	2 Ozs	14	11	0	160
Beef Heart	2 Ozs	17	3	0	105
Beef Kidney	2 Ozs	18	7	1	142
Beef Liver, Broiled	2 Ozs	11	2	3	80
Beef, Porterhouse Steak	2 Ozs	17	5	0	122
Beef Pot Pie	2 Ozs	5	8	10	137
Beef, Rib Roast	2 Ozs	16	28	0	148
Beef, Round Steak	2 Ozs	11	6	0	100
Beef, Short Ribs, Braised	2 Ozs	11	6	0	100
Beef, Sirloin Tip	2 Ozs	18	6	0	124
Beef Steak	2 Ozs	11	6	0	100
Beef Steak, Flank	2 Ozs	11	6	0	100
Beef Stew	2 Ozs	3	2	3	50
Beef, T-bone Steak	2 Ozs	17	5	0	122
Beef, Tenderloin Steak	2 Ozs	17	6	0	120
Beef Tongue	2 Ozs	9	8	T	112
Beer	12 Ozs	T	0	13	125
Beet Greens	1 Cup	2	T	4	25
Beet, Sugar	1 Tbsp	0	0	4	18
Beets	4 Ozs	2	T	10	50
Beets, Cooked	4 Ozs	1	T	8	35
Benedictine	1 Oz	0	0	7	75
Bitter Chocolate	1 Oz	3	14	8.	170
Black Beans	1 Serv	12	2	34	150
Blackberries, Canned	1 Cup	1	T	13	60
Blackberries, Fresh	1 Cup	1	1	13	60
Blackberry Brandy	1 Shot	0	0	0	75
Blackberry Pie	1 Serv	3	12	38	275
Bleu Cheese Salad Dressing	1 Serv	T	7	1	70
Blintzes, Cheese	1 Av	20	6	8	175
Blintzes, Jelly	1 Av	4	6	35	210
Bloody Mary	1 Serv	1	T	5	95

	AMT	PRO	FAT	CARB	CAL
Blueberries, Fresh	1 Cup	T	T	17	60
Blueberries, Frozen, Sweetened	4 Ozs	1	T	37	120
Blueberries, Frozen, Unsweetened	4 Ozs	1	T	22	60
Bologna	2 Ozs	8	14	T	165
Bonbons	1	T	T	9	35
Bouillon, Clear Condensed	4 Ozs	4	T	0	30
Bouillon Cubes	1	T	T	0	2
Boysenberries, Canned	4 Ozs	T	T	10	40
Boysenberries, Frozen, Sweetened	4 Ozs	T	T	27	110
Boysenberries, Frozen, Unswtnd	4 Ozs	1	T	13	55
Bran	1 Cup	8	2	32	111
Bran Flakes (40% Bran)	½ Cup	5	1	39	145
Brandy	3 Ozs	0	0	0	225
Brandy Fruit Cake	Av Serv	3	9	64	350
Bread, White (See Type)	1 Sl	2	T	12	65
Brewer's Yeast, Dry	1 Tbsp	5	T	3	50
Brioche, French	1	5	10	13	150
Broccoli	4 Ozs	3	T	5	30
Broccoli, Frozen	4 Ozs	5	T	6	35
Broccoli Soup	1 Serv	3	T	5	25
Broth, Clam	4 Ozs	3	T	T	20
Brussels Sprouts	1 Cup	5	T	9	50
Butter	1 Tbsp	T	11	T	100
Butter Cake	1 Serv	3	8	10	200
Butter, Salted	1 Tbsp	T	11	T	100
Butter, Sweet	1 Tbsp	T	11	T	100
Butterscotch Candy	1	1	3	24	120
Butterscotch Cookies	1	3	8	15	140
Cabbage, Baked	1 Serv	1	T	5	20
Cabbage, Chinese	4 Ozs	1	T	3	15
Cabbage, Cole Slaw	4 Ozs	1	9	7	110
Cabbage, Raw, Shredded	1 Cup	1	T	5	25
Cake, Angel Food	1 Sl	3	T	22	110
Cake, Flour	1 Cup	9	T	85	380
Cake, Gingerbread	Av Serv	2	6	21	180
Cake, Pound	1 Sl	3	6	35	380
Cantaloupe	½ Melon	1	T	8	35
Caper Sauce	1 Tbsp	T	2	T	20
Capon	2 Ozs	12	12	0	160
Caramel Candies	1 Med	1	3	8	60
Caramel Choc. Nut Candy	1 Av.	2	3	32	165
Caramel Ice Cream Sundae	4 Ozs	5	10	28	215
Caramel Pudding	4 Ozs	3	5	29	170
Carbonated Water, Quinine	4 Ozs	0	0	9	35
Carbonated Water, Seltzer	4 Ozs	0	0	0	0
Carrot Juice	1 Cup	T	T	13	50
Carrot Soup	1 Serv	T	T	10	45
Carrots, Canned	1 Cup	1	1	10	45
Carrots, Cooked	1 Cup	1	T	10	45
Carrots, Frozen	½ Cup	T	T	5	25

	AMT	PRO	FAT	CARB	CAL
Carrots, Raw, Grated	½ Cup	1	T	3	20
Carrots, Raw, Sticks	3	T	T	3	14
Catsup	1 Tbsp	T	T	4	15
Cauliflower	1 Cup	3	T	5	30
Cauliflower, Frozen	1 Cup	4	T	8	50
Cauliflower, Soup	1 Cup	5	T	8	50
Celery, Cooked	4 Ozs	1	T	3	15
Celery, Raw	4 Ozs	1	T	4	20
Cereal, Bran Buds	1 Cup	7	1	44	144
Cereal, Cheerios	1 Cup	3	1	18	99
Cereal, Cornflakes	1 Cup	2	T	21	95
Cereal, Cream of Wheat	1 Cup	5	1	40	180
Cereal, Dry (Average)	1 Cup	2	T	15	100
Cereal, Oatmeal, Cooked	1 Cup	4	2	21	120
Cereal, Raisin Bran	1 Cup	5	T	33	160
Cereal, Shredded Wheat	1 Biscuit	3	1	23	105
Cereal, Wheat, Bite Size	2 Ozs	6	1	30	200
Cereal, Wheat Germ	2 Ozs	17	6	28	220
Cereal, Wheat Whole (Average)	4 Ozs	2	T	11	50
Cereal, Whole Bran	1 Cup	4	T	32	120
Cereals: Check labels, many variations					
Champagne	1 Glass	T	0	14	80
Cheddar Cheese, Grated	½ Oz	4	5	T	60
Cheddar Cheese, Processed	1 Oz	7	9	T	105
Cheese, American	1 Oz	6	9	T	100
Cheese, Bleu	1 Oz	5	8	T	100
Cheese, Camembert	1 Oz	4	6	T	80
Cheese, Cheddar	1 Oz	8	10	T	120
Cheese, Cheddar, Grated	½ Oz	4	5	T	60
Cheese, Cottage, Skim	1 Oz	5	T	1	25
Cheese, Cream	1 Oz	1	3	T	35
Cheese, Dry Grated	1 Tbsp	5	3	T	50
Cheese, Edam	1 Oz	9	13	2	125
Cheese, Fondue	1 Serv	20	21	9	315
Cheese, Limburger	1 Oz	6	8	T	100
Cheese, Parmesan, Grated	1 Oz	10	7	T	105
Cheese Sauce	½ Cup	11	18	5	225
Cheese Soufflé	½ Cup	11	19	6	240
Cheese Spread	1 Oz	6	8	2	100
Cheese Spread, Bacon	1 Oz	10	9	2	130
Cheese Sticks	2 Ozs	6	16	3	240
Cheese, Swiss	1 Oz	8	8	T	105
Cheese, Swiss Gruyère	1 Oz	8	8	T	110
Cheese, Velveeta	1 Oz	6	9	T	105
Cheeseburger Sandwich	1 Av	28	37	22	540
Cherries, Candied, Choc.	2 Ozs	T	T	43	180
Cherries, Canned	1 Cup	1	T	19	90
Cherries, Fresh Pitted	1 Cup	1	T	20	85
Cherries, Maraschino	2 Av	T	T	2	10
Cherry Pie	1 Pc	3	15	41	350
Cherry Soda	8 Ozs	0	0	28	110

	AMT	PRO	FAT	CARB	CAL
Chestnuts, Dried	8 Med	1	1	11	50
Chestnuts, Fresh	4 Ozs	3	2	47	220
Chicken, Baked	2 Ozs	10	9	0	125
Chicken, Barbecued	2 Ozs	12	7	T	112
Chicken, Boiled	2 Ozs	11	7	0	112
Chicken, Canned, Boned	2 Ozs	17	5	0	114
Chicken, Creamed	½ Cup	32	26	6	385
Chicken Fat	1 Tbsp	0	5	0	45
Chicken Giblets	2 Ozs	9	1	T	55
Chicken Giblets, Fried	2 Ozs	70	6	2	135
Chicken Gizzard, Cooked	2 Ozs	15	2	0	77
Chicken Gravy	2 Tbsps	T	9	4	100
Chicken Gumbo	4 Ozs	1	T	3	25
Chicken Heart, Cooked	2 Ozs	13	4	T	97
Chicken Liver, Chopped	2 Ozs	6	28	4	290
Chicken Pot Pie	2 Ozs	3	6	10	170
Chicken, Roasted	2 Ozs	17	3	0	105
Chicken Soup and Matzoh Balls	1 Cup	1	5	34	175
Chicken Soup, Creamed	1 Cup	1	3	4	45
Chicken Soup, Noodle	1 Cup	3	2	6	55
Chicken Soup w/Rice	1 Cup	2	1	6	45
Chipped Beef	2 Ozs	19	4	0	110
Chitterlings, Fried	1 Serv	16	20	0	250
Chives	1 Oz	T	T	1	5
Choc. Bar	1 Oz	2	9	16	150
Choc. Bar w/Nuts	1 Oz	3	10	17	170
Choc., Bitter	1 Oz	3	14	8	170
Choc. Butter Frosting	1 Tbsp	3	4	6	70
Choc. Cake, Iced	1 Sl	5	8	45	275
Choc. Candies, Sweet	1 Oz	1	11	18	170
Choc. Chiffon Pie	1 Pc	5	11	33	250
Choc. Chip Cookies	3 Med	2	6	22	150
Choc. Cookies	3	2	6	22	150
Choc. Covered Almonds	1 Oz	3	10	14	160
Choc. Covered Ice Cream	Av. Scoop	6	14	23	245
Choc. Cream Cookies	1 Oz	4	5	20	140
Choc. Cream Peppermint Candies	1 Oz	4	5	8	110
Choc. Cream Pie	1 Pc	10	15	47	360
Choc. Creams	1 Av	2	2	12	60
Choc. Cup Cakes	1	2	7	20	155
Choc. Filling	1 Serv	5	12	25	240
Choc. Finger Cookies	1 Serv	5	8	6	115
Choc. Frosting	1 Tbsp	T	3	6	50
Choc. Fudge	1 Oz	T	5	27	125
Choc. Kisses, Candies	1	2	2	2	20
Choc. Layer Cake	1 Pc	5	5	64	320
Choc. Marshmallow Cookies	1	2	3	9	65
Choc. Marshmallow Pudding	4 Ozs	5	13	37	280
Choc. Mint Sauce	1 Serv	1	2	53	230
Choc. Mints	8 Sm	2	5	21	140
Choc. Mints, Cream	1 Bar	4	6	23	160

	AMT	PRO	FAT	CARB	CAL
Choc. Pudding	½ Cup	5	12	31	250
Choc. Sauce	1 Tbsp	1	1	5	25
Choc. Semi-sweet	1 Bar	6	12	17	200
Choc. Skim Milk	1 Cup	7	5	26	170
Choc. Soda	8 Ozs	0	0	15	75
Choc. Syrup	1 Tbsp	T	T	10	35
Choc., Unsweetened	1 Sq	3	15	8	180
Choc. Wafer Cookies	1	2	1	6	40
Chop Suey, Beef	½ Cup	20	20	4	275
Chop Suey, Chicken	½ Cup	12	8	4	135
Chop Suey, Pork	½ Cup	12	8	4	135
Chow Mein, Beef	½ Cup	14	4	2	115
Chow Mein, Chicken	½ Cup	14	4	2	110
Chow Mein, Pork	½ Cup	14	4	2	110
Chutney	1 Tsp	1	T	6	25
Cider	1 Cup	T	T	25	100
Cider, Apple	4 Ozs	T	T	13	55
Cider, Apple Hard	Shot	T	T	19	100
Cider, Sweet Apple	1 Cup	T	T	25	110
Cinnamon	⅛ Tsp	0	0	0	0
Cinnamon Bread	1 Sl	5	T	16	90
Cinnamon Bun	1	3	3	19	115
Cinnamon Cake	1 Sl	3	3	28	150
Cinnamon Muffin	1	2	4	23	135
Cinnamon Raisin Buns	1	2	4	29	160
Cinnamon Roll	1	5	4	11	100
Cinnamon Stick	1	0	0	0	0
Cinnamon Toast	1 Sl	2	1	12	65
Clam Chowder, Manhattan	½ Cup	0	0	2	30
Clam Chowder, New England	1 Cup	2	6	4	95
Clam Dip, Sour Cream	3 Tbsps	14	16	T	200
Clam Juice	4 Ozs	3	T	0	20
Clam & Tomato Broth	1 Serv.	1	1	8	40
Clam & Tomato Soup	4 Ozs	1	1	6	35
Clams, Broiled	6	10	6	5	115
Clams, Broiled, Stuffed	1 Serv	10	8	8	145
Clams, Canned, Drained	4 Ozs	17	3	2	105
Clams, Cherrystone (Meat Only)	6	15	2	5	100
Clams, Fried	6	12	15	5	200
Clams, Raw	4 Ozs	15	2	4	90
Clams, Roasted	6	15	6	5	135
Clams, Steamed	4 Ozs	12	3	4	100
Clams, Stuffed, Baked	6 Sm	5	5	10	100
Clams, Stuffed, Deviled	6	5	5	10	100
Cobblers, All	1 Serv	1	2	44	200
Cocoa, Powder	1 Tbsp	T	T	8	32
Cocoa, Skim Milk	1 Cup	7	T	12	100
Cocoa Syrup	1 Tbsp	T	T	12	40
Cocoa, Whole Milk	1 Cup	7	7	18	165
Coconut Cake	Av Serv	3	7	29	200
Coconut Dried, Sweetened	2 Ozs	2	20	27	280

	AMT	PRO	FAT	CARB	CAL
Coconut, Dried, Unsweetened	2 Ozs	4	35	13	385
Coconut, Fresh	2 Ozs	2	20	11	210
Coconut Fudge	1″ Sq	2	3	22	120
Coconut Macaroons	2 Sm	3	5	14	100
Coffee, Black	1 Cup	T	T	T	2
Coffee Cake	1 Pc	3	4	14	105
Coffee Cake Iced w/Nuts	1 Pc	4	10	33	240
Coffee Cream	1 Tbsp	T	3	1	30
Coffee, Expresso	2 Ozs	0	0	0	0
Coffee, Instant	1 Cup	T	T	0	2
Coffee, Turkish	1 Cup	T	0	20	100
Coffee, Viennese	1 Cup	T	2	8	50
Coffee w/Sugar, 1 Tsp	1 Cup	T	T	4	20
Coffee w/1 Tbsp. Condensed Milk	1 Cup	3	3	16	100
Coffee w/1 Tbsp. Evaporated Milk	1 Cup	1	1	2	20
Coffee w/1 Tbsp. Milk	1 Cup	T	T	T	10
Coffee w/1 Tbsp. Skim Milk	1 Cup	T	T	T	7
Coffee w/Cream	1 Cup	T	3	1	30
Coffee w/Sugar & Cream	1 Cup	T	3	5	50
Cognac	1 Oz	0	0	0	75
Cola	8 Ozs	0	0	25	100
Collards	½ Cup	2	2	5	45
Condensed Milk, Sweetened	4 Ozs	9	9	60	330
Consommé (Clear)	1 Cup	4	T	0	30
Cookies, Plain	1 Med	T	3	7	55
Cooking Fats	1 Tbsp	0	12	0	110
Cooking Oils (Vegetable)	1 Tbsp	0	14	0	125
Cooler, Rum	8 Ozs	4	6	19	150
Cooler, Vermouth	1 Serv	2	2	15	85
Cooler, Wine	8 Ozs	8	8	11	150
Cordials	Av Gl	0	0	7	75
Coriander	½ Tsp	0	0	0	0
Corn	2 Ozs	4	1	24	95
Corn Bread	1 Slice	4	5	22	170
Corn, Canned	1 Cup	5	1	41	190
Corn Cereal, Puffed	2 Ozs	4	2	50	240
Corn, Cream of, Soup	1 Cup	5	15	18	225
Corn Flour, Dry Sifted	4 Ozs	9	3	85	405
Corn Fritters	4 Ozs	9	24	43	425
Corn, Frozen	4 Ozs	4	1	23	115
Corn Meal	½ Cup	5	2	45	230
Corn, Mexican Style	½ Cup	1	2	16	85
Corn Oil	1 Tbsp	0	14	0	125
Corn on the Cob	1 Sm	3	1	20	100
Corn Pone	2″ Sq	4	3	40	210
Corn Starch	1 Tbsp	1	1	9	50
Corn Syrup	1 Tbsp	T	T	12	50
Corned Beef	2 Ozs	20	5	0	125
Corned Beef Hash	2 Ozs	8	4	4	73
Cotton Seed Oil	1 Tbsp	T	14	0	125
Crab, Canned	2 Ozs	10	T	0	56
Crab, Deviled	2 Ozs	9	1	0	52

	AMT	PRO	FAT	CARB	CAL
Crab Meat	2 Ozs	13	2	T	70
Crab, Shelled	2 Ozs	10	1	T	50
Crabapples	1 Lg	T	1	7	90
Cranberries	4 Ozs	T	T	11	50
Cranberry Juice Cocktail	4 Ozs	T	T	18	75
Cranberry Relish	1 Tbsp	T	T	15	65
Cranberry Sauce	1 Tbsp	T	T	9	35
Cream, Half & Half	½ Cup	4	13	5	160
Cream, Heavy	½ Cup	2	42	3	410
Cream, Heavy	1 Tbsp	T	5	T	50
Cream, Light	½ Cup	2	23	5	235
Cream, Light	1 Tbsp	T	3	T	30
Cream Pie	1 Pc	22	13	50	405
Cream Pie, Boston	1 Pc	6	11	55	325
Cream Pie, Cherry	1 Pc	20	20	55	480
Cream Puff	2 Ozs	4	7	12	130
Cream Sauce	2 Tbsps	3	4	2	50
Cream Soda	6 Ozs	0	0	21	75
Cream, Sour	1 Tbsp	T	3	T	30
Cream, Whipped	2 Tbsps	1	12	1	115
Creamer, Nondairy	1 Tsp	T	T	1	10
Crème de Cacao	Shot	0	0	7	75
Crème de Menthe	Shot	0	0	7	75
Crêpe Suzette	1 Av	10	12	22	235
Crisco	1 Tbsp	0	14	0	125
Croutons	6 Av	2	2	3	35
Crullers	1 Med	3	10	19	180
Crumb Cake	1 Sl	2	4	20	125
Crumb Cake, Apple	1 Pc	T	1	49	200
Crumbs, Bread	1 Tbsp	6	2	4	60
Crust, Pie, Graham Craker	Bottom	4	19	64	450
Cucumber	8″	T	0	3	14
Cumin	⅛ Tsp	0	0	0	0
Cupcake	1 Med	2	6	33	95
Currants, Dried	4 Ozs	5	2	74	160
Currants, Fresh	2 Ozs	1	T	5	30
Curry Powder	1 Tsp	0	0	0	0
Custard	½ Cup	3	3	24	130
Custard, Banana	1 Serv	6	6	24	175
Custard, Butterscotch	1 Serv	5	5	12	125
Custard, Canned, Instant	1 Serv	6	3	23	125
Custard, Egg, Baked	½ Cup	10	6	14	160
Custard, Frozen	4 Ozs	5	12	20	210
Custard Pie	1 Sl	6	12	23	225
Custard Sauce	1 Tbsp	6	6	2	85
Custard, Vanilla, Frozen	4 Ozs	5	12	20	210
Daiquiri	Cktl Glass	0	0	7	75
Dandelion Greens	4 Ozs	3	T	9	55
Danish Pastry	2 Ozs	4	13	25	240
Date Cookies	2	4	3	15	110
Date & Nut Bread	1 Sl	2	1	21	100

	AMT	PRO	FAT	CARB	CAL
Dates, Dried	1 Cup	4	1	13	560
Dates, Pitted	½ Cup	2	T	67	275
Dates, Pitted Candies	1 Bar	2	3	20	110
Devil's Food Cake	1 Sl	2	8	32	210
Deviled Egg	2	20	15	2	225
Deviled Ham	1 Tbsp	10	10	T	130
Deviled Ham Spread	1 Serv	5	10	T	110
Diet Dressings	1 Tbsp	T	2	1	25
Dill Pickles	1 Av	T	T	2	5
Dixie Cup	1 Cup	6	14	20	230
Dixie Cup Sundae	1 Serv	6	14	53	365
Doughnut, French	1 Oz	4	14	21	225
Doughnut, Iced	1 Oz	3	10	37	230
Doughnut, Jelly	1 Oz	3	10	37	245
Doughnut, Plain	1 Oz	3	10	19	180
Doughnut, Sugared	1 Oz	3	10	21	185
Duck Eggs	1 Med	6	5	1	75
Duck, Roasted	2 Ozs	11	4	0	95
Dumplings	1 Med	1	2	19	100
Eclair, Choc., Creamed	1 Av	7	15	15	225
Eclair, Choc., Custard	1 Av	7	15	20	240
Eels, Raw	2 Ozs	9	10	0	130
Eels, Smoked	2 Ozs	10	15	0	183
Egg	1 Med	6	6	T	80
Egg, Poached	1 Av	6	6	1	80
Egg White	1	3	0	T	10
Egg Yolk	1	3	6	T	80
Eggplant	1 Sl	1	T	7	35
Eggs, Deviled	2	20	15	2	225
Eggs, Dried	1 Tbsp	3	3	T	40
Eggs, Duck	1 Med	6	5	1	75
Eggs, Florentine	1 Serv	14	14	4	200
Eggs, Fried	1 Med	6	8	T	95
Eggs, Scrambled	2	11	12	T	155
Endive	4 Ozs	1	T	4	25
English Toffee	1 Pc	T	T	13	56
Escarole	4 Ozs	1	T	4	25
Eskimo Pie	Av	3	6	32	205
Fennel	⅛ Tsp	0	0	0	0
Feta Cheese	1 Oz	6	8	T	100
Fig Bars	1 Lg	1	1	19	90
Fig Newton	2	1	1	22	100
Figs, Canned	4 Ozs	T	T	19	75
Figs, Dried	1	1	T	12	55
Figs, Fresh	4 Sm	1	T	24	100
Filet Mignon	2 Ozs	18	4	0	125
Fish, Abalone	2 Ozs	10	T	1	50
Fish, Blue, Baked	2 Ozs	12	5	0	115
Fish, Blue, Fried	2 Ozs	11	2	0	112

	AMT	PRO	FAT	CARB	CAL
Fish Cakes, Fried	2 Ozs	8	4	5	95
Fish Chowder	1 Cup	1	2	12	65
Fish, Cod	2 Ozs	9	T	0	40
Fish, Cod (Cakes)	2 Ozs	8	4	5	94
Fish, Flounder	2 Ozs	9	T	0	45
Fish, Gefilte	1 Serv	3	2	1	75
Fish, Haddock	2 Ozs	10	3	4	90
Fish, Halibut	2 Ozs	10	3	0	70
Fish, Herring	1 Sm	26	8	0	190
Fish, Herring, Kippered	1 Sm	22	13	0	190
Fish, Lobster	½ Avg	16	2	T	90
Fish, Lobster, Canned	2 Ozs	10	1	T	55
Fish, Mackerel, Canned	2 Ozs	10	6	0	95
Fish, Salmon	2 Ozs	9	9	0	125
Fish, Salmon, Canned	2 Ozs	10	7	0	110
Fish, Sardines, Canned	2 Ozs	15	6	0	115
Fish, Shad	2 Ozs	10	5	0	90
Fish, Shrimp, Canned	2 Ozs	15	1	0	70
Fish, Sole	2 Ozs	18	7	0	90
Fish, Swordfish	2 Ozs	15	4	0	100
Fish, Tuna. See Tuna	2 Ozs	15	4	0	102
Flour, All Purpose	1 Cup	12	1	84	400
Flour, Arrowroot	2 Ozs	8	1	40	200
Flour, Buckwheat	1 Cup	6	1	80	350
Flour, Cake	1 Cup	9	T	85	380
Flour, Corn Meal	1 Cup	11	4	90	460
Flour, Rye, Dark	1 Cup	20	3	76	410
Flour, Rye, Light	1 Cup	11	1	98	440
Flour, Soy Bean (Full-Fat)	½ Cup	41	23	41	505
Flour, Soy Bean (Low-Fat)	½ Cup	49	7	34	425
Flour, Wheat	1 Cup	13	1	84	400
Flour, White	1 Cup	12	1	84	400
Fondue, Cheese	1 Serv	20	21	9	315
Frankfurter	1 Av	5	11	T	120
Frankfurter, All Beef	1 Av	7	14	0	170
Frankfurter Rolls	1 Av	7	6	12	160
Frankfurters & Sauerkraut	1 Serv	8	14	5	200
Frappé, Ice Cream	10 Ozs	12	19	35	360
French Fried Potatoes	6 Av	1	5	12	100
French Onion Soup	½ Cup	5	2	5	60
French Pastry	Med	4	9	40	260
French Rolls	1 Av	5	2	20	120
French Toast	1 Sl	4	4	15	115
French Toast w/Maple Syrup	1 Sl	4	4	23	150
Fruit Cocktail, Canned	1 Cup	1	T	47	190
Fruit Cocktail, Fresh	1 Cup	T	T	35	135
Fruit Drop Candies	3	T	T	10	40
Fruit Punch	6 Ozs	T	T	33	135
Fruit Syrups	1 Tbsp	T	T	14	60
Fudge	1 Oz	T	3	23	120
Fudge, Almond	1 Sq	1	4	22	130

	AMT	PRO	FAT	CARB	CAL
Fudge, Brown Sugar	1 Sq	T	3	22	115
Fudge Cake	1 Serv	6	10	35	255
Fudge, Choc. Candies	1 Pc	T	3	23	120
Fudge Frosting	1 Tbsp	T	3	6	50
Fudge Popsicle Ice Cream	1	3	6	13	120
Fudge Sauce	1 Tbsp	T	T	18	75
Fudge Sundae, Hot	1	7	25	53	465
Garbanzos (Chick Peas)	4 Ozs	23	5	60	390
Garlic Clove	1	1	T	T	5
Garlic Sauce w/Butter	2 Tbsps	T	33	1	200
Gelatin	2 Ozs	47	T	0	185
Germ, Wheat	1 Oz	7	3	12	100
Gin	2 Ozs	0	0	0	150
Gin Collins	1 Serv	0	0	14	225
Gin Fizz	6 Ozs	0	0	4	125
Gin Rickey	1 Serv	0	0	3	200
Gin & Tonic	6 Ozs	0	0	11	210
Ginger Ale	6 Ozs	0	0	16	75
Ginger Root, Fresh	4 Ozs	2	1	8	50
Ginger Snaps	5	1	10	6	165
Gingerbread	1 Sl	2	6	21	180
Goose, Roasted	2 Ozs	13	20	0	240
Goulash, Hungarian	4 Ozs	24	31	4	360
Grape Juice	½ Cup	T	T	18	75
Grape Soda	6 Ozs	T	T	28	110
Grapefruit	½ Sm	1	T	11	50
Grapefruit, Canned	½ Cup	T	T	18	75
Grapefruit, Canned, Swtnd	½ Cup	T	T	22	90
Grapefruit Juice, Canned, Unsw	½ Cup	T	T	32	65
Grapes	1 Cup	2	2	16	90
Gravy, Chicken	1 Tbsp	T	4	2	50
Green Beans, Canned	4 Ozs	2	T	6	30
Green Beans, Fresh Cooked	1 Cup	2	T	6	30
Green Beans, Frozen	½ Cup	2	T	8	40
Green Beans, Raw	½ Cup	2	T	8	40
Griddle Cakes	1 Av	2	3	11	80
Grits, Corn	4 Ozs	1	T	12	55
Grits, Hominy	½ Cup	2	T	28	120
Gum	1 Stick	0	0	2	8
Gum, Candy Coated	1 Stick	0	0	3	12
Ham	2 Ozs	9	13	0	150
Ham, Baked	2 Ozs	12	12	0	160
Ham, Boiled	2 Ozs	10	12	0	150
Ham, Canned Boneless	2 Ozs	10	7	0	107
Ham, Deviled	1 Tbsp	10	10	T	130
Ham Steak	1 Serv	15	5	0	115
Ham, Virginia, Baked	2 Ozs	11	12	0	157
Hamburger, All Beef	2 Ozs	13	11	0	160
Hamburger Rolls	1	3	2	21	120

	AMT	PRO	FAT	CARB	CAL
Hamburger Steak	2 Ozs	13	17	0	276
Hash, Corned Beef	2 Ozs	8	3	4	80
Herbs	1 Tsp	0	0	0	0
Hollandaise Sauce	1 Tbsp	T	8	T	70
Honey	1 Tbsp	T	0	17	65
Horseradish	1 Tsp	T	T	1	5
Hot Dog (No Roll)	1	7	14	0	170
Hot Dog Roll	1	7	6	12	160
Ice Box Cake	1 Sl	3	4	26	165
Ice Box Cookies	3 Med	1	5	19	125
Ice Cream	½ Cup	3	9	14	150
Ice Cream, Choc. Cov. Pop	1	3	9	15	150
Ice Cream, Coconut Cov. Pop	1	3	9	18	165
Ice Cream Cone (Cone Alone)	1	2	3	19	110
Ice Cream Fudge Pop	1	3	6	13	120
Ice Cream, Ices	1 Scp	T	T	27	120
Ice Cream Parfait	1	6	15	20	300
Ice Cream Sodas	8 Ozs	3	9	71	285
Ice Cream Sundae	1 Av	7	25	50	450
Ice Cream Sundae (Banana Split)	1 Av	8	25	75	560
Ice Cream Sundae (Hot Fudge)	1 Av	7	25	53	465
Ice, Lemon, Lime, etc.	1 Scp	T	T	27	120
Ice Pop	1	T	T	24	100
Iced Tea (No Sugar or Cream)	1 Gl	T	T	T	2
Icing	1 Tbsp	T	1	11	55
Italian Bread	1 Sl	2	T	12	60
Jams (Most)	1 Tbsp	T	T	14	55
Jellies (Most)	1 Tbsp	T	T	13	55
Jell-O	1 Serv	2	0	17	75
Kale	1 Cup	5	0	6	43
Kidney Beans, Cooked	1 Cup	14	T	37	225
Kidney Beans, Raw	1 Cup	26	2	67	380
Kumquats, Candied	1 Oz	T	T	6	25
Kumquats, Fresh	4 Ozs	1	T	17	75
Lamb, Leg, Roasted	2 Ozs	15	10	0	160
Lamb Liver	2 Ozs	18	7	1	140
Lamb, Loin Chops	2 Ozs	13	15	0	192
Lamb Roast	2 Ozs	12	16	0	195
Lamb Shish Kebab	1 Serv	5	4	6	67
Lamb Stew	1 Serv	7	6	7	118
Lard	1 Tbsp	0	12	0	125
Layer Cake	1 Sl	4	5	55	185
Layer Cake, Round w/Icing	1 Sl	6	15	61	400
Leeks	1 Pc	1	T	1	7
Lemon	1	T	T	5	20
Lemon Chiffon Pie	1 Pc	8	14	35	350
Lemon Drops	1 Oz	0	T	28	110

	AMT	PRO	FAT	CARB	CAL
Lemon Frosting	1 Tbsp	T	1	11	55
Lemon Juice	1 Tbsp	T	T	1	5
Lemon Juice, Canned, Swtnd	½ Cup	T	T	10	40
Lemon Juice, Canned, Unswtnd	½ Cup	T	T	7	30
Lemon Meringue Pie	1 Pc	4	12	45	300
Lemon Peel, Candied	1 Oz	T	T	24	90
Lemon Pudding	1 Serv	3	3	26	140
Lemon Sauce	1 Tbsp	T	1	5	25
Lemon Soda	6 Ozs	0	0	19	80
Lemon Sponge Cake	1 Pc	3	6	54	280
Lemonade	1 Cup	T	T	25	100
Lentil Soup	1 Serv	4	2	40	180
Lentils	½ Cup	9	T	17	105
Lettuce	2 Leaves	T	T	1	7
Lettuce Hearts	½ Cup	1	T	3	15
Lettuce, Romaine	½ Cup	2	T	4	25
Lettuce, Shredded	1 Cup	T	T	2	15
Lettuce & Tomato Salad	1 Serv	2	T	6	30
Lichee Nuts, Dried	1 Oz	1	T	15	65
Life Savers (All Flavors)	1 Roll	0	T	30	120
Lima Beans, Canned	4 Ozs	4	T	15	80
Lima Beans, Fresh	4 Ozs	8	T	27	135
Lime	1	T	T	5	20
Lime Juice, Fresh	1 Cup	0	T	18	60
Lime Juice, Frozen, Diluted	4 Ozs	T	T	11	45
Lime Soda	6 Ozs	0	0	19	80
Liver, Beef, Fried	2 Ozs	15	6	3	130
Liver, Calves', Fried	2 Ozs	15	7	2	140
Liver, Chicken	2 Ozs	15	2	1	92
Liverwurst	2 Ozs	8	15	2	170
Lobster, Baked or Broiled	1 Av	35	11	1	245
Lobster, Canned	2 Ozs	10	1	T	52
Lobster Newberg	1 Serv	19	11	3	195
Lobster Salad	½ Cup	11	7	5	125
Lobster, Steamed	½ Av	19	2	T	95
Lobster, Steamed w/2 Tbsp Butter	1 Av	38	26	1	390
Lobster Tails	2 Ozs	10	1	T	50
Loganberries, Canned	½ Cup	T	T	20	80
Loganberries, Fresh	½ Cup	T	T	11	45
Lollipops	1 Med	0	0	28	115
London Broil Steak	2 Ozs	17	4	0	105
Lox	1 Oz	5	5	0	60
Macadamia Nuts	2 Ozs	4	40	9	390
Macaroni au Gratin	1 Serv	10	12	30	250
Macaroni & Cheese	1 Cup	18	24	43	465
Macaroni, Cooked	4 Ozs	4	T	39	125
Macaroni Salad	1 Cup	4	20	26	260
Mace	⅛ Tsp	0	0	0	0
Malt, Cocoa	1 Cup	10	14	22	255
Mangos, Raw	4 Ozs	T	T	19	75

	AMT	PRO	FAT	CARB	CAL
Manhattan Cocktail	1 Gl	T	T	3	190
Marble Cake	1 Pc	3	5	30	185
Margarine	1 Tbsp	T	11	0	100
Marmalade	1 Tbsp	T	T	14	55
Marshmallow Candy	1 Oz	1	1	23	100
Marshmallow Sauce	1 Tbsp	T	0	6	25
Marshmallow Topping	1 Tbsp	T	0	12	50
Marshmallows	1 Av	T	0	6	25
Martini	3 Ozs	0	0	T	165
Martini, Dry	3 Ozs	0	0	0	205
Matai, Fresh	4 Ozs	2	T	21	90
Mayonnaise	1 Tbsp	T	10	T	90
Meatballs	2 Ozs	9	8	2	115
Meatballs & Spaghetti	2 Ozs	4	2	22	75
Meat Gravy	1 Tbsp	T	3	5	50
Meat Loaf	2 Ozs	8	7	1	112
Melba Toast	1 Sl	1	T	4	30
Melon Balls, Frozen	1 Cup	1	T	12	55
Melon, Cantaloupe	½	1	T	8	35
Melon, Honeydew	Wedge	T	0	13	50
Milk, Acidophilus	¾ Cup	8	9	6	145
Milk, Buttermilk	1 Cup	9	T	12	85
Milk, Choc. Flavored	1 Cup	8	8	25	200
Milk, Coconut	1 Cup	4	27	10	300
Milk Condensed, Undiluted	1 Oz	3	3	21	125
Milk, Dry, Nonfat	1 Tbsp	3	T	2	30
Milk, Dry, Whole	1 Tbsp	2	2	3	40
Milk, Goat	½ Cup	4	5	5	90
Milk, Skimmed	1 Cup	9	T	13	85
Milk, Skimmed, Choc.	1 Cup	8	T	26	130
Milk, Soy Bean	1 Cup	8	3	5	80
Milk, Whole	1 Cup	9	10	12	175
Mince Pie	1 Sl	3	9	52	300
Minestrone	1 Cup	4	3	10	80
Mint, Chopped	1 Tbsp	0	0	0	0
Mint Leaves	1 Tbsp	0	0	0	0
Mixed Vegetables, Canned	4 Ozs	4	T	15	75
Mixed Vegetables, Frozen	4 Ozs	4	T	16	75
Molasses, Blackstrap	1 Tbsp	T	T	11	45
Molasses, Cane Syrup	1 Tbsp	T	T	13	50
Molasses Cookie	1	T	1	5	35
Mousse	1 Serv	4	30	17	355
Muffins	1 Av	4	5	19	135
Muffins, Blueberry	1 Av	4	5	23	150
Muffins, Bran	1 Av	4	5	24	150
Muffins, Cinnamon	1 Av	2	4	23	135
Muffins, Date	1 Av	4	5	41	140
Muffins, English	1 Av	4	5	21	150
Muffins, Raisin	1 Av	4	4	27	160
Muffins, White	1 Av	3	2	21	120
Muffins, Whole Wheat	1 Av	2	3	19	115

	AMT	PRO	FAT	CARB	CAL
Mushroom Soup, Creamed	1 Cup	2	13	13	180
Mushrooms	½ Cup	3	T	5	35
Mushrooms, Broiled w/Tsp. Butter	½ Cup	2	11	3	65
Mushrooms, Button	½ Cup	2	T	3	20
Mushrooms, Canned	½ Cup	2	T	3	20
Mushrooms, Cooked, Fresh	½ Cup	2	1	3	30
Mushrooms, Creamed	½ Cup	3	2	3	42
Muskmelon	Av Serv	1	T	8	30
Mussels	2 Ozs	5	1	0	37
Mustard	1 Tbsp	T	T	T	10
Mustard, Dry	1 Tbsp	T	T	T	10
Mustard Greens	1 Cup	3	T	5	30
Mustard, Prepared	1 Tbsp	T	T	T	10
Mustard Sauce	¼ Cup	2	6	6	85
Mutton, Boiled	2 Ozs	13	15	0	187
Mutton Chop	2 Ozs	13	15	0	187
Mutton Chops or Roast	2 Ozs	12	16	0	195
Mutton, Leg, Roast	2 Ozs	10	14	0	162
Napoleons	1 Av	7	15	30	300
Nectarine	1	1	T	12	50
Noodles, w/Butter & Cheese	1 Serv	9	13	10	195
Nut Bread, Date	1 Sl	2	1	21	100
Nut Brittle	2 Ozs	4	6	45	250
Nutmeg	⅛ Tsp	0	0	0	0
Nuts, Brazil, Shelled	2 Ozs	8	35	6	365
Nuts, Butter	5 Av	2	4	1	50
Nuts, Cashew	7 Av	2	6	4	75
Nuts, Hazel	2 Ozs	8	37	9	380
Nuts, Hickory	10 Av	2	9	2	100
Nuts, Macadamia	2 Ozs	4	40	9	390
Nuts, Peanuts	10	6	11	3	175
Nuts, Pine	2 Ozs	17	27	7	310
Nuts, Pistachio	16	2	5	2	50
Oat Cereal, Ready to Eat	½ Cup	4	1	13	75
Oatmeal, Cooked	1 Cup	5	3	25	150
Oatmeal Cookies	1 Lg	2	3	15	90
Oil, Salad	1 Tbsp	T	14	0	125
Oil, Unsaturated, Vegetable	1 Tbsp	0	14	0	125
Oil & Vinegar Dressing	1 Tbsp	T	14	0	125
Okra	1 Cup	3	T	10	50
Okra, Cooked	8 Pods	2	T	6	30
Olive Oil	1 Tbsp	T	14	0	125
Olives, Green	2 Ozs	T	7	1	65
Olives, Ripe	2 Ozs	T	8	1	75
Omelet	2 Eggs	11	12	T	150
Omelet, Asparagus	2 Eggs	16	12	6	220
Omelet, Cheese	2 Eggs	18	21	1	260
Omelet, Mushroom	2 Eggs	12	12	2	160
Omelet, Onion	2 Eggs	11	12	1	160

	AMT	PRO	FAT	CARB	CAL
Omelet, Plain	2 Eggs	11	12	1	155
Omelet, Spanish	2 Eggs	12	13	8	200
Onion Roll	1	3	2	23	130
Onion Soup	1 Cup	5	1	4	50
Onion Soup, French	4 Ozs	5	2	5	60
Onions, Boiled	1 Cup	1	T	7	30
Onions, Creamed	½ Cup	3	4	8	65
Onions, French Fried	1 Lg	2	15	10	175
Onions, Fried	1 Lg	2	15	10	175
Onions, Green	6 Sm	T	T	T	25
Onions, Raw	1	2	T	11	50
Onions, Raw (Bermuda)	4 Ozs	2	T	10	40
Onions, Raw, Chopped	1	2	T	11	50
Orange	1 Med	1	T	17	70
Orange Juice, Canned, Swtnd	1 Cup	2	T	31	140
Orange Juice, Canned, Unswtnd	1 Cup	1	T	26	110
Orange Juice, Florida	1 Cup	2	T	26	110
Orange, Mandarin	1 Med	1	T	10	50
Orange Marmalade	1 Tbsp	T	T	14	55
Orange Peel, Candied	2 Ozs	T	T	48	190
Orange Sections	½ Cup	1	T	11	50
Orange-Grapefruit Juice	1 Cup	3	2	20	110
Orangeade Juice	½ Cup	1	T	19	80
Oregano	⅛ Tsp	0	0	0	0
Oyster, Blue Point	12	12	2	7	100
Oyster, Cape Cod	6	12	2	5	100
Oyster Cocktail, Raw	6 Med	9	1	6	75
Oyster Crackers	½ Oz	1	2	10	60
Oyster, Fried	2 Ozs	5	8	10	135
Oyster Stew w/Milk	1 Cup	5	5	21	150
Oysters on the Half Shell	6 Med	10	2	6	75
Oysters, Scalloped	6	12	8	6	150
Pancakes, Blueberry	2	8	8	29	250
Pancakes, Buckwheat	1	6	8	21	175
Pancakes, Choc.	2	2	8	16	200
Pancakes, Griddle	1	2	3	11	80
Pancakes, Wheat	1	2	3	11	80
Pancakes, Wheat (Enriched Flour)	1	2	3	11	80
Papaya	4 Ozs	T	T	11	45
Papaya Marmalade	1 Tbsp	T	T	15	55
Parfait	1 Av	6	15	14	215
Parsley	1 Tbsp	T	T	T	1
Parsnips, Cooked	1 Cup	2	1	21	95
Passion Fruit	4 Ozs	2	1	35	155
Pastry, Danish	1 Pc	4	13	25	240
Pâté de Fois Gras	1 Tbsp	2	8	1	85
Pate Maison	1 Oz	3	13	T	130
Pea Beans, Dried, Cooked	4 Ozs	4	T	18	90
Pea Soup	1 Cup	3	1	16	85
Peach Brandy	Shot	T	T	7	100

	AMT	PRO	FAT	CARB	CAL
Peach Pie	Av Serv	3	11	70	390
Peach Shortcake	Av Serv	6	12	41	300
Peaches, Canned	2 Hlvs	T	T	11	45
Peaches, Canned in Water	2 Hlvs	T	T	9	35
Peaches, Dried	2 Hlvs	4	T	76	300
Peaches, Fresh	1 Med	1	T	11	50
Peanut Bar Candy	2 Ozs	5	8	17	160
Peanut Brittle	2 Ozs	3	6	46	140
Peanut Butter	1 Tbsp	4	8	3	100
Peanut Cookie	1	1	2	9	65
Peanuts	10	6	11	3	175
Pear	1 Av	1	T	18	75
Pear Juice Nectar	4 Ozs	T	T	12	50
Pears, Canned	2 Hlvs	T	T	17	70
Pears, Canned (Water-packed)	2 Hlvs	T	T	9	35
Peas, Black-Eyed, Canned, Drained	4 Ozs	8	1	17	110
Peas, Canned	1 Cup	5	T	19	100
Peas, Chick (Garbanzos, Dry)	½ Cup	23	5	60	390
Peas, Fresh	Av Serv	3	T	10	55
Peas, Green	Av Serv	4	T	14	75
Pecan Pie	1 Av Sl	6	25	58	470
Pecans	6	1	7	2	75
Pecans, Chopped	1 Tbsp	T	3	1	35
Pecans (Halves)	2 Ozs	5	40	8	290
Pepper	⅛ Tsp	0	0	0	0
Pepper, Cayenne	⅛ Tsp	0	0	0	0
Peppermint Candy, Choc. Covered	1 Oz	T	3	21	115
Peppermint Patties	1 Oz	T	1	25	105
Peppers, Fresh	1 Med	1	T	4	20
Peppers, Stuffed	1	14	6	11	155
Perch	2 Ozs	11	2	0	60
Perch, Sea	2 Ozs	11	0	0	50
Persimmons	1 Av	1	T	24	100
Pheasant, Roasted	1 Serv	24	5	0	150
Pickles, Dill or Sour	1 Lg	T	T	3	10
Pickles, Sweet	1 Sm	T	T	5	20
Pie. See By Name	Av Pc	T	6	75	350
Pig Brains	Av Serv	6	5	1	70
Pig Liver	Av Serv	11	2	1	65
Pig's Feet, Pickled	2 Ozs	9	8	T	112
Pike	Av Serv	21	1	0	95
Pimiento, Hot	½ Cup	1	T	6	30
Pimientoes	½ Cup	1	T	6	30
Piña Colada	1	6	0	31	245
Pineapple, Candied	1 Sl	T	T	30	120
Pineapple, Canned	1 Sl	T	T	12	50
Pineapple, Canned, Low Calorie	½ Cup	T	T	11	45
Pineapple, Crushed, Canned	½ Cup	5	8	15	150
Pineapple, Fresh	1 Cup	T	T	16	60
Pineapple Upside-down Cake	1 Pc	7	10	38	275
Pinto Beans	½ Cup	25	1	72	390

	AMT	PRO	FAT	CARB	CAL
Pita, Shell	1	4	1	13	70
Pizza Pie w/Cheese	1 Pc	14	9	25	240
Pizza, Sausage	1 Pc	9	10	23	265
Plums, Fresh	1	1	T	7	30
Popcorn, Air-popped	1 Cup	1	T	10	50
Popcorn, No Butter	1 Cup	2	1	11	55
Popcorn, Sugar-coated	1 Cup	1	T	11	55
Popcorn w/1 Tbsp. Butter	1 Cup	2	12	11	155
Popovers	Av	3	3	11	75
Poppy Seeds	⅛ Tsp	0	0	0	0
Pork Chop	1 Med	30	16	0	275
Pork Chop, Fried	1 Med	30	41	0	375
Pork Chop, Loin Ctr Cut, Broiled	1 Med	30	16	0	275
Pork, Cured, Bacon	2 Ozs	4	38	T	375
Pork, Cured Ham	2 Ozs	10	6	0	107
Pork, Heart	2 Ozs	9	2	T	65
Pork, Kidney	1 Serv	9	2	1	57
Pork, Leg Roast	2 Ozs	7	19	0	225
Pork, Liver	Av Serv	11	2	2	75
Pork, Loin, Roasted	Av Serv	13	16	0	202
Pork, Spiced	2 Ozs	8	14	0	157
Pot Roast	4 Ozs	32	17	0	290
Potato au Gratin	4 Ozs	6	9	16	165
Potato, Baked	4 Ozs	4	T	28	125
Potato, Boiled	4 Ozs	4	T	28	125
Potato Chips	½ Cup	1	8	7	100
Potato, French Fried	6 Av	1	5	12	100
Potato, Idaho, Baked	1 Med	4	T	28	125
Potato, Irish, Boiled	1 Med	4	T	28	125
Potato Julienne	1 Med	8	6	30	225
Potato, Mashed	½ Cup	2	3	16	90
Potato, Pan Browned	4 Ozs	2	13	33	260
Potato Salad	4 Ozs	3	11	16	175
Potato Soup, Cream of	4 Ozs	4	5	8	100
Potato, Sweet, Baked	5 Ozs	3	1	45	200
Potato, Sweet, Boiled	5 Ozs	2	1	44	160
Potato, Sweet, Candied	6 Ozs	2	5	60	295
Potatoes, Fried	½ Cup	4	16	12	285
Potatoes, Hash Brown	4 Ozs	3	13	33	260
Potatoes, Scalloped	½ Cup	3	4	14	120
Potatoes, Sweet, Canned	1 Cup	5	1	45	285
Pound Cake	1 Sl	3	6	35	380
Prune Juice	4 Ozs	1	T	23	94
Prunes, Cooked (Sugar Added)	4 Ozs	1	T	50	205
Prunes, Dried	4	1	T	24	100
Prunes, Stewed (No Sugar)	4 Ozs	1	T	40	165
Pudding, Bread	½ Cup	6	7	32	210
Pudding, Butterscotch	½ Cup	3	3	23	140
Pudding, Cornstarch	½ Cup	3	3	24	135
Pudding, Date	½ Cup	4	5	16	125
Pumpkin, Canned	1 Cup	2	1	18	90

	AMT	PRO	FAT	CARB	CAL
Pumpkin Pie	1 Pc	8	23	47	430
Pumpkin Seeds	1 Oz	8	13	4	155
Quail, Broiled	2 Ozs	14	4	0	95
Quince, Fresh	1	T	T	12	50
Quinine Water	6 Ozs	0	0	12	50
Rabbit	2 Ozs	34	11	0	120
Rabbit Stew	2 Ozs	7	6	7	117
Radishes	4 Sm	T	T	2	8
Raisin Bran Flakes	1 Cup	4	T	40	140
Raisin Bread	1 Slice	2	1	12	65
Raisin Cookies	¼ lb.	5	6	90	430
Raisins	¼ Cup	1	T	29	120
Raspberries	1 Cup	2	2	16	80
Raspberry Pie	Av Sl	T	6	57	280
Relish, Pickle, Sweet	1 Tbsp	T	T	3	12
Rhubarb	1 Cup, Diced	1	T	5	18
Rhubarb, Frozen	½ Cup	1	T	20	80
Rice, Boiled White	1 Cup	4	T	49	223
Rice, Brown	1 Cup	3	T	38	178
Rice, Spanish	1 Cup	4	4	40	210
Rice, Wild, Cooked	1 Cup	6	2	30	70
Roast Beef	2 Ozs	16	5	0	114
Roast Beef, Canned	2 Ozs	14	6	0	125
Roast Beef Hash	2 Ozs	5	6	6	102
Roll, Plain	1	3	2	21	120
Root Beer	6 Ozs	0	0	15	75
Rosemary	⅛ Tsp	0	0	0	0
Rum	1 Shot	T	T	T	100
Rutabaga	½ Cup	1	T	9	40
Ry-Krisp	3	2	T	10	50
Rye Bread	1 Sl	2	T	12	55
Rye Flour, Dark	1 Cup	20	3	76	410
Rye Flour, Light	1 Cup	11	1	98	440
Rye Wafer Crackers	1	T	T	2	8
Sage	⅛ Tsp	0	0	0	0
Salami	2 Ozs	14	22	T	240
Sauerkraut	½ Cup	1	T	5	25
Sausage, Canned, (Pork)	2 Ozs	10	18	1	212
Sausage, Frankfurter, Cooked	1	6	15	1	165
Sausage, Knockwurst	1 Av	12	16	1	185
Sausage, Liverwurst	1 Sl	5	7	T	90
Sausage, Polish	2 Ozs	9	14	0	170
Sausage, Pork	1	10	25	0	265
Sausage, Pork, Dried	2 Ozs	18	21	0	242
Sausage, Vienna, Canned	2 Ozs	8	11	0	135
Scallions	5	1	T	5	20
Scallops	2 Ozs	14	1	1	70
Scallops, Broiled	2 Ozs	14	1	1	70

	AMT	PRO	FAT	CARB	CAL
Scallops, Fried w/Butter	3-4	20	9	15	230
Scotch	Shot	0	0	0	100
Scotch & Soda	1 Drink	0	0	0	100
Seltzer (Carbonated Water)	4 Ozs	0	0	0	0
Seltzer Water	8 Ozs	0	0	0	0
Sesame Seeds, Whole	1 Oz	5	14	6	165
Shad, Roe	2 Ozs	12	1	0	65
Sherbet Ice Cream, w/Water	¼ Pt	1	1	35	130
Shoofly Pie	1 Pc	5	8	48	285
Short Bread	1 Sl	2	7	19	140
Shortcake, Banana	1 Sl	4	7	44	250
Shortcake, Biscuit	1	4	10	27	210
Shortcake, Peach	Av Serv	6	12	41	300
Shortcake, Plain	Av Serv	5	11	31	255
Shortcake, Raspberry	Av Serv	69	12	47	325
Shortcake, Strawberry	Av Serv	6	12	43	300
Shortening, Crisco	1 Tbsp	0	14	0	125
Shrimp, Boiled	2 Ozs	10	0	1	45
Shrimp, Canned	2 Ozs	14	0	T	66
Shrimp Cocktail	6 Med Size	16	1	1	75
Shrimp Creole	2 Ozs	10	4	2	92
Shrimp, French Fried	10 Av	23	12	11	240
Shrimp, Fried	3 Jumbo	8	4	8	100
Shrimp Salad Sandwich	1	14	2	26	180
Shrimp Salad w/Celery	1 Serv	10	1	5	70
Shrimp Scampi in Garlic Butter	6	20	24	T	300
Snails	6 Med	16	13	2	190
Soda, Cherry	6 Ozs	0	0	21	80
Soda, Chocolate	6 Ozs	0	0	15	75
Soda Crackers	6	5	6	35	215
Soda, Cream	6 Ozs	0	0	21	75
Soda, Ginger Ale	6 Ozs	0	0	16	75
Soda, Grape	6 Ozs	0	0	28	110
Soda, Ice Cream	10 Ozs	3	9	71	285
Soda, Lemon	6 Ozs	0	0	19	80
Soda, Lime	6 Ozs	0	0	19	80
Soda, Orange	6 Ozs	0	0	19	80
Sorghum Syrup	3 Ozs	T	T	58	230
Soufflé, Almond	½ Cup	17	6	40	280
Soufflé, Cheese	½ Cup	11	19	6	240
Sour Balls	6	0	T	28	110
Sour Cream	1 Tbsp	T	3	T	30
Soy Beans	½ Cup	11	6	6	120
Soy Sauce	1 Tsp	T	T	1	4
Soybean Curd	1 Oz	2	1	3	20
Soybean Milk	8 Ozs	8	3	5	80
Soybean Sprouts, Raw	½ Cup	7	2	3	70
Soybeans, Mature, Dried	½ Cup	25	T	25	180
Spaghetti, Cooked	1 Cup	7	1	46	200
Spaghetti w/2 Meatballs	4 Ozs	8	5	45	150
Spaghetti w/Butter	4 Ozs	4	9	20	210

	AMT	PRO	FAT	CARB	CAL
Spaghetti w/Clam Sauce	4 Ozs	8	1	43	220
Spaghetti w/Meat Sauce	4 Ozs	5	3	47	235
Spaghetti w/Tomato Sauce	4 Ozs	3	1	47	210
Spareribs, Barbecued	6 Av	24	47	0	505
Spareribs, Pork	2 Ozs	11	22	0	247
Spinach	½ Cup	3	T	3	25
Spinach, Canned	1 Cup	6	1	6	55
Spinach, Frozen	1 Cup	7	1	6	60
Spinach, Raw	1 Cup	7	1	6	60
Spinach Soufflé	Av Serv	9	12	6	170
Sponge Cake	Av Pc	2	2	22	115
Squab	1	20	8	0	160
Squash, Acorn	½ Cup	T	T	12	50
Squash, Butternut	½ Cup	1	T	12	55
Squash, Hubbard	½ Cup	1	T	10	50
Squash, Summer	½ Cup	1	T	4	20
Squash, Winter, Boiled	½ Cup	1	T	10	45
Squid	2 Ozs	9	0	1	45
Steak, Chopped	¼ Lb	31	13	0	245
Steak, Chuck w/Bone	2 Ozs	20	5	0	125
Steak, Cubed	2 Ozs	12	23	0	260
Steak, Flank	2 Ozs	11	6	0	100
Steak, Ham	2 Ozs	16	5	0	115
Steak, Pepper	2 Ozs	15	6	2	125
Steak, Porterhouse	2 Ozs	11	23	0	260
Steak, Rib	2 Ozs	16	9	0	142
Steak, Round	2 Ozs	11	6	0	100
Steak, Salisbury	2 Ozs	19	11	T	122
Steak, Sirloin	2 Ozs	18	4	0	112
Steak, Swiss	2 Ozs	17	4	7	105
Steak, T-bone	2 Ozs	11	24	0	260
Steak, Tenderloin	2 Ozs	17	6	0	120
Steak, Veal	2 Ozs	20	7	0	132
Stew, Beef	2 Ozs	3	2	3	50
Stew, Beef & Vegetable	2 Ozs	3	2	3	50
Stew, Irish	2 Ozs	7	6	7	117
Strawberries	1 Cup	1	1	12	55
String Beans	½ Cup	2	T	6	30
Stroganoff, Beef	2 Ozs	19	10	3	182
Stuffed Cabbage	Av Serv	15	6	7	140
Stuffed Peppers	1	14	6	11	155
Stuffing, Bread	½ Cup	5	14	28	280
Stuffing, Chestnut	½ Cup	4	7	26	185
Succotash	½ Cup	5	T	21 ·	110
Sugar, Beet	1 Tsp	0	0	4	18
Sugar, Brown	1 Tsp	0	0	4	18
Sugar, Cane	1 Tsp	0	0	4	18
Sugar Cookie	1	1	2	7	50
Sugar, Granulated	1 Tsp	0	0	4	50
Sugar, Maple	1 Oz	0	0	12	100
Sugar, Powdered	1 Tbsp	0	0	24	90

	AMT	PRO	FAT	CARB	CAL
Sunflower Seeds	1 Oz	7	14	6	159
Syrup, Brown Sugar	1 Tbsp	0	0	15	60
Syrup, Caramel	1 Tbsp	0	0	16	65
Syrup, Choc.	1 Tbsp	T	T	10	35
Syrup, Corn	1 Tbsp	T	T	12	50
Syrup, Maple	1 Tbsp	0	0	13	50
Syrup, Molasses	1 Tbsp	T	T	11	55
Tangerine	1 Lg	1	T	8	35
Tangerine Juice, Fresh	½ Cup	1	T	10	50
Tapioca, Pudding	½ Cup	6	6	24	175
Tapioca, Ready-to-Serve	½ Cup	5	5	19	150
Tarragon	⅛ Tsp	0	0	0	0
Tartar Sauce	1 Tbsp	T	8	T	75
Tarts, Apple	1	2	7	26	175
Tarts, Blueberry	1	2	7	21	150
Tea	1 Cup	T	T	T	2
Tea, Iced, No Sugar or Cream	1 Glass	T	T	T	2
Thyme	⅛ Tsp	0	0	0	0
Toast, French, 1 Tbsp. Maple Syrup	1 Pc	4	4	23	150
Toddy, Hot	1 Cup	2	3	24	150
Tofu	4 Oz	10	6	1	90
Toll House Cookie	3 Med	2	6	22	150
Tomato Consommé	1 Serv	3	3	6	65
Tomato, Fresh	Med	1	T	4	20
Tomato Juice	1 Cup	2	T	10	50
Tomato & Lettuce Salad	1 Serv	2	T	6	30
Tomato Soup, Clear	1 Serv	T	T	4	15
Tomato Soup, Creamed	1 Serv	6	6	18	155
Tomatoes, Stewed or Canned	1 Cup	3	T	10	50
Tortilla	1	1	1	10	55
Tortoni, Biscuit	1 Sm	2	12	14	175
Tuna	2 Ozs	12	4	0	85
Tuna, Canned in Oil, Drained	2 Ozs	11	3	0	79
Tuna, Canned in Water	2 Ozs	14	T	0	63
Tuna Salad	½ Cup	16	12	2	180
Turkey	2 Ozs	18	5	0	125
Turkey, All Dark	2 Ozs	16	4	0	115
Turkey, All White	2 Ozs	18	2	0	100
Turkey, Canned, Boned	2 Ozs	12	7	0	112
Turkey Soup, Cream of	1 Cup	16	10	12	200
Turkey Hash	2 Ozs	7	6	4	72
Turkey, Roasted	2 Ozs	18	5	0	125
Turkey Soup	1 Cup	2	1	13	70
Turnip Greens, Canned	1 Cup	3	1	11	55
Turnip Greens, Cooked	1 Cup	4	T	8	45
Turnips, Cooked	1 Cup	2	T	12	55
V-8 Juice	1 Cup	2	T	9	45
Vanilla Extract	1 Tsp	1	T	0	5
Vanilla Ice Cream	1 Scp	3	9	14	150

	AMT	PRO	FAT	CARB	CAL
Vanilla Malted w/Ice Cream	1 Cup	10	10	53	235
Vanilla Soda w/Ice Cream	8 Ozs	3	9	71	285
Vanilla Wafer Cookie	1 Av	T	1	4	25
Veal Chop	1 Med	30	15	0	260
Veal Cutlet, Breaded	2 Ozs	12	5	4	115
Veal Cutlet, Broiled	2 Ozs	16	6	0	116
Veal Loaf	2 Ozs	10	6	1	117
Veal & Peppers	2 Ozs	8	6	0	90
Veal Roast	2 Ozs	15	9	0	122
Veal Steak	2 Ozs	20	7	0	132
Vermicelli	½ Cup	3	4	8	80
Vermouth	2 Ozs	0	0	3	60
Vichyssoise	1 Cup	6	20	15	275
Vienna Bread	1 Sl	2	1	10	60
Vinegar	1 Oz	T	T	1	5
Vodka	1 Oz	0	0	T	70
Waffle, Blueberry	1 Med	9	10	35	300
Waffle, Choc.	1 Med	11	17	48	380
Waffle, Ham	1 Med	18	20	28	325
Waffle, Plain	1 Med	10	12	28	225
Walnuts	10	11	28	8	355
Water	1 Cup	0	0	0	0
Watercress	1 Bunch	2	T	3	20
Watermelon	Med Sl	1	T	22	100
Welsh Rarebit	½ Cup	18	30	22	430
Wheat, Cream of	½ Cup	2	T	15	65
Wheat Flour, All Purpose	1 Cup	13	1	85	400
Wheat, Thin, Cracker	4	1	2	5	55
Whipped Cream	1 Cup	3	45	4	420
Whiskey	1 Shot	T	T	T	100
White Sauce, Med	1 Tbsp	1	2	1	25
Wine, Red	1 Glass	T	0	4	75
Wine, White	1 Glass	T	0	2	75
Worcestershire Sauce	1 Tbsp	T	0	2	10
Yam, Canned	8 Ozs	2	T	54	225
Yam, Baked	1 Sm	1	T	23	105
Yam, Candied	1 Med	2	5	60	300
Yeast, Baking, Dry	1 Oz	10	T	3	85
Yeast, Dry, Brewers	1 Tbsp	5	T	3	50
Yogurt (Read All Containers)	1 Cup	7	8	13	140
Zucchini	8 Ozs	2	T	8	40
Zwieback	1 Av	T	T	5	30

Bibliography

Abraham, S.; Carroll, M.; Najjar, M.; and R. Fulwood. "Obese and Overweight Adults in the United States." National Center for Health Statistics, *Vital and Health Statistics* 11, no. 230 (1983): 83–1680.

Asher, W. and R. Dietz. "Effectiveness of Weight Reduction Involving Diet Pills." *Current Therapy and Research* 14 (1972): 510–524.

Berkow, R., ed. *Merck Manual of Diagnosis and Therapy.* 15th ed. New Jersey: Merck Sharp and Dohme Research Laboratories, 1986.

Bistrian, B. "Clinical Use of a Protein-Sparing Modified Fast." *Journal of the American Medical Association* 240 (1978): 2299–2302.

Bjorntorp, P. "Regional Patterns of Fat Distribution." *Annals of Internal Medicine* 103 (1987): 994–5.

Bjorntorp, P.; Varnausakas, E.; and B. Lindholm. "Lipid Mobilization in Relation to Body Composition." *Metabolism* 18 (1969): 841–51.

Blackburn, G. and I. Greenberg. "Multidisciplinary Approach to Adult Obesity Therapy." *International Journal of Obesity* 2 (1978): 133–42.

Blackburn, G. "Obesity." *Conn's Current Therapy* (1983): 444–9.

———. "Obesity from Fallacies to Facts." Nutritional Management Inc., Center for Nutritional Research, Boston (1983).

Boston University Alumni House. "Stress: An In-depth Issue." *Boston Magazine* 56, nos. 4–5 (1985).

Bray, G. "The Energetics of Obesity." *Medicine and Science in Sports and Exercise* 15, no. 1 (1983): 32–40.

Brownell, K.; Marlatt, G.; Lichtenstein, E.; and G. Wilson. "Understanding and Preventing Relapse." *American Psychology* 41 (1986): 765–82.

Cahill, G. "Starvation in Man." *New England Journal of Medicine* 282 (1970): 668–75.

Center for Nutritional Research. *Rx Weight Control.* Boston: December 1982–June 1985 iss.

Chatton, M. and P. Ullman. "Nutrition, Nutritional and Metabolic Disorders." *Current Medical Diagnosis and Treatment* (1981): 763–86.

Danforth, E. "Diet and Obesity." *American Journal of Clinical Nutrition* 41 (1985): 1132–45.

————. "The Role of Thyroid Hormones and Insulin in the Regulation of Energy Metabolism." *American Journal of Clinical Nutrition* 38 (1983): 1006–17.

Department of Health and Human Services, Public Health Service, Food and Drug Administration. *FDA Consumer* (1980–90).

Eaton, S. and M. Konner. "Paleolithic Nutrition." *New England Journal of Medicine* 312, no. 5 (1985): 283–89.

Epstein, L.; Wing, R.; and B. Valoski. "Effects of Diet Plus Exercise on Weight Change in Parents and Children." *Journal of Clinical Psychology* 52 (1984): 429–37.

Fixx, J. *The Complete Book of Running.* New York: Random House, 1977.

Flatt, J. "Dietary Fat, Carbohydrate Balance and Weight Maintenance, Effects of Exercise." *American Journal of Clinical Nutrition* 45 (1987): 296–307.

————. "The Metabolic Costs of Nutrient Storage." *Obesity and Weight Regulation* (1983): 5–18.

Food and Nutrition Board. *Toward Healthful Diets.* Washington, D.C.: National Academy of Science/National Research Council, 1980.

Gonzalez, E. "Studies Show Obese May Prefer Fats to Sweets."

Journal of the American Medical Association 250, no. 5 (1983): 579–83.

Gormally, J.; Rardin, D.; and S. Black. "Correlates of Successful Response to a Behavioral Weight Control Clinic." *Journal of Counseling Psychology* 27, no. 2 (1980): 179–91.

Gortner, W. "Nutrition in the United States." *Cancer Research* 35 (1975): 3246–53.

Harper, A. "Healthy People." *American Journal of Clinical Nutrition* 33 (1980): 1703–12.

Health Living Institute. *International Obesity Newsletter.* North Dakota, 1989–90.

Henderson, J.; Hall, S.; and H. Lipton. "Changing Self-Destructive Behavior." In *Health Psychology: A Handbook.* (1980); 141–60.

Hirsh, J. "Fatty Acid Patterns in Human Adipose Tissue." In Vol. 5, *Handbook of Physiology,* 181–89. Bethesda: American Physiology Society, 1965.

Institute for Aerobics Research. *The Strength Connection.* Dallas, 1990.

Keys, A. "Overweight, Obesity, Coronary Heart Disease and Mortality." *Nutrition Review* 38 (1980): 297–307.

Kreitler, S. and A. Chemerinski. "The Cognitive Orientation of Obesity." *International Journal of Obesity* 12 (1986): 403–15.

Marstan, R. "Nutrient Content of the National Food Supply." *National Food Review* 13 (1981): 19–22.

Mills, J. *Coping With Stress.* New York: John Wiley & Sons, 1982.

National Academy of Sciences. *Recommended Dietary Allowances.* Washington, D.C.: National Research Council.

Nutrition Search, Inc. *Nutrition Almanac.* New York: McGraw-Hill, 1979.

Rimm, A. and P. White. "Obesity: Its Risks and Hazards." *Obesity in America,* Pub. no. 80. U.S. Department of Health, Education, and Welfare, Public Service, National Institutes of Health, (1980): 103–24.

Select Committee on Nutrition and Human Needs, U.S. Senate.

Dietary Goals for the United States. U.S. Government Printing Office, 1977.

Simopoulos, A. and T. Van Itallie. "Body Weight, Height, and Longevity." *Annals of Internal Medicine* 100, no. 2 (1984): 285–95.

Wadden, T. and A. Stunkard. "A Controlled Trial of Very Low Calorie Diet, Behavior Therapy, and Their Combination in the Treatment of Obesity." *Journal of Consulting and Clinical Psychology* 54: 482–88.

Wadden, T.; Smoller, A.; and A. Stunkard. "The Treatment of Marked Obesity by Very Low Calorie Diet and Behavior Therapy." *Advances in Eating Disorders* 1 (1987): 57–116.

Weinsier, R.; Wadden, T.; Ritenbaugh, C.; Harrison, G.; Johnson, B.; and J. Wilmore. "Recommended Therapeutic Guidelines for Professional Weight Control Programs." *American Journal of Clinical Nutrition* 40 (1984): 865–72.

Index